BONE
BEHAVIOUR

KITTY LITTLE

BONE

BEHAVIOUR

1973

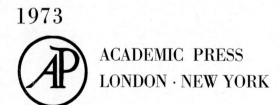

ACADEMIC PRESS
LONDON · NEW YORK

ACADEMIC PRESS INC. (LONDON) LTD.
24/28 Oval Road,
London NW1

United States Edition published by
ACADEMIC PRESS INC.
111 Fifth Avenue
New York, New York 10003

Library of Congress Catalog Card Number: 72–84359
ISBN: 0–12–452050–2

PRINTED IN GREAT BRITAIN BY
COX & WYMAN LTD., LONDON, FAKENHAM AND READING

PREFACE

There are various approaches to the study of bone, from the points of view of the anatomist, physiologist, pathologist, physician or surgeon. The understanding of each of these is dependent to a certain extent on their knowledge of the behaviour of the cells contained in the bone, of how they contribute to its growth and subsequent development, of how the properties of the intercellular matrices that the cells produce are modified, of how these cells react to applied stimuli, whether physical or chemical, and also of the vital role of the blood vessels and vascular endothelial cells. The bones are an important part of the framework of the body, and they protect vital tissues and organs. These include the brain, and the heart and lungs, and also the bone marrow, which manufactures the main components of the blood, red and white cells, and platelets. But, whereas the brain is a quite separate organ, the bone marrow is an integral part of the bone, and so needs to be considered together with the structural cells which produce the bone tissue. It is one of the purposes of this book to describe, and to a certain extent discuss, some of the more fundamental properties of the cells and vessels in bone, and to indicate how this knowledge can be applied to practical problems. Since the book is in no way intended to be a textbook of pathology, pathological conditions are considered only where a part of the process throws light on some aspect of cell behaviour. For as L. C. Johnson has said, "Disease processes never involve any strange or new reactions but only altered relationships in normal reactions. The alteration may, however, separate out and focus attention upon stages in reactions that are otherwise overlooked." The reaction of bone to infection, and here rheumatoid arthritis has many of the characteristics of a reaction to infection, will not be mentioned.

Bones are not isolated objects, but an integral part of the body, and so an attempt has also been made to indicate how they fit in with activities of other parts of the body, and with other connective tissues, both in health and disease. Muscles affect the behaviour of bone by the mechanical stresses they exert, while hormones affect it by a chemical mechanism. Here the bone plays an essential role in the reaction of the person to his environment, that person having both a mind and a body. Both the mind and to a lesser extent the body, in their reaction to the environment, can modify the hormones; and certain of these hormone modifications affect the bone, and in particular the marrow, with the production of abnormal megakaryocytes and platelets, and then thrombi, which in turn may cause alterations, more or less drastic, in other tissues and organs. An understanding of bone, therefore, is necessary for an adequate understanding of the major stress diseases, which during the last quarter of a century have become the dominant cause of ill-health.

The publishers have asked that this book shall be a book for the use of both medical students and junior doctors. This means that it needs to be more than a collection of facts. Many of the facts which it would be useful to know have not yet been discovered, while at the present time to "do some research" is being considered as increasingly important in medical education. For those junior doctors who embark on part-time research, two quite different mental approaches are required. When confronted with a patient the need is for an immediate decision, giving the best answer possible with the available evidence. Here the "opinion" of a senior colleague is frequently of value, that opinion being based on experience. When they turn their attention to research time is no longer a dominant factor. The essential requirement is to obtain sufficient evidence for a correct answer to be obtained. Here an "opinion" has only the value of a speculation, and should not be confused with a clinical opinion. It is the logical consideration of evidence that matters. Some indication is needed of the fields in which research may be pursued profitably, and an attempt has been made to do this throughout the book.

Too often it is imagined that "research" is the manipulation of some instruments in a laboratory, the more complicated the technique the more erudite being the research. This concept is quite erroneous; the only research tool that is absolutely essential is the mind of the investigator. In research, considered in general terms, the object of the exercise is to correlate a series of factual observations in order to obtain a better understanding of the subject. The method employed is to collect facts and observations on a topic (which may be large or small, simple or complicated); consider them, see if a hypothesis can be propounded which links them; look for other facts whose possible existence is suggested by the hypothesis; consider whether these should be cautiously accepted, modified or rejected; consider the modified hypothesis, seek more facts, and so on. Groups of related hypotheses are then considered, to see whether they fit together, whether some or all need modification or possibly rejection, and what possible new facts they suggest should be sought. These can then be investigated, until a sufficient number of correlated facts are available to form a theory. The hypotheses should never themselves be treated as facts, and when they are contradicted by factual observations it is the hypothesis which should be immediately abandoned, and not the fact. When seeking knowledge, it is a sign of weakness and not of strength to imagine that a modification of one's ideas with experience is in any way undesirable. One fact that is sometimes forgotten is that a valid fact remains a fact, whether it was discovered 2 years ago, or 2000 years ago.

November, 1972   Kitty Little
M.A., B.Sc., D.Phil.
Ridgeway Consultants Ltd.,
19 Victoria Road,
Abingdon, Berkshire

ACKNOWLEDGEMENTS

The assembling of facts and evidence necessary for the production of this book would not have been possible without the help and encouragement of many people, and the frequent discussion of both ideas and evidence. I am especially grateful to Professor Joseph Trueta, who for over a decade inspired a high standard of achievement in the Wingfield-Morris Hospital in Oxford. During Professor Trueta's time as Nuffield Professor of Orthopaedic Surgery in Oxford the Research Department was established as an integral part of the hospital, and after the generous gift of buildings and contents for the University Department by Lord Nuffield, together with the equipping of the research department, the name of the hospital was changed to the Nuffield Orthopaedic Centre, in his honour.

Professor Trueta's outstanding contribution to our understanding of bone has been to provide definitive evidence of the role of the vascular endothelial cells as osteogenic precursor cells, and to demonstrate beyond any possibility of doubt the importance of the blood vessels and blood flow in all the functions of the bone. I owe a great deal of my understanding of the properties of bone and cartilage to the many stimulating discussions I have had with him, and with the surgeons and research workers who came to the Department during his time as Professor.

In addition to those working on various aspects of the vascularization of bones I would mention Dr. W. M. Rigal, who came from Cape Town, South Africa, and made valuable contributions to our knowledge of the behaviour of bone and cartilage cells in tissue culture, the early stages of the mechanism of cell division, and the action of growth hormone; Dr. R. Scapinelli, from the University of Padova, Italy, for his work on tissue metaplasia; Mr. T. K. F. Taylor, now Professor of Orthopaedic Surgery in Sydney, Australia, who studied lumbar and thoracic disc lesions; Drs J. A. F. de Valderrama and L. Munuera, from Madrid, Spain, for their part in the early stages of our investigation of catabolic and anabolic steroids; Mr. H. B. S. Kemp, who added, to the observations already made by Professor Trueta, his contribution to our understanding of Perthe's disease and fracture healing; and, first in time, Mr. L. H. Pimm, who introduced me to the problems of osteoarthritis and Paget's disease. Professor J. L. Matthews, who visited us for a short time from Dallas, Texas, stimulated my interest in the modifications to the effects of radiation brought about by the simultaneous presence of excess oxygen. I would also express my gratitude to the surgeons and senior medical staff of the Nuffield Orthopaedic Centre who, during the period 1956 to 1966, introduced me to the problems facing orthopaedic surgeons and their patients.

My introduction to medical science was through the problems involved in calcification, and the properties of the intercellular matrices, and in this field I received a great deal of help and encouragement from Dr. J. Thewlis, Head of the Diffraction Branch at A.E.R.E., Harwell; Sir Edward Mellanby, Secretary of the Medical Research Council, and Lady Mellanby, whose work on the effects of vitamins on bones and teeth, respectively, was outstanding; and Dr. R. W. G. Wyckoff, who for two years was Science Attaché at the United States Embassy in London— and kept an electron microscope in his office. I have had many rewarding discussions with them, and also with Professor A. I. Darling of the Bristol Dental Hospital; Dr. S. L. Rowles from the Birmingham Department of Dental Pathology; Dr. F. Happey, now at the Department of Textile Industries, Bradford; and Dr. A. Courts, Director of the British Gelatin and Glue Research Association.

Soon afterwards Dr. H. Kramer introduced me to some of the problems of reticulin and the connective tissues, and without the knowledge of pathology gleaned from him, Drs R. W. Cox and W. A. Aherne, and other pathologists at the Radcliffe Infirmary, Oxford, during the period 1949 to 1956, it would hardly have been possible for me to proceed far in the more restricted field of bone pathology. Dr. J. Landells, from the London Hospital, also gave much sound advice during a three-month visit to the Nuffield Orthopaedic Centre. I am especially grateful to Dr. L. C. Johnson for the time he so generously gave in instructing me in the field of bone pathology, and for many stimulating discussions during a visit to the Armed Forces Institute of Pathology in Washington (and to Colonel G. W. Reid, R.A.M.C., who arranged that visit); and I would also thank Dr. T. S. Edgington of the University of California, Los Angeles, and Dr. L. Sokoloff, of the National Institute of Health, Washington, for their contributions to my understanding of bone pathology.

In the field of steroids and bone marrow Dr. A. M. White of CIBA Laboratories Horsham, has given me a great deal of practical help, in addition to advice and the benefit of his experience. I am most grateful to him, and also to Dr. D. Burley and other members of the staff of CIBA; to Dr. L. Goldman of Bayer Products, Surbiton-on-Thames; and to Dr. Alan Sharp of the Haematology Department, Oxford.

Dr. K. Williams, Head of the Medical Division, A.E.R.E. Harwell, first drew my attention to the dominant role of the vessels in the effect of radiation on bones, and since that time I have had valuable discussions on the mechanisms of radiation damage and sarcoma formation with Professor W. S. S. Jee and Professor T. F. Dougherty of the U.S.A.E.C. group at Salt Lake City; Dr. L. C. Johnson at the A.F.I.P.; Dr. C. H. G. Price and Mrs. Ada Joseph of the Bristol Bone Tumour Register; Dr. F. R. Wells of the Clinical Pathology Department in Oxford; and many others. Discussions with Dr. A. E. Sobel were especially fascinating, and it was a major set-back to our understanding of the malignant change when he died before his work on that subject was ready for publication.

During much of the time that I have been working on these topics I have been assisted by Mrs. Maureen Holdoway. While at A.E.R.E., Harwell, she helped in the assembling of the information on calcification which is recorded in Chapter 1, a topic which we inherited from Dr. J. Thewlis, who began work on it in 1930, while he was at the National Physical Laboratory. Later she worked with me at the Nuffield Orthopaedic Centre and at the Wantage Research Laboratory, and I have been most grateful for her loyal co-operation. She has very generously read the manuscript of this book and made many helpful suggestions, and has produced the illustrations for the Introduction.

I would also thank Mrs. Gillian Swaite, Mrs. E. S. Rogers and Mr. D. Drury for their help in the production of the book; and Mr. A. J. Gunning, Dr. L. C. Johnson, Dr. C. H. G. Price and Dr. L. Sokoloff for reading portions of the book and for much helpful advice.

I acknowledge with gratitude photographs lent to me for reproduction by Dr. G. D. Beaumont (2.7, 2.8, 7.1); Dr. A. Elkeles (8.48, 8.49, 8.52); Prof. W. S. S. Jee (4.25 to 4.28, 10.1 to 10.4); the late Prof. S. Jellinek (5.9); Mr. H. B. S. Kemp (5.32 to 5.35); Mr. J. D. Morgan (3.12); Dr. W. M. Rigal (2.16, 3.6, 4.3, 9.4); Mrs. C. Robinson (2.13); Prof. T. K. F. Taylor (1.19, 1.20, 1.60, 1.61, 8.41, 8.42); and Prof. R. W. G. Wyckoff (1.16). Material for photographs has been lent by Dr. V. Amato (3.11); Dr. F. J. Aumonier (1.4); Prof. W. F. Enneking (9.11, 9.12); the late Dr. D. I. Fryer (8.13, 8.14); Mr. J. R. P. Gibbons (5.36 to 5.38); Prof. W. S. S. Jee (3.27, 10.5, 10.8); Mr. H. B. S. Kemp (1.1, 2.17 to 2.19, 4.1, 4.14, 4.33); Dr. C. H. G. Price (9.8 to 9.10); Dr. W. M. Rigal (1.33, 3.8). Other photographs have appeared in papers in *Current Therapeutic Research* (2.31, 3.2, 3.14, 3.15, 3.17, 3.18, 3.19, 3.21, 3.22, 3.23, 3.24, 3.25, 3.26, 4.22, 6.5, 6.9, 6.10, 6.11, 6.12, 6.13, 6.15, 6.16, 6.17, 6.18, 6.20, 6.21, 6.22, 6.23, 6.25, 6.28, 6.29, 6.30); *Gerontologia* (2.32, 2.33, 2.34, 2.35, 2.36, 4.29, 5.25, 5.26, 6.21, 6.38, 6.39, 8.1, 8.3,

8.4, 8.5, 8.7); *Journal of Bone and Joint Surgery* (1.24, 1.26. 1.31, 3.12, 8.24, 8.25); *Journal of Pathology* (5.7, 5.8, 5.12, 5.17); *Journal of the Royal Microscopical Society* (1.56, 3.8, 9.1, 9.2, 9.3); and the *Lancet* (1.55, 4.5, 4.6, 4.30).

CONTENTS

O ye dry bones, hear the word of the Lord. . . .

There was a noise, and behold a stirring, and the bones came together, each at its proper joint; the sinews and the flesh came up upon them, and the skin covered them above . . . then the breath of life came into them, and they lived.

Ezekiel: Chapter 37

INTRODUCTION

This book is intended to fill the needs of two rather separate groups of individuals: medical students whose main object is to acquire knowledge of facts; and those junior doctors who wish to do some research.

The primary objective in doing research is to add to the accumulated knowledge of the subject—in this case cell mechanisms in bone. To fill the needs of this latter group some subjects have been discussed in more detail than is strictly necessary for those just entering the field, since before one can add to the pool of knowledge it is necessary to know where its frontiers are.

For beginners, whether to the subject, or to research in the subject, it is wise to start by investigating the scope of the problem. Accordingly, the first part of this Introduction gives a brief outline of the component parts of bone, and the names that will be used for them. Technical names—or jargon—tend to vary from time to time, so that different labels for the same thing tend to be found in the medical literature. One necessity, therefore, is to make quite sure that one understands the meaning of the terms that are being used. Similarly, in the second part of the Introduction the underlying purpose and methods of research will be outlined. It must be understood clearly, from the outset, that research is concerned with finding facts and searching for evidence, and is in no way concerned with "showing" something that for devious reasons one might want (e.g. that sugar causes dental caries, or that smoking causes whatever happens to be at the top of the list in the current causes of death), or with the manipulation of some fashionable equipment or experimental procedure.

Bone Structure and Function: Terminology

Since the primary purpose of the book is to give an account of the types and causes of different aspects of the behaviour of cells in bone, and it is not intended to be a manual on orthopaedics, anatomy or pathology, it will suffice if for most topics the femur and vertebrae provide the main illustrations of these characteristics. These are the bones most commonly affected by degenerative diseases.

In the foetus a cartilage model of the bone known as the *anlage cartilage* is formed, which is approximately the same shape as the final bone. These shapes are genetically determined, and Ward's comment (1838) on their form, in a footnote in his book on Osteology, is worth quoting:

> "I had never imagined that these slight undulations in the shafts of the cylindrical bones could play any important part in the mechanism of the limbs, until I happened to learn how greatly the durability of carriage wheels is increased by a scarcely perceptible curvature in their spokes. An experienced mechanic assures me that, when the spokes of a wheel are sufficiently slender to curve under the pressure exerted by the heated tire-iron in shrinking, though the deviation from perfect rectilinearity in each spoke does not exceed 2 or 3 sixteenths of an inch, they are found to remain firm and unloosened at the nave, when wheels, having straight and consequently rigid spokes, have opened at the joints, and become unsound . . . much greater absolute strength, entirely on account of the elastic play permitted by this seemingly trivial variation of form."

The anlage cartilage is made up of cartilage cells with a surrounding immature *intercellular matrix*. In the long bones, during the first stages of conversion into bone, cartilage cells in the central part of the *shaft* increase their rate of proliferation, enlarge, and become *hypertrophic*. *Blood vessels* penetrate into this altered cartilage, and in their wake there is *osteogenic* activity. The osteogenic cells have the capacity to change their function, and the name given to a cell depends on its activity at the time. Cells in the process of laying down an *osteoid* matrix, which rapidly *calcifies* are the *osteoblasts*. Some become buried in the bone they have produced and are then known as *osteocytes*. These osteocytes maintain the viability of the bone. They are interconnected with cell processes passing through *canaliculi* in the calcified matrix. Those nearest to the surface are also joined to the layer of osteoblasts. When the cells coalesce to form multinucleated cells which remove bone they are known as *osteoclasts*. Another group of cells, the *phagocytic* cells, can also coalesce to form multinucleated cells which remove tissue. When they are present in bone they are also known as osteoclasts. Their precursor cells have been given various names, the one used in this book being *macrophage*.

The process of replacing cartilage by bone, after vascular penetration, is known as *enchondral ossification*. This proceeds from the central regions of the shaft towards the ends, the *epiphyses*. When the advancing ossification front reaches the epiphyseal region, then ossification commences separately within the epiphysis, to form the *secondary bone nucleus*. The main regions in a developing bone are shown diagramatically in Fig. 1. During childhood a region of cartilage remains at either end of the long bones, between the epiphysis and the *metaphysis*. It is in a highly organized state, contains vigorously proliferating cells, and is

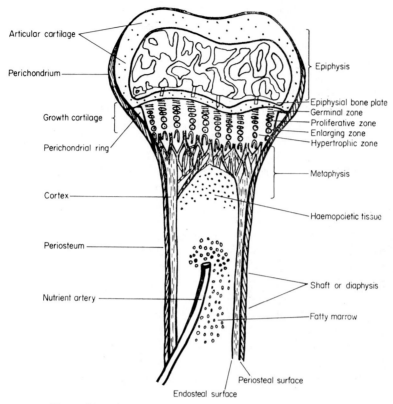

Articular cartilage

Perichondrium

Growth cartilage

Perichondrial ring

Cortex

Periosteum

Nutrient artery

Epiphysis

Epiphysial bone plate
Germinal zone
Proliferative zone
Enlarging zone
Hypertrophic zone

Metaphysis

Haemopoietic tissue

Shaft or diaphysis

Fatty marrow

Periosteal surface
Endosteal surface

FIG. 1. Diagram to show main features in developing long bone.

known as the *epiphyseal growth cartilage*, or sometimes the *epiphyseal growth plate*.

The zone of this growth cartilage nearest to the epiphysis is the *germinal* or resting zone. It is similar to the anlage cartilage. Then comes the *proliferative* zone with columns of active rapidly dividing cells. These enlarge and form a *calcifiable matrix* which is laid down over the main structural part of the intercellular matrix. In the stages of most rapid growth they enlarge further to form the *hypertrophic* zone. As enchondral ossification takes place each hypertrophic space is invaded by an advancing *sinusoid vessel*. When the rate of growth slows cartilage may be removed without enlargement of the cells to the hypertrophic state. The mode of removal is then by multinucleated cells known as *chondroclasts*. These coalesce from similar cells to those that formed the osteoclasts, the different name denoting the different function. In either case enchondral ossification takes place with the formation of bone *trabeculae*. They may be very regularly arranged during the period of rapid growth, and are rather less regularly arranged when growth is accompanied by chondroclast activity. These trabeculae occupy the *metaphyseal* region of the bone. The epiphyseal growth cartilage will be considered in detail in Chapter 3.

During growth, while the epiphyseal growth cartilage provides for the growth in length, there is also an increase in diameter of the shaft of the long bones. New bone is laid down on the outer part of the *cortex*, the *periosteal* surface, while at the same time bone is removed from the inner surface of the cortex, the *endosteal* surface. In the case of periosteal bone formation cartilage is not formed as an intermediate stage in the process. Changes in the shape and distribution of the bone tissue occur both before and after growth has ceased, by the process of *remodelling*. One of the main factors regulating this process is the application of physical forces, which may either act directly on the walls of sinusoid vessels in the bone, or act indirectly by altering blood flow and pressure. In the former case the remodelling consists of the removal of trabeculae followed by the formation of new ones in rather different positions. The latter frequently leads to the formation of *osteones* in the *cortical* bone in the shaft. More generally, this type of bone is known as *compact* bone. During osteone formation there is a proliferation of vessels, with accompanying osteoclasts, that bore a channel through the bone tissue. This channel—a *Haversian canal*—is then partly filled with new bone laid down concentrically around the vessels.

Trabecular bone is also known as *cancellous* bone, and again we can quote Ward's description of its function (1838).

"The arrangement of the cancellous bone in the ends of the femur is very remarkable; and, as it illustrates the general mechanical principles which determine the structure of this tissue throughout the skeleton, it should engage our particular attention. In the lower extremity of the bone, it consists of numerous slender columns, which spring on all sides from the interior surface of the compact cylinder, and descend, converging towards each other, so as to form a series of inverted arches, adapted, by their pointed form, to sustain concussion or pressure transmitted from below. These converging columns not only meet, but decussate each other, and they are further strengthened by innumerable connecting filaments and lamellae, which cross them in all directions, so that no single arch could break without those in its neighbourhood also giving way. Hence, notwithstanding the tenuity and brittleness of each several fibre, the reticular structure possesses great strength as a whole . . .

The cancellous tissue in the upper extremity of the shaft presents a similar arrangement—the convexities of the arches being here, however, directed upwards."

When cortical or trabecular bone is laid down the osteoblasts arise from the vessel walls, and are arranged in rows. Cortical bone that has been so formed in a regular array is known as *lamellar* bone. It is present in children, but when they take sufficient exercise it is all converted to osteonal bone by the time the adolescent changes are complete. Small animals, such as the rabbit, tend to retain a lamellar bone structure throughout life.

When bone is first formed after injury and local cell death it is irregularly arranged and has different properties. This type of bone is known as *woven bone*. Available evidence shows that cells of the sinusoid vessel walls are the source of osteogenic cells, for both ordinary bone and woven bone. The various types of bone formation and removal will be discussed in Chapter 4.

When bone tissue is formed it is accompanied by *bone marrow*. Marrow is of two main types. One is red marrow, containing *haemopoietic tissue*, which is found in those parts of the bone where there is cell activity, either growth or turnover. This tissue contains the precursors of the circulating blood cells, red cells or *erythrocytes, leucocytes* (white cells) of various types, and *platelets*. These platelets are formed from large cells known as *megakaryocytes*. The proportion and properties of the components of haemopoietic tissue are under *hormonal* control. In the more quiescent regions of bone *fatty marrow* is found.

Throughout the bone, both in the marrow, among the trabeculae and in *Haversian canals* in compact bone are *sinusoid* vessels, which are of varying diameter. In normal marrow only about 1 in 10 of these is open at any given time. These blood vessels have a sheath of *basement membrane* or *reticulin*, and flattened *endothelial* cells are seen at intervals on their walls. Wherever these sinusoid vessels are found in the body, whether in bone or in the spleen and liver, there haemopoietic activity is possible. Their cells only act as bone precursors in the presence of a substance known as the *osteogenic factor*. Other blood vessels, whether *arteries* or *veins*, have more substantial walls. Even small *capillaries* tend to have a continuous layer of cells over their basement membrane. During proliferation, sinusoid vessels and capillaries display similar characteristics. *Nerves* are found accompanying many arteries.

The ends of the long bones are covered by *articular cartilage*, while between the two articular surfaces in a *joint* is the *synovial fluid*, the remaining surfaces of the fluid-containing cavity being occupied by the *synovial membrane*. Cells on the surface of the synovial membrane secrete the synovial fluid. The shaft of the bone is covered by a sheath of connective tissue called the *periosteum*, and outside this again there are usually *muscles*. Points of attachment of muscles to bone are known as *muscle insertions*. The tissue surrounding the growth cartilage is known as the *perichondrial ring*, and fibrous tissue surrounding those parts of the articular cartilage which are not in contact with the synovial fluid is called the *perichondrium*.

Arrangements around other bones are of a related type. Between the *vertebral bodies* in the *spine* are the *intervertebral discs*. In these there is at each side a *cartilage end plate*, which in the growing child acts as a growth cartilage, while in the adult it has many of the characteristics of articular or *hyaline* cartilage. The central part of the disc is a type of *fibrocartilage* known as the *nucleus pulposus*, and surrounding it is an orientated fibrous tissue known as the *annulus fibrosus*. Of the bone in the vertebral bodies a part (the shaded area in the top vertebra shown in Fig. 2) is originally formed by enchondral ossification, while the re-

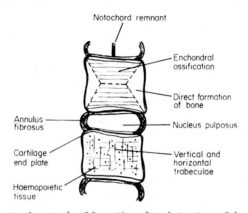

FIG. 2. Diagram to show mode of formation of, and structure of, bone in vertebrae.

mainder is formed by *periosteal ossification*. The whole area of a normal vertebral body is occupied by trabecular bone surrounded by haemo-poietic tissue.

Ward (1838) says of the spine:

"The vertebral column is a remarkable piece of mechanism. Strong enough to support several hundredweight, yet pliant and elastic; furnished with levers and muscles, by which it is bent in every direction, yet lodging an organ susceptible of injury from the slightest pressure: formed for lightness, of a loose and reticular tissue, yet capable of sustaining without fracture, shocks and strains and contortions of considerable violence: this column certainly combines the most opposite qualities, and performs functions apparently incompatible."

The properties of the cells in bone are primarily controlled by agents which affect cell membranes. These membranes are of two main types: *rough membranes* which are known as the *endoplasmic reticulum*, called rough because of an array of *ribosome* particles on the surfaces of the membranes; and *smooth membranes* which comprise the *cell surface, nuclear envelope* and their connecting membranes. The endoplasmic reticulum is responsible for the production of intercellular matrices, the surface membranes for cell mobility, and the smooth membranes for cell division. The stages of division are the *pre-division* or *antephase*, followed by the more spectacular *prophase, metaphase, anaphase* and *telophase*.

Since the remainder of the division process is dependent upon the pre-division stage, which is the only one that requires a source of energy, this is clearly the most important stage when one is considering the tissue as a whole, rather than the fate of an individual cell. At the start of meta-phase, membrane connections are formed between the nucleus and the outside of the cell, and raw materials for the daughter nuclei are taken in. These are then *polymerized* and at the end of this chemical synthesis the cell is ready to proceed to the actual business of division.

There are a variety of controls and requirements for the proper functioning of the two sets of cell membranes, which in turn are res-ponsible for the proper construction and functioning of the whole tissue. These include a supply of raw materials for *proteins, polysaccharides* and *nucleic acids*; energy producing materials for *glycolysis*, and particularly *carbohydrates*; trace compounds which control such properties as the quality of the intercellular matrices, *vitamins* and *fluoride*; *oxygen* and *carbon dioxide*; *polypeptide* and *steroid hormones*; and so on, together with the direct action of mechanical forces on cells and tissues. It is the primary purpose of this book to describe these mechanisms for control-ling and modifying the structure and function of the different bone constituents, and the pathological consequences of their malfunction. These include the effects of an excess or deficiency of vitamins and fluoride, *osteoporosis, osteoarthritis, intervertebral disc lesions, osteo-genesis imperfecta, sarcoma* formation and *thrombus* formation. The various consequences of *stress*, and particularly that mechanism which leads to a raised *cortisol* production by the *adrenal cortex*, account for a high proportion of present day illnesses. The bone and bone marrow are closely involved in many of the sequelae of stress.

Methods of Investigation

Since this book is intended for those who wish to add to knowledge, as well as for those who want to acquire available information, it is necessary to consider what research is, what aspects are relevant to the present subject, what the fundamental methods of conducting research are, how to seek evidence oneself, and how one assesses evidence compiled by other people.

Categories of research. The greater part of research effort is devoted to acquiring and integrating information in some particular field, where in-creased information and understanding have a forseeable practical use. In the present instance a knowledge of the properties and behaviour of bone is likely to result in the better treatment of or prevention of illnesses which involve the bone either directly or indirectly. The type of information sought includes a knowledge of the mechanisms of bone formation and removal, matrix formation and cell division, the action of vitamins, fluoride, hormones, peptides and steroids, the effect of varying blood flow and the partial pressure of oxygen and carbon dioxide in the blood. What emerges is some understanding of the mechanisms of osteoporosis, osteoarthritis, disc lesions, Paget's disease and osteosarcoma. Few of the biological mechanisms investigated could be known beforehand to be directly concerned with the pathological conditions whose mechanisms have been elucidated, but there was a reasonable probability that a sufficient knowledge of bone behaviour would result in a better understanding of the diseases. This type of fundamental research has been called "strategic" research.

In addition to the main body of research there are two rather different fields of investigation known as pure (or basic) and applied (or tactical) research. Pure research involves the pursuit of knowledge for its own sake, with no preconceived ideas (except occasionally in very general terms) about any possible use to which the information might be put. As examples from the study of bone might be taken:

(a) The crystal structure of the calcium phosphates.

In Chapter 1 it will be shown that the properties of bone tissue and connective tissues are very largely dependent upon the physical properties of the intercellular matrices, and it will also be shown that the type of mineralization depends upon the nature and structure of the underlying organic matrix. To recognize what is normal and what is abnormal there is no need to know the crystal structure of the deposited mineral crystals. At the most, knowledge of their identity and crystal size and habit gives all that is required to understand the biological mechanisms involved in both normal bone behaviour and pathological aberations. To investigate the crystal structures of these mineral compounds would therefore be an exercise in pure research, the acquisition of knowledge for its own sake.

(b) The detailed chemistry of the polysaccharides in articular cartilage, and its modification by steroids.

The essential property of these polysaccharides is their ability to form a stable gel. Cells in the cartilage are at risk when the gel structure is broken down, whether as a result of excessive pressure, the presence of blood in the synovial fluid or an infection. Observations that will be described in Chapter 6 show that steroids, and particularly corticosteroids, render the gel more stable if they are present at the time it is being formed. For both normal and pathological states the observations of greatest relevance are those involving the mechanisms whereby articular cartilage maintains or loses it structural integrity. Its actual chemical composition, and the minor variations in its composition when it is formed in the presence of different steroids are again matters of purely academic interest.

Sometimes, of course, a discovery made while the investigator is engaged in pure research may have a practical application. One dramatic example of this was the splitting of the atom by J. D. Cockcroft and E. T. S. Walton. This academic exercise led to the timely discovery of how to utilize atomic energy—timely, because there are only coal and oil supplies available for another 50 years or so, and these need to be conserved for use as chemical raw materials or for applications where other sources of energy are impractical. Plastics, for example, are mostly made from oil. Because of the comparatively short time available there has been the need to amass a wide variety of information, particularly in the fields of chemistry and materials science, and the effects of radiation on metals and other materials, together with the physical and engineering knowledge required for the construction of reactors for power stations, marine engines, and those other applications where coal or oil must be replaced as a source of energy, and of nuclear batteries for applications where less energy is required. All this information, for which Harwell and other Atomic Energy Establishments were created, comes into the fundamental (strategic) research category, of assembling and integrating knowledge, putting the jigsaw puzzle together, and so finding the gaps that need to be filled. In the medical field such large-scale integrated research efforts are rarely needed, one of the few examples being the requirements for an investigation of the biological effects of radiation. This problem and the information so far available will be discussed in Chapter 10. One reason that this is the only major topic which requires such a concentrated effort is because the information and evidence required in the greater part of medical science has been accumulating, at a gradually accelerating rate, for over 2000 years whereas atomic energy only dates from the 1930s.

The other wing of the research field is that of applied (tactical) research. Here the activity is neither the pursuit of knowledge for its own sake, nor putting together the jigsaw puzzle of information in a given, fairly wide field, but the application of information gained from the main stream of research to a narrow specific end. In medicine this usually means a clinical application. Examples of such problems would be:

(a) Choice of the best operative procedure for a particular condition, e.g. an arthritic hip, or a condition necessitating a bone graft.

(*b*) Choice of the most suitable anabolic agent, and its correct dose, for a patient with post-menopausal or senile osteoporosis.

(*c*) Adaptation of methods of treatment of rickets and osteomalacia to Asian patients who have a different fat metabolism from the British.

In the atomic energy field the type of problem which would come under the heading of applied (tactical) research would be: the adaptation of a suitable category of reactor to a specific purpose, e.g. an aircraft carrier, passenger liner, or cargo ship; the use of ionizing radiations for sterilizing medical equipment or preparing tissue grafts, or the choice of isotopes and preparation of labelled compounds to use in tracer work, in biology or industry.

The first step in embarking on research is to choose a problem. Since this book is intended for doctors the question of pure (basic) research does not arise—that is a matter for the academic scientist. The choice is between fundamental (strategic) research, where the application to clinical problems may not be so immediately apparent, and a simple applied problem. The difference between these two must be clearly recognized. Without the answers to fundamental questions one cannot rationally start on the applied problems, so that even if the results do not show immediate returns, or if their application is still several decades hence, fundamental (strategic) research is an essential part of the foundation of applied research. A specific example may help to clarify this point:

Osteoporosis is a word that means too little bone tissue. Sometimes the cause is fairly obvious, a deficiency of vitamin C prevents the formation of bone matrix, the presence of a metastatic soft tissue tumour is preceded by a loss of bone, or a lack of muscular movement (e.g. a paralysed limb) causes some bone loss. Other cases, particularly in the elderly, have had no such obvious cause, and have been called idiopathic osteoporosis. There was therefore the need to find the mechanisms involved in this idiopathic osteoporosis, in order to ascertain if or how it could be prevented or cured, and there have been three types of approach to the problem.

(*a*) The first did not come into the category of either science or research. It consisted of the unreflecting assumption "there is too little calcium in the bone, therefore the cause is too little calcium in the body", and a series of meaningless activities based on that assumption.

(*b*) The next approach was to consider it as a problem of applied (tactical) research, that could be considered in isolation. This approach leads to a description of the condition, but little more. It can be observed that there are two dominant groups of cases; that there are active and passive phases; that in the active phases there is haemopoietic tissue in areas of bone resorption; that this haemopoietic tissue contains abnormal looking megakaryocytes; that in the inactive phases there is a very high proportion of fatty marrow; that in, say, the osteoporotic head of femur the trabeculae that are present contain prominent arrest lines, while the articular cartilage is unusually stable; and so on. Each of these observations raises more questions, so that the attempt to treat it as a problem in applied research has only succeeded in asking more questions than it has answered, without providing a mechanism of the changes.

(c) This leaves the approach from the angle of fundamental (strategic) research, of fitting together the pieces of the jigsaw puzzle. Adjoining pieces give a knowledge of some of the effects of stress, of the action of the steroids when present in excess, when present in combination, and so on. Study of combinations of steroids produces appearances similar to those which have been observed for osteoporosis, and the way then lies open for an approach on a broad front, with stress and steroids at the centre of the picture. Temporarily abandoning osteoporosis, per se, and concentrating on an investigation of the steroids, and the effects of stress as manifested by a raised cortisol level, in due course leads to the mechanism of both the types of osteoporosis which have been observed (see Chapter 8). But it also leads to other results which can themselves act as foci for further investigation. Among these are the mechanism of thrombus formation; the group of diseases which are primarily due to emotional stress (including osteoporosis, vascular disease, asthma and chronic bronchitis); undesirable side-effects of contraceptive steroids, particularly among adolescents; differences between races in emotional reactions and temperament that cannot be modified by environment; and so on. Once the mechanisms of all these are known, the methods of dealing with these problems, osteoporosis included, becomes a matter of applied research.

This distinction is well understood by physical scientists, and in the case of atomic energy, where there is an urgent need for a great deal of information to be acquired and integrated in the course of 50 years or so, led to the establishment of the atomic energy research organizaton based on Harwell. The scientists who recommended this realized that a great deal of fundamental information was needed, and that to expect, say, financial returns within a decade, was nonsensical, so they made provision for the necessary strategic research to be carried out. Very frequently, however, in the biological and medical fields this distinction is overlooked, so that the correct choice of a problem must be looked on as an integral part of one's research. Various areas where sufficient information is still lacking are indicated in the book.

Research procedure. Having decided on a problem, next comes the question of how to tackle it. The analogy of a jigsaw puzzle has been used. Pieces of information are available; some may be on the surface, and only require to be seen, while others need to be sought. The primary method of research, then, is the acquisition of information, and its assembly in a logical manner—the pieces of the puzzle must fit together accurately. In practice, one makes observations, sometimes performs experiments, and generally assembles evidence.

The next stage is to formulate a hypothesis. The rules here are that *all* the facts must be accounted for by the hypothesis, and that any further requirements of the hypothesis should be in accord with further observations. Having formulated the hypothesis, one should then look for further facts and evidence, and particularly those observations which might be suggested by the hypothesis. Should any of this further evidence fail to be in accord with the hypothesis, then it must be modified, or else abandoned and a new hypothesis considered. Further evidence is then required to test the new hypothesis . . . and so on. Always, if there is any discord, it is necessary to keep to the facts and abandon the hypothesis. In this book, a number of topics that are frequently taught will not be mentioned. This is partly because they give the appearance of being superstitions built upon incorrect hypotheses or speculation. The process of reasoning, and of fitting the information together, piece by piece, has been followed in the account of vascular disease given in Chapter 2, and in less detail in the account of carcinogenesis given in Chapter 9.

There are various pitfalls that must be avoided if one is to do good and sound work. One should never treat speculations as if they were facts, while it is always wisest to seek the biological mechanisms involved in any given process, and avoid facile correlations. In this regard it must be remembered that the use of statistics has very severe limitations. Most important of these is that it nearly always seems to give an answer, but that answer will only be the correct answer if all the relevant information has been fed into the system. Thus, there are several different causes of lung cancer, or possible causes, and in recent years statistics has been used as a method of "proof" that smoking is the primary cause. But an adequate mechanism has not been demonstrated, while a probable mechanism involving diesel fumes has been ignored. Until this and other possible causes have been adequately investigated, statements concerning smoking and lung cancer remain invalid.

A good rule is never to start out to "show" something, but always aim to acquire more information about the system in question. Thus, it is well known that tetracyclines are taken up into the bone, so that there might be a temptation in an animal experiment merely to take some bones and discard the rest of the corpse. One would thus fail to notice that in young animals and with comparatively high doses, there is a very considerably splenomegaly, and abnormal formation of haematopoietic tissue (Little and Edgington, 1963)—a relevant fact when one is choosing an antibiotic for premature or young babies. There is also the need to actually see what one is looking at and not what one expects to find. This can best be illustrated by an example.

A fallacy that is quite widely taught is that the bone in Albers-Schonberg Disease (Marble Bone) cannot be resorbed or involved in bone turnover or remodelling, whereas in fact the bone is resorbed normally and it is the calcified cartilage that cannot be resorbed (Little, 1969a). On one occasion I was being assured by a pathologist who had learnt it from the textbook that no osteoclasts were found in Marble Bone. He took a section to illustrate his point, looked round it and said, "Look, no osteoclasts". The field he had left under the microscope contained no fewer than five osteoclasts!

When one approaches a problem, it is always best to have a look at the material, and see for oneself, before turning to the record of other people's work. Where new work is involved there will only be a small number of references. The accounts of the actions of steroids and anabolic agents in Chapter 6, and of the effects of irradiation in Chapter 10 are two such topics, and in these accounts emphasis has been placed on factual observations. Other topics have been the subject of an immense amount of work, and one consideration in the choice of references has been to introduce the beginner to the range of information available. No one journal or group of journals can be considered adequate, neither can one ignore publications before, say, 1950 or 1955. A great deal of valuable information is present in the earlier literature. The stress diseases (Chapter 7) and carcinogenesis (Chapter 9) are two examples.

The medical literature. The medical literature has tended to come in fairly well-defined phases, partly because the types of observation reported depend to a certain extent on the available techniques. The first phase was the longest, and it may be taken as the period before printing came into general use. Copying manuscripts was laborious, and few books were written. Peter Lovve, "a Scottishman" (who announced that fact at the beginning of every chapter—he worked in Paris) wrote what is probably the first major text in the English language (Lovve, 1634). His book was published in 1634, and a list of 180 names covered all the material available to him from Hippocrates onwards.

These early works were manuscripts and tended to vary with copying. The earliest known text of the Hippocratic Oath, for example, is a fragment of Papyrus from Oxyrhynchus in Middle Egypt, and dates from the third century, A.D. (Barns, 1964). It was a working document, complete with spelling errors, and written on the back of some agricultural accounts. The next earliest text is from the eleventh century, and there are minor textual differences (apart from the spelling mistakes). Added to this, there are possible ambiguities which can arise from translation, and from differences between jargon at the time of translation and the present day. Two translations of a portion of the Oath may help to illustrate this. Both were translated direct from the Greek.

Lovve's translation of 1634 (Hippocrates, B.C. *b*) reads:

". . . Also that in practising and using my science towards the sicke, I shall use onely things necessary, so farre as I am able, and as my spirit and good understanding shall give unto mee, and that I shall not doe any thing against equitie, for hatred, anger, envie, or malice, to any person what forever: Morever, that I shall minister no poyson, neither councell nor teach poyson, nor the composing there of, to any. Also, that I shall not give, nor cause to be given, nor consent that anything be applyed to a woman breeding, or bigge with childe, to destroy, or make her voyde her fruit . . ."

Adams translation in 1849 (Hippocrates, B.C. *a*) renders this passage as:

". . . I will follow that system of regimen which, according to my ability and judgement, I consider for the benefit of my patients, and abstain from whatever is deleterious and mischievous. I will give no deadly medicine to anyone if asked, nor suggest any such counsel; and in like manner I will not give to a woman a pessary to produce abortion . . ."

Even with Adam's translations of Hippocrates works linguistic problems arise where different words are used to describe the same thing. Two descriptions of the spine, in different parts of the book read:

"In the first place, the structure of the spine should be known, for this knowledge is requisite in many diseases. Wherefore, on the side turned to the belly the vertebrae are in a regular line, and are united together by a pulpy and nervous band of connection, originating from the cartilages, and extending to the spinal marrow. There are certain other nervous cords which decussate, are attached, and are extended from both sides of them".

"The vertebrae on the inside are regularly placed upon one another, but behind they are connected by a cartilaginous ligament."

Hippocrates had obviously done careful dissections, but his description of the smooth white fibrous tissue has in one place been translated as nervous cords and in another as ligaments—and it does not mean that he thought ligaments were nerves.

All the early medical literature has as its two dominant themes the many infectious diseases and infections, and the treatment of wounds and injuries. In his introduction to the translation of Hippocrates works Adams (1849) was able to say:

"The parts which relate to dislocations at the shoulder and the hip-joint, and more especially the latter, in which, as it appears to me, he has given a fuller and more complete history of everything relating to the subject than is to be found in any single work, even at the present day".

Other conditions are mentioned in the ancient literature. Aretaeus, the Cappadocean, for instance, who lived in the perhaps somewhat dusty regions of Asia Minor, was clearly familiar with lung cancer. His works have also been translated from the Greek by Francis Adams, and in Chapter XII of his book on the "Causes and Symptoms of Chronic Diseases" (Aretaeus, B.C.), with a heading translated as Pneumodes, he says:

"Pneumodes is a species of asthma . . . the disease is protracted for a time yet not longer than one year. They have this as peculiar, they cough as if going to expectorate, but their effort is vain, for they bring up nothing . . . though the lungs be free from suppuration, they are filled with humours which are, as it were, compacted. The intervals of the paroxysms in this affection are greater. Some, indeed die speedily of suffocation before anything worse is transferred to the general system".

Until the latter part of the nineteenth century there was no standard nomenclature for the description of cancer. Lovve (1634) in Lib. IIII Chapter XVI has the heading "Of cancer, which the Greekes called Carcinoma", and in Lib. V Chapter XXV uses either Sarcoma or Polypus to describe tumours in the nose, but a century later few published case histories made use of any of these terms.

The next phase of medical development and publications is that from the general use of printing until the general use of the microscope and the realization of the importance of cells, in the nineteenth century. Single lenses, with a limited magnifying power had been used for some considerable time, and simple microscopes using the sun's rays as a light source were available in the middle of the eighteenth century. As early as 1740 Miles (1740–41) was describing the motion of red cells in circulating blood.

"In the lesser vessels . . . I several times saw the Globules of an oblong form . . . gliding along one after another." "Another thing I observed, more than once, with Pleasure, that the globules would, in some Places, gradually slacken their motion, at length seem to be about to stand still; in an Instant, a globule would be compressed, . . . and then, as if it had squeezed through a narrow Passage, resume its former shape, and pass on with great Swiftness . . ."

During this period the publications of the Royal Society, the first technical scientific journals, made possible the more rapid dissemination of knowledge, and so paved the way for a more orderly process of assembling knowledge. Thus, Belchier (1735–36 a) discovered that blood circulates not only within bones, but also in the compact bone of the shaft, "the Circulation is universally and intimately distributed through the most solid and compact Substance of the Bones." This he did by staining with Madder, a red dye, mixed with the food of animals or birds, These original observations were on pig's bone, and soon afterwards he reported the results of some experiments using cocks (Belchier, 1735–36 b), and was surprised to find that within 16 days of the commencement of the diet one already had all its bones dyed red. Du Hammel (1737–38) read these accounts and initiated experiments of his own. He used pullets, turkeys and pigeons. With these birds he was able to view the red colouring of bones in the wing, where they were close to the surface. He fed the pullets on the Madder-containing diet until their bones were red, and then found that after a month they lost the colour again. With young growing birds he showed that at 24 h the uptake of dye was just starting, and that more was taken up in 36 h and more again by 3 days. He also found that the bones of adult birds took up far less dye. Also: "Upon viewing these Bones with a good glass, their smoothest Surface appears bored with a vast number of small Holes in which the colouring . . . is perceived." Finally, he experimented with the effect of the dye on fracture callus and ascertained that as well as being taken up in the newly laid down bone it interfered with subsequent development of the callus.

The use of the microscope in the nineteenth century enabled immense strides to be made in the acquisition of knowledge, and the medical history of that period is primarily of the acquisition of new knowledge and facts. The earlier observations had often been accurate, e.g. "Chemical analysis resolves the bones into an animal matter, chiefly gelatin, and an earthy matter, principally phosphate and carbonate of lime. They owe their elasticity and toughness to the former, and hardness and rigidity to the latter" and "The cartilage is formed from a soft jelly which becomes opaque immediately before calcification" (Ward, 1838), but these observations could now be expanded and extended.

The period 1895 to 1910 saw the assembly of many facts into hypotheses, and since then the problems of disentangling facts, observations and hypotheses have assumed an increasing importance. The period since 1950 has shown a mushrooming of the number of papers, which has sometimes defeated its own end. Many minor experimental techniques are mentioned as assisting in the understanding of the subject, but at the same time over-indulgence in a technique or overdependence on a hypothesis can hinder the advance of knowledge. Before proceeding to a discussion of the modern literature, it is of some interest to take a specific topic and trace its development—osteoporosis (post-menopausal and/or senile) is suitable for the purpose.

Senile osteoporosis tends to be a disease of the elderly, and so one must remember that the average life span has varied. In his Aphorisms Hippocrates (B.C. *a*) says in III 31 that apoplexy is a disease of old age, and then in VI 57 "Persons are most subject to apoplexy between the ages of 40 and 60".

At the end of the sixth century Paulus Aegineta wrote a comprehensive treatise on medicine (this may appear in library catalogues under either Paulus or Aegineta). He refers to what we now know as osteoporosis in two places, and quite obviously it never occurred to him to connect the two. On the one hand he considers low back pain, and describes a number of related conditions under the general heading "On Gout and Arthritis" (Book 3, Sect. LXXVIII). Of the type of arthritis in which the vertebrae and various other sites are affected he says the disease is occasioned by a "preternatural humour" and a "weakness of the parts" meeting together. In a quite different section he deals with the special problems of fractures at the head of the thighbone.

Lovve (1634) also realizes that the "passions" can cause illness, and cites sadness and fear, anger, envy and hatred as the causes of a variety of symptoms. He also deals with the fractures in the hip quite separately:

> "All fractures in hard and dry bones, as in old people, are more difficile and are longer in healing, than such as are soft and humide, as in young people. Avicen saith, that fractures in chollericke and old people are very difficile, and in very old people be very unpossible."
>
> "Some (fractures) are longer in healing, some shorter, according to the greatness, hardness and dryness."

Without modern diagnostic aids, and particularly clinical radiographs, it proved difficult to distinguish between the different types of pathology in the hip. Bell, as late as 1824, in describing the sequence of events in osteoarthritis of the hip, which at that time still did not have a definite name, was at considerable pains to distinguish it from the intracapsular fractures found in soft bones:

> "The bone possesses a proper degree of density, and sometimes appears on dissection to be even more compact in its structure than the osseous structure generally is."

He also made the point that the hip tends to be the only joint affected. The characteristic which impressed him most was the shortening of the neck of the femur, it being this that could cause confusion with intracapsular fractures, but:

> "The neck of the bone, in some of these cases, seems as if it were incased in a sheath of ossific matter, which is sometimes of a loose and spongy texture,

c

and penetrated by numerous small holes, while in other instances it is dense, and presents an irregular stalactic surface".

Ward (1838) comments:

"The length of the neck has also been observed to diminish with advancing years, so that the head gradually sinks below the level of the trochanter major . . . Benjamin Bell, indeed, who first drew attention to the process of interstitial absorption upon which these progressive metamorphoses depend, describes it not as a healthy action natural to the senile period of life, but . . ."

Hips were discussed and described, low back pain was discussed, but it was not until the advent of clinical radiography in the present century that it was realized that the intracapsular fracture of a bone-deficient head of femur and the progressive shortening of the spine were two manifestations of the same condition, characterized by a rarefaction of bone, and particularly of the cancellous bone. Again, it had been realized from very early times that the unpleasant emotions could cause physical symptoms, but it was not until after the development of organic chemistry in the last 150 years or so, that the stage was reached in the 1930s, when those symptoms could be related to hormonal changes. It then took only another year or two for Albright to distinguish post-menopausal osteoporosis and produce convincing evidence (Albright, Bloomberg and Smith, 1940; Albright, Smith and Richardson, 1941) that the bone changes were of hormonal origin.

For the next 25 years after Albright's evidence was published the literature on osteoporosis was very confused. A diversity of speculations were published, then treated as fact, and it is only recently that the detailed evidence necessary to give a coherent picture has emerged. This exemplifies the main problem in reading the modern literature. One must be careful to distinguish between observations, fact and evidence, and speculations or hypotheses developed from fragmentory or half-understood evidence, and contrary to known facts. In the same way that one applies the rules of evidence to one's own work, they must be applied to the information available in the literature. The stress diseases (Chapter 7) and carcinogenesis (Chapter 9) have been described from this point of view.

Since 1950 in particular, a problem has been gradually emerging, that has now reached acute proportions. It is the increasing tendency for information to be scattered among a large number of journals, some apparently dealing with quite different problems. To acquire information about bone, therefore, it is not sufficient to read journals primarily devoted to the recording of facts about bone. There are abstract journals, publications listing current papers, and the Medical Index. Papers covering various topics may be found in the Subject Index, while the Name Index can be used to check papers by people who have been found to be working in a given field. Other relevant papers can be found in the references given in papers already found. This book contains more references than is usual in a textbook, and many of these have been chosen to give an indication of the scope of the literature, and to provide a starting point for a literature survey. It need hardly be said that before a paper is quoted, it should actually be read, with an open mind, to consider what the author says, and what evidence he has for what he says.

Experimental methods. Another very obvious statement, that should hardly need to be made, is that the use of some particular piece of equipment or method of investigation does not in itself count as research. Research is the name now given to the activity involved in solving problems or seeking facts. When one is doing research on bone there is a considerable range of techniques which are useful for isolated aspects of the problem, but not for general use. Examples of some that will be quoted in this book are given below.

(*a*) Tissue culture—cells or fragments of tissue are grown in a variety of media to investigate their properties, and their behaviour under different conditions, and a great deal of valuable information has been obtained by A. Carrel, J. C. Mottram, H. Fell and many other workers. The method has one very definite limitation. Osteogenic cells are derived from cells of the vessel walls, bone activity is regulated by the distribution of vessels and the flow of blood through those vessels, radiation damage to bone is primarily damage to vessel walls—while there is no blood supply to the fragments of tissue in culture. The significance of this must not be overlooked during the course of tissue culture experiments.

(*b*) X-ray diffraction—this has been used to identify the mineral components of bones, teeth and pathological calcifications. Once the type of compound and its crystal size and habit are known for each set of conditions met with there is no further use for the technique in the investigation of bone, except for pure research. Similarly X-ray fibre diffraction has been used to distinguish the different proteins that may be met with—two collagen structures, several beta-proteins, a dense beta-protein and elastic tissue—and also some of the polysaccharides. Once these have been sorted out the information gained can be used for future more detailed interpretation of histological sections and the method is no longer required.

(*c*) Electron microscopy—a similar state of affairs pertains to the use of electron microscopy. Some very useful information can be gained about the nature of the intercellular matrices, for example, but afterwards this information is best used as an aid in the more complete interpretation of histological sections, which are of a more useful size— electron microscope sections are limited to about a millimetre across. A limited amount of useful information has also been obtained about the detailed structure of cells, but the greater part of the electron microscope examination of cells is primarily of academic interest, and therefore in the province of the pure (basic) research scientist.

Various other exotic techniques are of transient use, but they come and go, so that it is unwise to let a research programme revolve around a technique instead of around a problem. Two techniques, however, tend to be perennials, and are regularly and consistently used for a wide variety of problems. These are histology and radiography. For the present subject, the behaviour of cells in bone, the more relevant technique is histology, and so the majority of illustrations in the book are of histological sections.

Animal and human experiments. The material used for investigation comes from three main sources: tissue taken at operation, post mortem tissues, and tissues from animal experiments. In these animal experiments the effects of adjusting or modifying a variety of parameters can be followed. Conditions vary for each investigation, but there are a number of general principles which should be observed.

In the first place it is most unwise to plan in detail a large-scale experiment involving many animals. The object of the exercise is to obtain new information, and planning of large-scale experiments implies that one is sure one knows what the answer will be. The only time these could be justified, and only with a minority of problems, is to dot the i's and cross the t's when a qualitative answer is already known. One partial exception to this rule are some of the experiments which will be described in Chapter 10, where several variables are allowed for simultaneously. More usually the best plan is to initiate a pilot experiment or experiments with small groups of animals, to see what happens. The findings usually suggest various modifications to the experimental procedure to make it more informative. In fact, it is usually best to do the experiment with small groups of animals, examining each group of animals carefully before proceeding to the next. Since the intention is to obtain information about mechanisms, there is no point in using large numbers of animals. Consistent findings in three or four animals for each modification is adequate. If the findings are so variable that one might be tempted to think in terms of "statistically significant", then the experiment should be abandoned or redesigned.

Particularly when using isotopes, or performing other experiments where there is a potential risk, it is advisable to consider a number of pertinent questions. For instance, whether the experiment is really capable of giving the type of information that is needed; whether it is the best way of obtaining that information, or whether there are simpler, easier or more reliable methods. One factor that needs to be considered is the species of animal. If one is interested in the mechanisms of action in the epiphyseal growth cartilage, with every zone under the influence of one or more hormones, the choice of rats, with a quite different hormonal system from the human could lead to very dubious results. Similarly, rats cannot be used if potential carcinogenic agents are under investigation—false positives are easily obtained.

Experiments upon patients present another type of problem. These same two considerations apply—that the experiment should be capable of giving a useful answer, and that there should be no other more desirable way of obtaining that answer. There are others. Limited investigations are necessary for improvements in treatment, trying out potentially better operating procedures, or drugs, but these experiments should be restricted to the fields of diagnosis or treatment. General experiments, not concerned directly with the patient's welfare, but only with adding to existing knowledge of a condition or for reasons even more remotely connected with the patient's personal problems are almost always completely unjustifiable.

There can be very little excuse, for example, for the young doctor who came to "do research", but had no interest either in joining in the investigations current in the department, or starting an investigation of his own. He merely wanted to practice a technique on patients, that had not only no connection with diagnosis or treatment, but also no connection with any viable investigations into physiological or pathological problems. The reason was that the technique was fashionable, and he felt that to be able to say he had used it would be of help to his career. There can be no excuse at all for the eminent clinician who wrote to me on one occasion, professing to be bewildered because I had refused to co-operate in some experiments, since "they would only cause pain and perhaps infection in some cases, but should not actually endanger the lives of the patients". These experiments again were unconnected with either diagnosis or treatment, and were not designed in a manner which could have led to any increase in knowledge. Quite apart from moral or ethical considerations, such experiments are almost always scientifically unjustifiable, and should not be embarked on if the object is to seek evidence for the purpose of increasing our knowledge of normal tissues and of pathological processes.

1. INTERCELLULAR MATRICES AND CALCIFICATION

The property which most clearly distinguishes bone from other connective tissues is its mineral content. Because of this bones are hard, and rigid enough to support the body and to provide mechanical protection for the more vital tissues, the brain, bone marrow, and the heart and lungs. In recent years there has been a tendency to concentrate on this different aspect when bone is described and investigated but, as with all other tissues in the body, it is the cell behaviour that matters. At the same time, in order to understand bone fully, it is useful to have some knowledge of the intercellular components, the mineral, and the mechanism of calcification. It is not necessary to have a detailed and complete knowledge of the crystal properties of each possible mineral component, or of the precise chemical composition of each type of intercellular matrix, in order to follow the course of the various normal or pathological changes which may occur. In this first chapter some aspects which are relevant to the main theme of the book will be considered.

At a first reading it will be more useful to skim through this chapter with the intention of finding what it contains rather than assimilating it completely, and then to come back to the various points as the need arises.

Intercellular Matrices

Connective tissue cells

The cells which produce bone belong to the connective tissue series. Closely related cells form tendons and ligaments, reticulin, fibrous tissue, cartilage and bone. They have in common the property of forming intercellular matrices. These cell products are composed primarily of polymeric compounds which form the structural framework of the body. There are also muscle cells, in which the fibrous polymeric components remain within the cells. The products of connective tissue cells are gels and rubbers, of varying degrees of firmness and resilience, which are responsible for the mechanical properties of the tissues.

Attempts have been made to classify these cells according to the chemical nature of their products, how they are formed or arranged, and so on. A major difficulty is that the cells tend to change their behaviour according to their surroundings, so that the same cell may, for instance, function consecutively as an osteoblast (which produces matrix), and osteocyte (which maintains it) and an osteoclast (which produces enzymes that destroy the matrix), and may even reverse these functions. One of the more useful attempts at classification has been that of Willmer (1960, 1970). He describes cells of the connective tissue and muscle series as behaving as either mechanocytes or amoebocytes. The former tend to be elongated and progress by creeping over a substrate, while the latter are rounded and can exist free in a liquid medium. Figs 1.1, 1.2 show cells of these two types as seen in fracture callus. The cartilage cells have spread through a fluid space, while the granulation tissue cells (mechanocytes) are advancing through a blood clot. The group of mechanocytes is subdivided into precursors of bone, fibrous

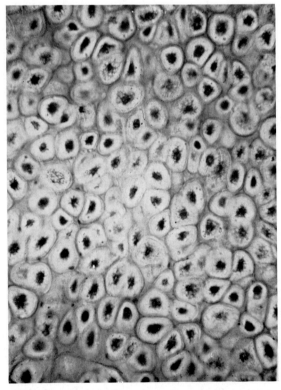

Fig. 1.1. Fracture callus in a young rabbit. These cartilage cells have proliferated into a space caused by displacement at the time of fracture. ×400.

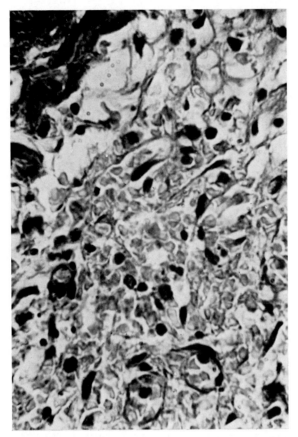

Fig. 1.2. Granulation tissue cells (dark and elongated) progressing through an organized clot in the bone of a young child. At the top left is some surviving bone tissue. ×400.

tissue and fibrocartilage, which together produce the dominant components of the connective tissues, and muscle cells. In tissue culture Willmer found that proliferating muscle cells which were not producing muscle fibrils had a close morphological resemblance to proliferating fibroblasts.

In the bones and their surrounding tissues cartilage may arise from amoebocytes or mechanocytes or from a mixture of the two. Matrices which are commonly regarded as typical of cartilage, with a tangled array of protein filaments, are formed from cells of either group. Although sometimes they may present virtually indistinguishable appearances, at other times tissues from the two types retain their characteristic appearances, as may be seen in the healed disc cartilage from a fracture at the junction of the nucleus pulposus and cartilage end

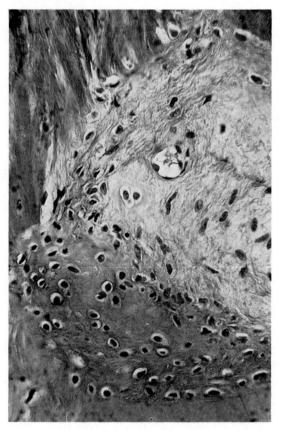

Fig. 1.3. Healed microfracture at the junction of the cartilage end plate and nucleus pulposus near a Schmorl's node. From lumbar disc of an elderly man. Cells derived from the two tissues show different characteristics, and their intercellular matrices resemble those of the tissues from which the cells were derived. × 200.

plate shown in Fig. 1.3. The cells on either side of the new tissue resemble the adjacent cells from which they were derived.

Cells of mechanocyte type found in bone tissue are responsive to their surroundings and may have more than one mode of development. Those described by Willmer were grown in tissue culture, and much of the detailed work on osteogenesis by Fell (1933) and her collaborators was on foetal bone also grown in culture media. Differences in protein content of the media alter cell behaviour, so that cultured cells, although they have been investigated in considerable detail, must not be regarded as typical. In particular, it must be remembered that one of the most outstanding characteristics of bone is its vascularity. Various nineteenth century workers, and more recently J. Trueta and his colleagues have

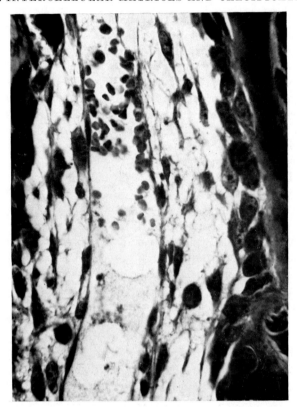

FIG. 1.4. Metaphyseal vessel in long bone of puppy. On either side there are direct inter-cellular connections from cells in the vessel wall, through intermediate cells to the osteoblasts on the bone surface. The region occupied by the intermediate osteogenic cells has a high fluid content, resulting in empty spaces (white) in the dried specimen. ×400.

produced a great deal of evidence to show that the major source of osteoblasts is from cells of sinusoid vessel walls (Fig. 1.4). These cells are normally interconnected and show other differences in behaviour from cells grown in many culture media. This question of the origin of osteoblasts will be considered in greater detail in Chapter 4.

Matrix production

To return now to the intercellular matrices produced by these cells: the main components which are responsible for the mechanical properties of the matrices are proteins and polysaccharides. These are polymeric compounds. That is, their molecules are long chains built up from subunits, of amino acids or sugars, joined together by covalent bonds. The individual sugar residues are rings, and two of the amino acids (proline and hydroxyproline) in the proteins are ring structures, but the predominant structure is a long molecular chain, sometimes with a certain amount of branching. Other examples of long chain polymers are textile fibres and plastics such as nylon, polyethylene terephthalate (Terylene or Dacron), PTFE (polytetrafluoethylene, Teflon or Fluon), polyethylene and polypropylene; the natural and synthetic rubbers and the silicone rubbers. Materials such as the epoxyresins or bakelite have more random links which give a three-dimensional structure. In polymers, whether natural or synthetic, some regions are more ordered than others. These ordered regions often show a quite regular crystal structure. The degree of crystallinity is usually in the range 10% up to 60% or 70%.

There has been a certain amount of confusion in the literature over nomenclature of the polymeric matrices in the connective tissues. The word "collagen" for instance has been given a variety of meanings, often without adequate definition. Sometimes it means a whole bundle of tissue, containing many collagen fibrils, polysaccharides, lipids, cells, possibly surrounding reticulin, and even blood vessels. Most frequently, perhaps, it means a fibril or group of fibrils with their associated poly-saccharides and lipids, while to the chemist or crystallographer it means the protein component of those fibrils. It is in this stricter sense that the word will be used here. The term "matrix" has also been used with different concepts present in the minds of different authors. Sometimes it is the non-protein components of the intercellular mixture of sub-stances that is meant, sometimes it is the non-fibrillar components, and sometimes it is the whole of the intercellular material, including not only the polymeric proteins and polysaccharides but also the lipids which may be present. Here the whole of the intercellular mixture will be referred to as the intercellular matrix.

Within connective tissue cells the matrix components are produced in those regions of the cell occupied by membranes of the endoplasmic reticulum (Fig. 1.5). These membranes tend to be parallel and can extend to the ends of cell processes (Fig. 1.6). There is evidence that unless they are intact any matrix that is formed is faulty. In the absence of vitamin C, for example, the endoplasmic reticulum is scanty and poorly formed, although other intracellular membranes remain intact. The matrix that is produced in scurvy is also scanty and imperfectly formed.

Having been polymerized from its low molecular weight precursors, the matrix is extruded from the cells through segments of the cell sur-faces which protrude and then retract. This is best seen in ciné-pictures, as in those of cartilage cells taken in Smith's laboratory (1965) and of fibroblasts taken by T. F. Dougherty, D. L. Berliner and M. L. Berliner (Dougherty, Berliner and Berliner, 1961; Berliner, 1965; Berliner and

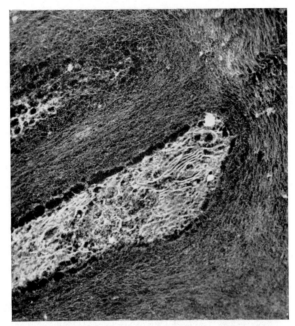

Fig. 1.5. Cartilage cell in the proliferative zone of the epiphyseal growth cartilage in a child $2\frac{1}{2}$ years of age. The cell is surrounded by a matrix containing immature non-collagenous protein, with some fibrillar collagen at the top right of the photograph. Membranes of the endoplasmic reticulum may be seen in the cytoplasm. E.M. 100kV. ×3500.

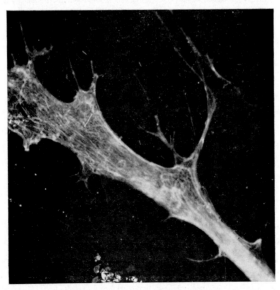

Fig. 1.6. Section of fibroblast process in loose connective tissue. Membranes of the endoplasmic reticulum extend to the ends of the cell processes. E.M. 100kV. ×3500.

Ruhmann, 1966) and others, but a very good idea of the process may be gained by comparing the appearance of cells in different stages of activity in histological sections. From each protruding segment of the cell there is extruded a bundle of collagen fibrils with their associated polysaccharide. Figure 1.7 shows an early stage of the process, in human

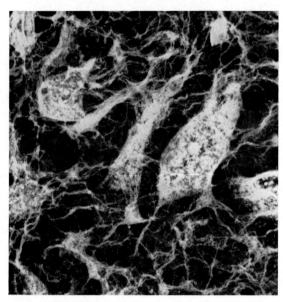

Fig. 1.7. Fibrous tissue in human foetus. There is a low proportion of cytoplasm in cells as compared with those in more mature tissue. A small quantity of matrix has been extruded from protruding segments of the cell surfaces. E.M. 100kV. ×2000.

foetal tissue, when only a little of the intercellular matrix had been formed. After extrusion from the ends of cells bundles of collagen fibrils often remain separated. Figure 1.8 shows bundles of mature collagen fibrils which had been extruded from a single cell in the skin. The characteristic banding of the collagen shows in this photograph because treatment of the specimen had resulted in some degradation of the muco-polysaccharide which normally surrounds each individual collagen fibril. The banded structure has been exaggerated by "shadowing" the specimen. That is, a small amount of metal has been evaporated in a vacuum and allowed to fall on it at an angle, so that small irregularities on the surface, in this case the bands on the fibrils, are brought into relief. When the motion of the surface membrane of a cell is made more sluggish by the action of cortisol (Dougherty et al., 1961) even unorientated non-fibrillar matrix may be found in discrete patches, as seen in the section of growth cartilage shown in Fig. 1.9, instead of showing the more homogeneous texture which is usually found (e.g. Fig. 1.5).

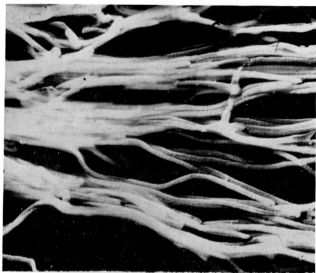

Fig. 1.8. Bundles of mature collagen fibrils extruded from a cell in the skin of a young adult. The section has been metal "shadowed" so that the 640 Å bands may be seen in some fibrils. The bands on many fibrils are masked by the polysaccharide-containing component of the matrix which surrounds them and holds the fibrils together within the bundles. E.M. 100kV.

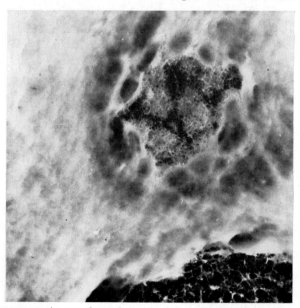

Fig. 1.9. Transverse section near base of growth cartilage in rabbit treated with cortisone for two weeks. The section passes through the non-fibrillar matrix close to a cell. Matrix extruded by each cell process has remained as a discrete patch. Normally the motion of cell surfaces would have resulted in a more uniform distribution of matrix. The fibrous matrix surrounding this area is partly calcified. E.M. 100kV. ×3500.

When matrix is extruded from the central regions of a cell the fibrils are not orientated and the fibroblast then functions as a fibrocartilage cell. It is possible in this case that the matrix is extruded in liquid form and precipitated a little way away from the cell. Figures 1.10–1.12 are

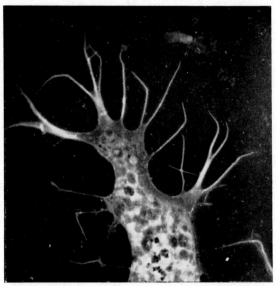

FIG. 1.10. Whole fibroblast (skin), on formvar membrane which had been placed in cell culture. Portions of cell surface are protruding at end of cell. E.M. 100kV.

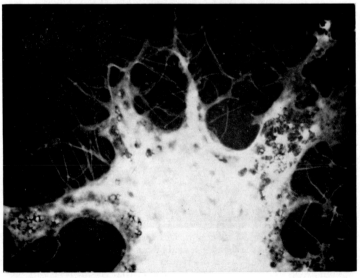

FIG. 1.11. Another whole fibroblast. A few collagen fibrils may be seen. E.M. 100kV.

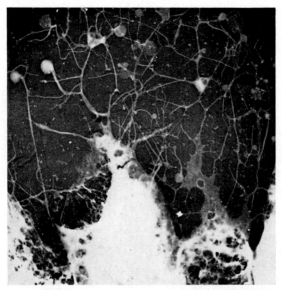

FIG. 1.12. Another whole fibroblast. Portions of the cell surface are protruding from the side of the cell, and some strands of collagenous matrix may be seen. Their appearance as a network suggests that they were precipitated after extrusion rather than having been extruded in fibrillar form. Several "blobs" of non-fibrillar matrix may also be seen. E.M. 100kV.

electron microscope photographs of whole fibroblasts grown in cell culture, in which was placed a formvar membrane. Figures 1.10, 1.11 show portions of the cell surfaces protruding, while Figures 1.12 shows the beginning of matrix precipitation. It has sometimes been imagined that these appearances of protruding sectors of cell surfaces are due to shrinkage or other preparation artefact, and some workers go to considerable trouble to choose for photography cells that do not show protrusions. However, quite apart from the evidence provided by observation of living cells, when one sees the protruding parts of the cells trapped in the matrix they have made (Fig. 1.13) or the configuration of fully formed matrix following that typical of the tails of fibroblasts (Figs 1.14, 1.15), it seems that in such instances a slowing down of the dynamic mechanism is being portrayed. As the proportion of the surrounding space occupied by matrix is increased there is no longer room for free movement of the cell walls.

Characterization of matrix components

The dominant components of the intercellular matrices are the proteins and polysaccharides. They are extruded from the cells together, and in general each protein has its associated polysaccharide. Lipids and

D

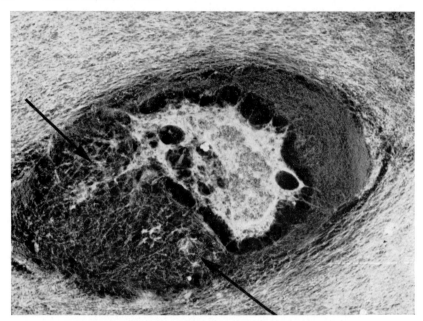

Fig. 1.13. Cell in anlage cartilage in rabbit epiphysis. Protruding portions of the cytoplasm (arrowed) have been trapped by the matrix they produced. E.M. 100kV. ×3500.

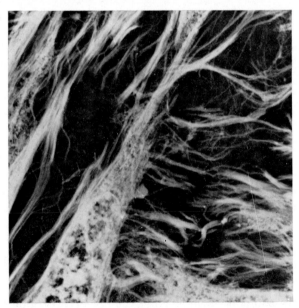

Fig. 1.14. Fibroblast in newly formed fibrous repair tissue on surface of osteoarthritic bone. Long cell processes with their extruded collagen give the appearance of a "tail". E.M. 100kV. ×3500.

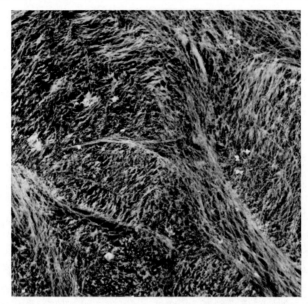

FIG. 1.15. Fibrous tissue near bone surface in osteoarthritis. The configuration of the matrix is typical of that shown by the "tails" of elongated fibroblasts. E.M. 100kV. ×3500.

possibly other minor components are also present. Citrates are nearly always found associated with collagen, particularly in bone where they adsorb onto mineral crystals and so are not leached away. There is some evidence to suggest that their presence is necessary to induce fibril formation in collagen (Courts and Little, 1963). To understand the function of the different types of matrix in bone, cartilage and connective tissues no detailed knowledge of their chemistry is necessary. It will suffice if they are classified into a few groups according to their main physical properties.

The best known of the structural proteins are the collagens. In the foetus and infant collagens are more soluble and less chemically stable than in the elderly. The increase in stability with age of the individual is not a change which takes place in the protein during the years after it has been extruded from the cell that synthesized it, but a change in the behaviour of the cells manufacturing the collagen in the older individuals. The differences are due to the hormones present (Davidson, 1964). Growth hormone is responsible for the more labile compounds present in the young, and the steroids for the more stable compounds in adults (Davidson and Small 1963). Detectable physical ageing of individual filaments usually take place within five days of extrusion, and most of this change is in the first hour or so. After that, unless it is subjected to chemical degradation, the collagen remains unchanged for literally millions of years. Figure 1.16 shows intact collagenous matrix in the decalcified femur of a Pleistocene horse. That the collagen fibrils are still held firmly together indicates that at least a part of the polysaccharide component, acting as a glue between the fibrils, is still intact. In this photograph the bands in the collagen fibrils are prominent, not because of shadowing as in Fig. 1.8, but because the specimen was stained with phosphotungstic acid. This fossil bone was preserved in a tar pit (Shackleford and Wyckoff, 1964). Usually in the examination of

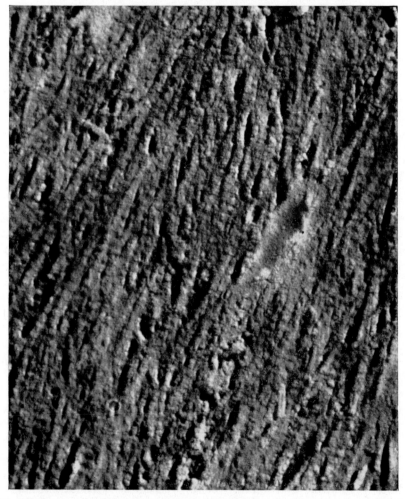

Fig. 1.16. Intact collagenous matrix in the decalcified femur of a Pleistocene horse. Staining with 0·5% phosphotungstic acid in 50% ethyl alcohol has revealed the banded structure of the collagen. E.M. ×40,000.
The author thanks Prof. R. W. G. Wyckoff for providing this photograph.

fossils extraneous mineral inclusions and deposits (often silicates and manganese phosphate) are a hindrance, since the chemicals required to remove the mineral also degrade the matrix. Manganese phosphate, in particular, is closely adherent to fossil bones in sedimentary deposits. However, Isaacs, Little, Currey and Tarlo (1963) have succeeded in obtaining fragments of collagen from a dinosaur (200 million years) and a cellulose-like compound lining dentine tubules from the heterostracan ostracoderm (400 million years).

The crystalline portions of the collagen fibril give a characteristic X-ray diffraction pattern, by which it may be distinguished either alone or in mixtures with other proteins. All crystalline materials have this property of diffracting X-rays. When a monochromatic X-ray beam is used a single crystal diffracts the beam in such a manner as to form a regular array of spots, while multicrystalline materials provide rather more complex patterns. The diffracted X-ray beams originate in planes of atoms in the material (Fig. 1.17), and each plane of atoms gives a

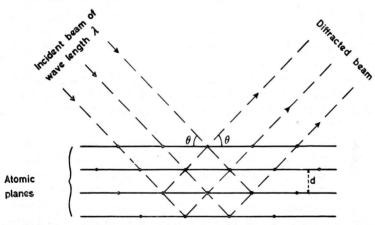

FIG. 1.17. Diagram to illustrate diffraction of a parallel beam of X-rays by the planes of atoms in a crystal. The distance between the planes which produces each spot (or ring for a multi-crystalline specimen) is given by the function $d = \dfrac{n\lambda}{2 \sin \theta}$, where n is an integer denoting the order of the reflection, λ is the wavelength of the incident X-ray beam and θ is the angle of incidence of the X-ray beam on the set of planes in question (Bragg and Bragg, 1913). This is known as Bragg's law.

separate diffracted spot (Thewlis, 1940; pp. 10–14). The more atoms in a plane the more intense is the diffracted beam. Additionally, the more orderly the arrangement of these atoms the more well-defined is the beam. When taking a photograph of the array of diffracted beams from a specimen one may place a cylindrical X-ray film around the specimen, as is commonly done to record the spots from a single crystal; or a thin strip of film is placed around a multi-crystalline specimen, to obtain lines in the so-called powder diffraction pattern; or the diffracted beam may be allowed to impinge on a flat plate. This last is the method commonly used for polymeric compounds, such as proteins or textile fibres, and the pattern obtained from these is referred to as a fibre diffraction pattern. Each compound or element can have one or more crystal structures, and the differences in the arrangement of planes of atoms within these crystals allows X-ray diffraction to be used as a "finger-print" method for their identification. X-ray diffraction is used for both polymeric and mineral components of the tissues as a rapid and usually more accurate substitute for chemical analysis

This use of X-ray diffraction as a "finger-print" method for the identification of components in a sample does not require more than a superficial acquaintance with the technique. When the actual structure of a material is required then a considerable understanding of diffraction and crystallographic techniques is essential. Very occasionally with a simple compound an "inspired guess" can give the structure, which can then be more easily verified, but usually there is no alternative to exact and time-consuming procedures. The elucidation of the structure of penicillin with its unexpected 5 membered ring, or of the structure of the DNA molecule with water molecules as an integral part of the crystal, would not have been feasible without precise crystallographic measurements. A textbook such as C. W. Bunn's *Chemical Crystallography* (O.U.P.) is recommended for those who would like to go into the subject more deeply.

X-ray reflections from very imperfect crystals are broadened, and some may be so dispersed as to be lost in the general background of scattered radiation. In these cases the "finger-print" method is less precise than for highly ordered crystals. For each reflection the distance apart of the planes of atoms which formed it may be calculated. This distance is sometimes used as a means of referring to a particular reflection as, say, the 4·65 Å ring which is shared by many proteins (1 Ångstrom unit = 10^{-8} centimetres). Figure 1.18 shows a typical fibre diffraction pattern of a partially orientated collagen. The other main proteins which may be found in the intercellular matrix are three that have the 4·65 Å reflection of a beta-protein dominating. The name beta-protein is a general name given to the group of proteins with extended molecular chains, to distinguish them from proteins with folded chains (e.g. alpha keratin in straight hair). Of the beta-proteins found in the connective tissue matrices two may be referred to as an immature beta-protein, present in the foetus and infant, and as a mature beta-protein, present in older children and adults. The sharpness of the crystalline reflection, an indication of the degree of ordering of the

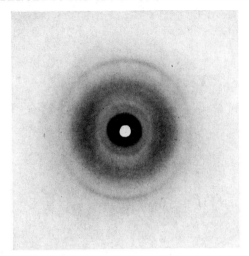

FIG. 1.18. X-ray fibre diffraction photograph of a partially orientated collagenous tissue. The clarity of rings K, E and F (see Fig. 21) as compared with their background is an indication that this tissue contains a high proportion of collagen. The longer an interplanar spacing, the closer is the diffraction ring it produces to the centre of the photograph.

molecules in the protein, increases with age. The comparison photograph of diffraction patterns of beta-proteins, taken from the intervertebral discs of a young and an elderly person, in Fig. 1.19 shows

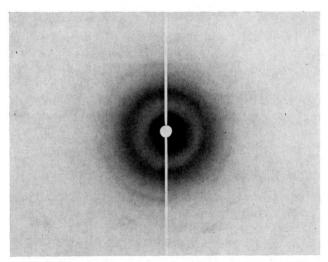

FIG. 1.19. X-ray fibre diffraction photographs comparing the beta-protein from prolapsed lumbar disc tissue (left) with dense beta-protein from the disc of an elderly person (right). Each is mixed with some collagen, so the collagen pattern is superimposed on the beta-protein patterns. The pattern on the left shows a side spacing of collagen alone (B—see Fig. 21), while that on the right shows two side spacings, of collagen (B) and the dense beta-protein (N). The author thanks Prof. T. K. F. Taylor for this photograph.

the mature beta-protein and the third of the beta-proteins which is denser than the others. Figure 1.20 is a comparison photograph of this

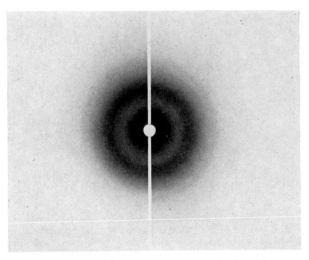

Fig. 1.20. X-ray fibre diffraction photographs comparing the dense beta-protein (left) and elastic tissue (right). The main interchain spacing of elastic tissue, at approximately 4·65 Å gives a broader and more diffuse ring than does that of the beta-protein. It has a somewhat shorter side spacing. Relative positions are shown diagrammatically in Fig. 21. Both specimens contained a little collagen, while very faint rings of magnesian whitlockite are superimposed on the elastic pattern. The author thanks Prof. T. K. F. Taylor for this photograph.

third dense beta-protein and elastic tissue. The dense beta-protein also gives sharper rings when specimens from older individuals are examined. The relative positions of these various diffracted rings are shown in the diagram in Fig. 1.21 in which each sector represents the rings given by a different protein. The ring A is the 2·86 Å reflection characteristic of collagen and not present in the beta-proteins, while L is the 4·65 Å ring of the beta-proteins.

Other properties by which these main structural proteins may be characterized are by means of their autofluorescence, either in the gross state or in section, their appearance in sections examined in the electron microscope, and their appearance in histological sections. These methods have the practical advantage that no attempt at chemical isolation is required. When viewed in ultra-violet light, each of the structural beta-proteins shows autofluorescence with a slightly different shade of blue (Moschi and Little, 1966), while associated lipids give a yellow colour. The advantage of the electron microscope over the light microscope is its increased resolution rather than the higher magnifications this increased resolution makes possible. Figure 1.22 shows two photographs, at the same magnification, of a three micron diameter quartz

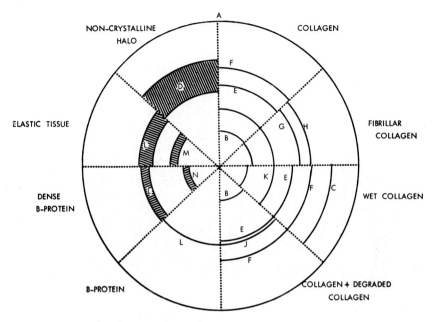

Fig. 1.21. Diagram in which each sector represents the rings given by a different protein diffraction pattern. The outer ring A is found in collagen and fibrillar collagen, whether wet or dry, but not in any other component. Rings in the vicinity of 4·65 Å (L, J, E, T, G) are common to many linear polymeric structures as well as to the proteins. The spacing B of the collagens varies in position according to whether they are wet or dry. As collagen degrades the rings become more diffuse, K being the first to be lost. With more complete degeneration the characteristic collagen rings are replaced by J (corresponding to an expanded chain). Spacings are:

A 2·86 Å	B 14·3–11·3 Å	C 3·37 Å
D 5·3–3·6 Å	E 4·72 Å	F 3·94 Å
G 4·56 Å	H 4·01 Å	J 4·65 Å
K 7·20 Å	L 4·65 Å	M 7·8 Å
	N 9·5–10·8 Å	

fibre, which illustrate the increased clarity resulting from the increased resolution. The disadvantage of the electron microscope is that, as a result of the geometrical requirements for obtaining this added resolution, only a small area can be examined or photographed at any one time.

In this book the light microscope photographs are being printed as dark objects on a white ground, while the electron microscope photographs are being printed as a light object on a black background. Figure 1.22 is one of the few exceptions. The scanning electron microscope photographs will also be printed as light objects on a black ground. In those cases where shadowing has been used this is necessary (otherwise a light shadow would cause confusion) and it would seem to be more

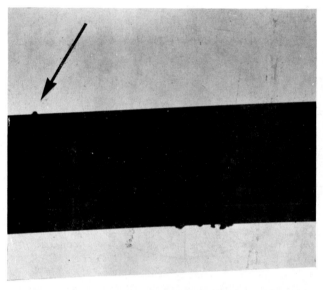

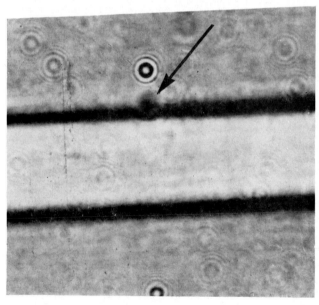

Fig. 1.22. Photographs of a three micron diameter quartz fibre, at the same magnification, to illustrate the difference in resolution between the electron microscope and light microscope (with oil immersion lens). Diffraction effects are always prominent when a source of illumination is being employed near the limit of resolution of which it is capable. The size of the dust particles on the fibre surface is at the limit of resolution of the light microscope.

logical to use the same printing convention for all photographs taken using similar techniques.

For adequate electron microscope characterization of the components of the intercellular matrices a necessary condition is that the embedding medium used for sectioning should be removed before examination in the microscope. This precaution is desirable for a number of reasons. Most important is that the various possible embedding media and these components scatter electrons to about the same extent, so that the scattered electrons from the medium would effectively mask many of the details of the matrix structure. Also relevant to the examination of intercellular matrices is the fact that in the act of sectioning the surface layer of the section suffers a certain amount of distortion (Farmer and Little, 1969). With too thin a section it consists of nothing but two distorted surface layers. Thicker sections are needed for the image from the unaltered central region of the section to dominate. The distorted surface layers scatter electrons more efficiently than the bulk of the specimen, and for too thin sections electron stains are sometimes used in an attempt to minimize this effect and increase contrast.

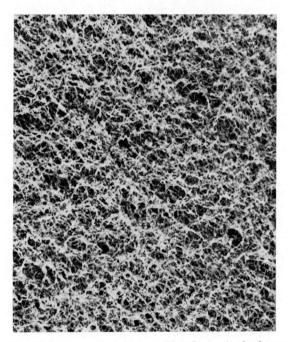

FIG. 1.23. The intercellular matrix in anlage cartilage. It was in the form of a gel, and on drying the polysaccharide-containing material between the network of fine collagen fibrils shrinks and clings to the fibrils, which also shrink. Dark spaces represent lost water. E.M. 100kV. ×6000.

When suitable sections of the connective tissues under investigation have been prepared the appearance of the various components are characteristic. It must be pointed out, however, that these characteristic appearances include some due to preparation artefacts. The tissues are gels or rubbers, and it is a dried material which is viewed. In the case of the gels this process of drying the components will not retain their exact spacial configuration. There is a tendency for the polysaccharides to cling to their underlying protein filaments or fibrils. Figure 1.23 shows the matrix in anlage cartilage, Fig. 1.24 is from mature articular cartilage, and Figs 1.25, 1.26 are of the matrix in decalcified lamellar

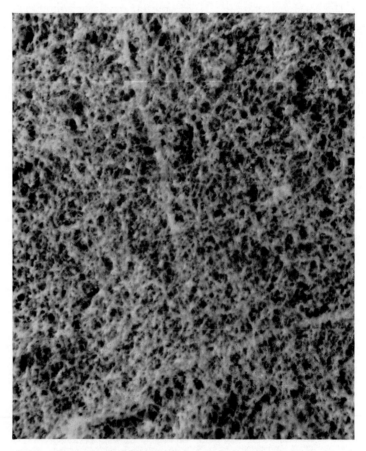

FIG. 1.24. The intercellular matrix in mature articular cartilage. Again the matrix was a gel, and during drying the polysaccharide-containing material between the network of collagen fibrils clung to those fibrils. In the mature cartilage collagen fibrils are of different diameters, and in this photograph two large fibrils are seen in the plane of the section. E.M. 100kV. ×10,000.

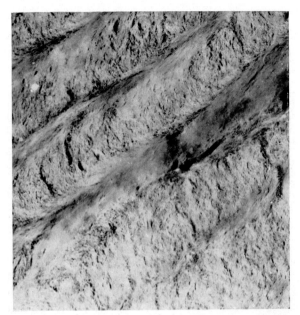

FIG. 1.25. Decalcified lamellar bone from a young child. The collagen fibrils are arranged in layers, with alternating orientation, and are surrounded by a mixture of non-collagenous substances. Tracks of canaliculi may be seen. 8% hydrochloric acid was used to remove the mineral component. E.M. 100kV. ×3500.

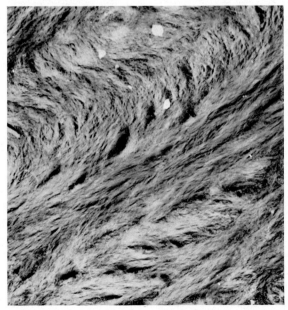

FIG. 1.26. Decalcified lamellar bone from a mature individual. This specimen was a fully mineralized bone, and the amount of non-collagenous material is considerably less than in the bone shown in Fig. 25. This enables individual collagen fibrils to be distinguished. 8% hydrochloric acid was again used as the decalcifying agent. Canaliculi are present. E.M. 100kV. ×3500.

bone (primary and secondary). Figure 1.27 shows collagen and the mature beta-protein present in the cartilage of the intervertebral disc, and Fig. 1.28 shows elastic tissue and the dense beta-protein together in

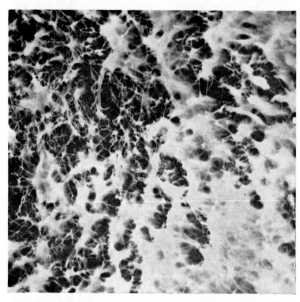

FIG. 1.27. Cartilage matrix in the nucleus pulposus of a lumbar intervertebral disc from a mature individual. There is a collagenous network, with dark spaces where fluid has been lost from the cartilage gel. The more uniform material surrounding the collagen (towards the right of the photograph) is the mature beta-protein. It has a lower water content than the gel, and less distortion has been caused by the drying process. E.M. 100kV. ×3500.

the wall of an artery. This contrast in density is best observed in a single section, since in a photograph the apparent density is affected by such factors as section thickness, aperture size, voltage and condenser settings in the electron microscope, and photographic techniques. Figure 1.29 is of elastic tissue in the cartilage of the ear, and in this print the apparent density is similar to that of the dense beta-protein in Fig. 1.28.

In practice it is found that use of the more time consuming techniques such as X-ray diffraction and electron microscopy sometimes gives information that could not readily be obtained by examination of ordinary histological sections: but that once this information has been gained it can then be used for the more complete interpretation of those sections. After this stage has been reached it is better to use the information already available in assisting to interpret further histological preparations, rather than unnecessarily continuing to use the more exotic and time-consuming techniques.

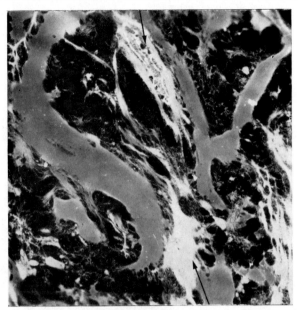

FIG. 1.28. Strands of elastic tissue and dense beta-protein in the wall of the aorta. The dense beta-protein closely surrounds very elongated cells (arrowed), while no evidence has yet been found to associate elastic tissue with any particular cell type. E.M. 100kV. ×3500.

Gels amd rubbers

The X-ray diffraction patterns and electron microscope photographs shown have all been of dried tissue, where the matrix is at its most ordered. When present in the body proteins tend to be in a swollen state. Collagen, for instance, would give an X-ray fibre diffraction pattern similar to that in Fig. 1.30. The molecules are much less ordered, and the physical state is that of a gel. The adequate functioning of many of the connective tissues is due to the fact that they are gels. All the poly-saccharides surrounding the proteins form gels, and it is the collagen fibrils contained within them, themselves in the state of a firmer gel, that provide the coherence. Immature tissues are in the form of looser gels, and as age increases the gels become firmer. Even calcified bone is better regarded as a very firm gel rather than as a rigid solid, though in this case a considerable proportion of the water in the polysaccharide between the collagen fibrils is replaced by small mineral crystals. In any consideration of the mechanical properties of bone it has to be remembered that it is the firm collagen-polysaccharide matrix that forms the continuous phase, and not the mineral crystallites. One

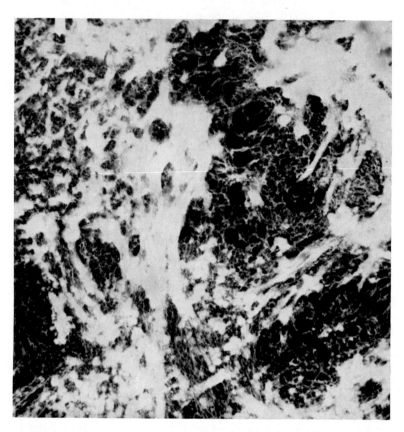

FIG. 1.29. Elastic cartilage in the ear of a stillborn child. Elastin surrounds collagen in the network of fibrils in the intercellular matrix, but there is none associated with the protein of the cell capsules. At a later stage of development dense sheets of elastin are found, with the collagen network acting as a fibrous reinforcement. E.M. 100kV. ×5000.

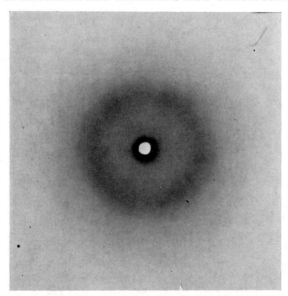

FIG. 1.30. X-ray fibre diffraction photograph of wet collagen. The 2·86 Å ring and the ring K remain. Diffraction rings representing intermolecular spacings are not present, but a diffuse ring with a spacing of 3·37 Å makes its appearance. The atomic groupings responsible for this reflection are not known. Within this ring a diffuse background represents all the possible sideways interchain spacings.

consequence of this is that healthy bone is resilient. Dead bone, on the other hand, is brittle and readily cracks.

Gels suffer from a mechanical disadvantage, in that severe pressure may cause a breakdown of the gel structure, while a less severe pressure, or a lack of adequate alternation between compression and relaxation may prevent circulation of acid waste products away from the cells. Such a build-up of acidity may also cause a breakdown of the gel structure. With a temporary breakdown of the gel, several days elapse before the cells have produced sufficient polysaccharides to provide a replacement gel. During this time the cells are at risk and may be killed by comparatively minor trauma. Figure 1.31 shows cartilage in the knee joint of a rabbit. The gel structure was damaged by injecting blood into the joint, and trauma near the tip of the meniscus has resulted in a patch of dead cells (Guicciardi and Little, 1967). In the parts of the body which are most at risk this danger is minimized by the presence, sometimes as the major component, of one or more of the proteins whose resilence is provided by a rubber-like texture and not by a gel structure. These are the mature and dense beta-proteins and elastic tissue. The mature beta-protein is the most flexible and the dense beta-protein the stiffest of the three. These two are formed directly by cells, under

E

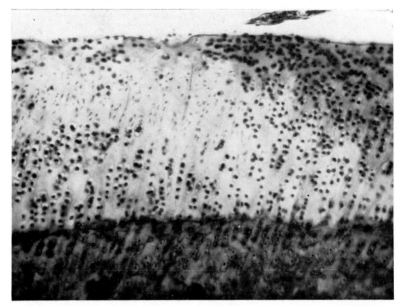

Fig. 1.31. Cartilage in the knee joint of a rabbit. The gel structure of the intercellular matrix was damaged by injecting blood into the joint. A patch of dead cells is seen in the cartilage underlying an area near the tip of the meniscus. Recent calcification of the base of the cartilage may also be observed. × 100.

conditions where those cells are subjected to a combination of pressure and rotational forces during the time of matrix formation. There is an increasing volume of evidence that they are formed as an alternative to collagen when the movements of the protruding segments of the cell surface are hindered by the applied mechanical forces. Figure 1.32 for example, shows a mass of mature beta-protein in the immediate vicinity of a cell in prolapsed lumbar disc tissue. Both the mature and the dense beta-protein are produced in a more ordered form in older individuals (as shown by the X-ray diffraction evidence).

The conditions for formation of elastic tissue are rather different. There is as yet no evidence that its formation is dependent on any particular cell while its texture varies little with age, although at all ages there are considerable variations in its physical form. The conditions for its formation seem to include a tensile combined with a cross force. It is found in the foetal aorta soon after the circulation is established; it is present in considerable quantities in the ligamentum nuchae of, say, sheep or goats, but in smaller quantities in the human ligamentum nuchae. The human ligamentum flavum, on the other hand, has a high proportion of elastic tissue. The aorta normally contains both elastic tissue and dense beta-protein. In many tissues the elastin is seen to engulf pre-existing collagen fibrils.

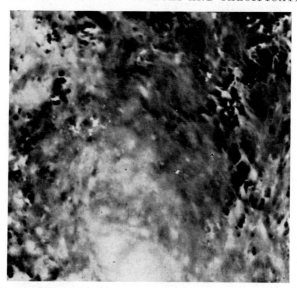

Fig. 1.32. Prolapsed lumbar disc tissue. Newly formed mature beta-protein in vicinity of cell. E.M. 100kV. ×3500.

The calcifiable matrix

The other main type of intercellular matrix is the calcifiable matrix. This is produced in the enlarging zone of the epiphyseal growth cartilage, and is laid down over the other matrix components. In tissue culture, where the conditions for its formation may be maintained for several days, large quantities (comparatively speaking) can be produced, as shown in Fig. 1.33. The X-ray diffraction pattern of such a specimen shows that this matrix also contains a beta-protein as a major component. Histochemical examination (Johnson, 1964; Wuthier, 1968) has shown that there are a number of other chemical compounds among the components. In bone, osteoblasts lay down first collagen and its associated polysaccharide, then the calcifiable matrix (Fig. 1.34). This calcifies (Fig. 1.35), and then another strip of collagen is laid down. This sequence is repeated several times by each osteoblast to produce a characteristic lamellar structure (Johnson, 1964), such as is shown in Fig. 1.36. Calcifiable matrix undergoes a physical change immediately before calcification takes place. This shows very clearly in the enamel matrix from an unerupted tooth in Figs 1.37, 1.38. In addition to providing nucleation centres for mineral to be deposited the calcifiable matrix also contains a component known as the "osteogenic factor". Wherever it is present cells from sinusoid vessels and granulation tissue differentiate as osteogenic cells and not fibroblasts.

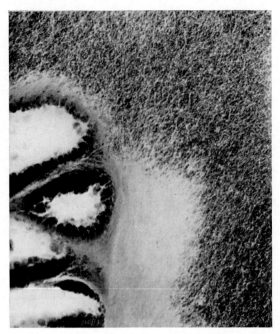

FIG. 1.33. Rabbit growth cartilage, maintained for 9 days in tissue culture (2/3 serum, 1/3 Hanks solution). In this medium cartilage cells are unable to divide, but are able to produce the calcifiable matrix. This has collected around the cells in abnormally large quantities. E.M. 100kV. ×2000.

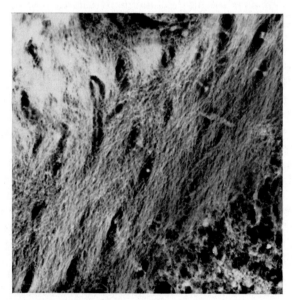

FIG. 1.34. Oblique section through edge of trabecula in metaphysis. A portion of an osteoblast is at bottom right. Above and to the left is newly laid down osteoid, the collagenous bone matrix, with canaliculi, through each of which passes a cell process joining the osteoblasts with osteocytes in the bone. Towards the top left is calcifiable matrix, with discrete patches of mineral deposited on it. E.M. 100kV. ×6000.

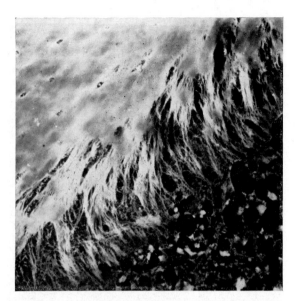

FIG. 1.35. Edge of trabecula, showing portions of an osteoblast at the bottom right, and bone with canaliculi containing cell processes at the top left. Apatite crystals in this primary calcification cannot normally be resolved in the electron microscope at 100kV because of electron scatter from the underlying calcifiable matrix. Between the bone and the surface is partially calcified matrix. E.M. 100kV. ×6000.

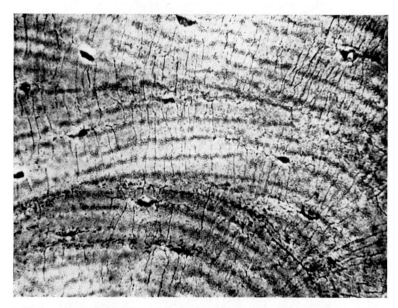

FIG. 1.36. Bone in cortex. Portions of the walls of three successive osteones are shown, each with the lamellae in slightly different directions. This appearance is caused by the fact that with each change in osteoblast function there is a change in the direction of the underlying collagen fibrils in the matrix they produce. The direction of canaliculi is predominantly perpendicular to the direction of the collagenous layers. ×35.

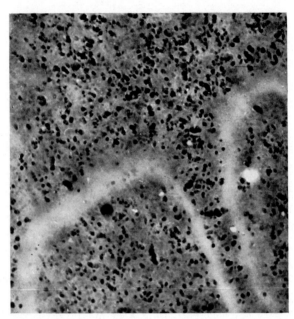

Fig. 1.37. Enamel matrix from an unerupted tooth. The walls of enamel prisms are of a denser protein than the remainder of the beta-protein containing matrix. These underlying components are covered by calcifiable matrix. The area shown is very near the surface. E.M. 100kV. ×6000.

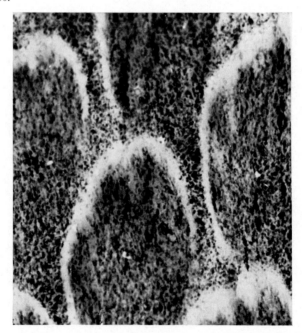

Fig. 1.38. Enamel matrix in unerupted tooth, close to the calcifying front. The calcifiable matrix has shrunk towards the underlying beta-protein network, and the small dark areas are spaces left by the evaporation of fluid. These would soon be filled by newly deposited mineral. E.M. 100kV. ×6000.

Mineralization

In normal development the calcifiable matrix is responsible for the main mineralization process in the body, that of cartilage, bone, dentine and dental enamel. In bone a secondary mineralization takes place, preceded by the loss of some of the original matrix which underlies the crystals of the primary calcification. This results in somewhat different properties of the bone. A further type of abnormal and pathological mineralization is found on some dead and necrotic tissues. Before discussing these processes of calcification or mineralization further, some of the properties of the deposited mineral salts will be discussed.

The calcium phosphates

The most widespread mineral present in the body is one of the calcium phosphates, hydroxyapatite $Ca_{10}(PO_4)_6(OH)_2$. Like most complex inorganic compounds it has a range of possible compositions, the "ideal" composition lying to one end of the range which is found in practice. In Fig. 1.39 is shown the constitutional diagram for the relevant portion of the calcium–phosphate system. In this triangular diagram the top corner represents water, the bottom left calcium oxide (CaO) and the bottom right corner phosphorus pentoxide (P_2O_5). A compound containing only a little water will be situated near the bottom of the diagram, while with higher calcium it will be towards the left and with higher phosphate towards the right. The oval marked A represents the range of compositions of the hydroxyapatite, that marked O, with its long axis corresponding to a greater or lesser amount of water of crystallization, is octacalcium phosphate ($Ca_4H(PO_4)_3.3H_2O$) and so on. Mineral names, hydroxyapatite, whitlockite, monetite and brushite are to be preferred, since it is more natural to think of them having a range of compositions. A chemical name might lead one to expect an exact composition with no deviations, and this is something that is practically never found in normal minerals.

To identify the mineral component present in any given tissue X-ray diffraction may be used as a "finger-print" method and, as for the fibre diffraction photographs of the proteins, without any attempt at chemical separation or analysis being necessary. To do this a powder diffraction pattern of a sample is taken, the sample is then heated to 900°C to 1000°C for an hour, cooled, and another diffraction pattern taken. Some of the patterns which have been obtained are shown in Fig. 1.40. The diagram in Fig. 1.41 shows the lines for a portion of the hydroxyapatite pattern, with relative positions of the main reflections from the other possible

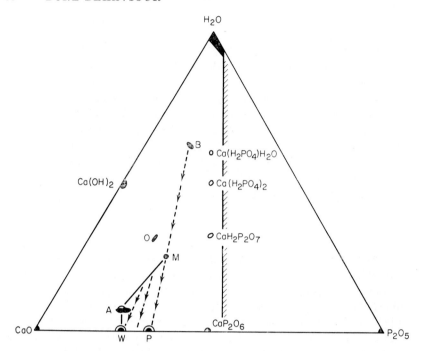

Fig. 1.39. Constitutional diagram of the system $CaO:P_2O_5:H_2O$. Compounds with higher calcium content are shown.

A Hydroxyapatite $Ca_{10}(PO_4)_6(OH)_2$
O Octacalcium phosphate $Ca_4(PO_4)_3H\ 3H_2O$
B Brushite $CaHPO_4\ 2H_2O$
M Monetite $CaHPO_4$
W Whitlockite $\beta-Ca_3(PO_4)_2$
P Pyrophosphate $Ca_2P_2O_7$

compounds indicated. If the lines on the first pattern were diffuse, then the crystallites were small, if they were sharp, then the crystallites were larger (with dimensions of over 1000 Å). If the diffraction patterns of both the unheated and heated specimens are of hydroxyapatite alone, then the original material was hydroxyapatite. If the lines on the first pattern were of hydroxyapatite, and after heating both hydroxyapatite and whitlockite were present, then there were hydroxyapatite crystallites present together with excess phosphate. Sometimes on a diffraction pattern from an unheated pathological calcification fairly sharp whitlockite lines may be seen. These have not quite the same interplanar spacing as the lines for the whitlockite obtained by heating hydroxyapatite with excess phosphate. It has been found that this whitlockite which is formed from the tissue fluids at body temperature is a magnesian whitlockite with 12–15% of the calcium atoms replaced by magnesium atoms (Tovborg-Jensen and Rowles, 1957 a, b; Rowles,

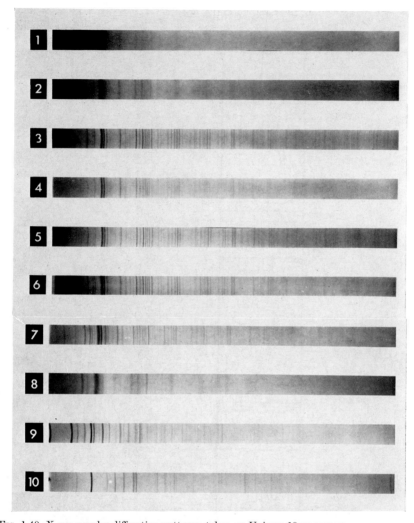

FIG. 1.40. X-ray powder diffraction patterns, taken on Unicam 19cm camera.
1. Very small hydroxyapatite crystallites (primary calcification).
2. Hydroxyapatite crystallites in mature bone (secondary calcification).
3. Heated bone, with large hydroxyapatite crystallites.
4. Dental enamel—weak 004 reflection due to slight orientation.
5. Pathological calcification heated: hydroxyapatite and CaO.
6. Heated bone from young animal: hydroxyapatite and trace of whitlockite.
7. Hydroxyapatite and whitlockite—heated specimen.
8. Hydroxyapatite and large whitlockite crystals in unheated specimen: patholo2ical calcification.
9. Brushite.
10. Calcite.

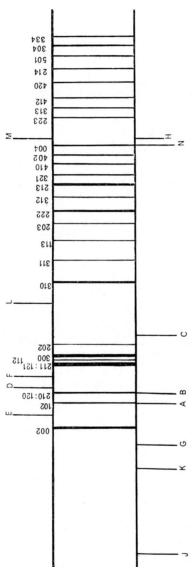

FIG. 1.41. Diagram of a portion of the hydroxyapatite pattern, giving indices of lines, and showing the positions of the main reflections from other possible compounds. Whitlockite: increased intensity of line A as compared with line B, due to superimposition of a whitlockite reflection. Line in position C. Calcite: main reflection in position D. Monetite: reflections in positions E and F. Octacalcium phosphate: pattern very similar to hydroxyapatite. Faint additional lines in positions G and H. There is also a strong reflection with long spacing not obtainable with the Unicam 19cm camera. Brushite: strong reflections in positions J and K. Calcium oxide: in mixtures with hydroxyapatite lines L and M are suitable for identification. Several minor components affect the intensity of the 004 reflection of hydroxyapatite (line N). It is also sensitive to orientation effects.

1968). Magnesium atoms have the effect of stabilizing the structure. Ordinary whitlockite is formed only at elevated temperatures.

The solubilities of the calcium phosphates are given in the diagram in Fig. 1.42. The corners of the triangle again represent H_2O, CaO and

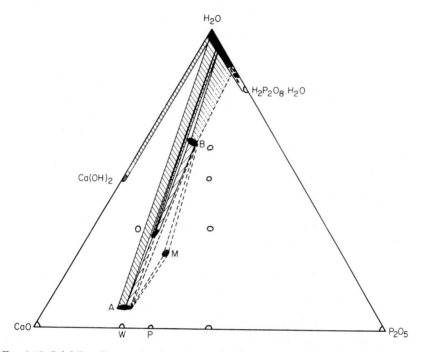

Fig. 1.42. Solubility diagram for the calcium-phosphate system. Black areas: single phase regions. Shaded areas: two phase regions. Those shown are: calcium hydroxide and solution; hydroxyapatite and solution; octacalcium phosphate and solution; octacalcium phosphate and brushite; brushite and solution. Dotted lines represent the most probable position of phase boundaries that have not yet been adequately studied.

A   Hydroxyapatite $Ca_{10}(PO_4)_6(OH)_2$
O   Octacalcium phosphate $Ca_4(PO_4)_3H\ 3H_2O$
B   Brushite $CaHPO_4\ 2H_2O$
M   Monetite $CaHPO_4$
W   Whitlockite $\beta -Ca_3(PO_4)_2$
P   Pyrophosphate $Ca_2P_2O_7$

P_2O_5. The solution is the strip from the top corner towards the first phosphoric acid on the H_2O–P_2O_5 side of the triangle. There is quite a wide range of conditions, with varying proportions of calcium and phosphate, and consequently also varying pH, under which hydroxyapatite is the component which crystallizes out of solution. The zone between the solution and the hydroxyapatite represents the range of conditions in which solution and solid compound can co-exist. The conditions under which octacalcium phosphate crystallizes out of solution are much more precise. With this narrow range, it is interesting that it was among the first of these compounds to be isolated, by Berzelius (1835, 1845). Little more was known of it until a century later Bjerrum (1936, 1949, 1958) worked out the solution chemistry of the calcium phosphates. This diagram (Fig. 1.42) has been derived largely from the results of his work. The three-phase regions where three components (solution, hydroxyapatite and octacalcium phosphate; or solution, octacalcium phosphate and brushite) can co-exist are bounded by straight lines. This is one of the requirements of the physical law known as the Phase Rule. A lack of knowledge of the Phase Rule and the chemistry of saturated and super-saturated solutions has been responsible for many of the confused statements on calcification which have appeared in the literature during the last 20 years. Because of the confusion, and also because most of the relevant papers are not found in the various medical Indexes, a fairly extensive Bibliography will be given for this topic at the end of the list of references.

It has been mentioned that X-ray diffraction may be used to identify the mineral components in tissues without it being necessary to have an understanding of the subject such as would be required by a crystallographer. Similarly, since for each type of underlying matrix which can act as a substrate for the deposition of mineral crystallites there is a characteristic mode of mineralization, with varying composition and crystal habits, this fact can be used for their identification without any detailed knowledge of the chemistry of the mineral or of the mechanisms of nucleation being required. For general purposes, including a knowledge of pathological processes involving calcification, the amount of information given in this chapter is ample; but for anyone who proposes to work on the mechanisms of calcification an adequate knowledge of physical chemistry, including the Phase Rule, saturated and super-saturated solutions, and chemical equilibria and kinetics is essential. In addition to S. Glasshouse's *Textbook of Physical Chemistry* (Macmillan and Co., London) or other work of similar standard, a specialist book on the Phase Rule should be consulted. In the application of thermodynamics it must also be remembered that equations derived from theories of dilute solutions cannot be applied to saturated solutions. There is no point in wasting time attempting to understand papers in which this elementary mistake has been made.

Calcification

One of the earliest investigations of calcification was by Andral whose observations on aortic calcification were published in 1827 and 1837.

Work continued steadily throughout the nineteenth century, and the information collected was reviewed by Wells in 1910. By that time there was abundant evidence that calcification was a physico-chemical process, that there were several types of calcification according to local conditions in the tissues, and that deposition of mineral salts from the tissue fluids occurred as a result of some change in the underlying matrix.

The calcium phosphates form very persistent supersaturated solutions (Bjerrum, 1936, 1949). By supersaturated is meant a solution in a thermodynamically unstable state, with high energy content, which persists because of the even higher energy barrier required to initiate precipitation. The reason for this energy barrier is simple. For the formation of a single unit of hydroxyapatite 18 ions have to come out of solution and arrange themselves in a specific order. Only when they are arranged in the correct configuration can other ions easily add on and form a crystal. For the initial ordered arrangement to occur in the short space of time before the first ones have returned to the solution is unlikely, unless there are a reasonably high proportion in the solution. Consequently there tend to be two values for the solubility of the compound, one for going into solution and a higher one for coming out of the solution. Above this solubility limit (the supersaturation limit) precipitation will occur on any available surface. Below this value for

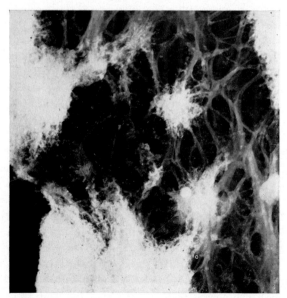

FIG. 1.43. Early calcification in the growth cartilage of the rat. A cluster of crystals forms around each nucleation centre. These crystals are larger than those of the primary calcification found in the human and other species. E.M. 100kV. ×12,000.

the total ionic concentration precipitation will only occur if there is a "nucleation centre" to hold the ions that first come out in the correct configuration for a long enough time for the rest of the 18, and then more, to arrive. Once a crystal has started, then it can act as a nucleating centre for neighbouring crystals. In this way clusters of crystals tend to be deposited (Fig. 1.43). The photograph in Fig. 1.44, of a single unit of hydroxyapatite in a crystal structure model which shows the spacial arrangement of the atoms and their interatomic distances, has been taken perpendicular to the axis along which crystals usually grow. It can be seen that in each group of 18 atoms which form the smallest unit of structure 10 of them (5 calcium and 5 phosphorus) lie in one plane. Normal crystal growth takes place a layer at a time by a process of a new layer starting from a specific active centre and spreading across the face of the crystal, so that a compound with active groups in the spacial arrangement shown in Fig. 1.45 could use these groups as a nucleation centre.

In the body, ionic concentrations of calcium and phosphate in the tissue fluids are in the middle of the supersaturated range (Fig. 1.46). Even in pathological conditions involving changes in these ionic concentrations the abnormal values still lie well within the supersaturation limits. Before the limit is reached a state of tetany supervenes. It follows, then, that all calcification in the body, whether physiological or pathological, takes place on components of the intercellular matrix which can provide nucleation centres. When one eliminates from consideration dental calculus and renal and urinary calculi formed from solutions of quite different composition from the ordinary tissue fluids (Figs 1.47–1.49 show early calcification in renal tubules) the range of compounds found is small. Examination of a large number of specimens has shown that each type of crystalline deposit is upon a characteristic underlying matrix.

The most important is the calcifiable matrix. This matrix is produced in cartilage as the first stage of the process that leads to enchondral ossification. It is also produced by connective tissue cells that have been stimulated to differentiate into osteoblasts by one of its components (previously produced by cartilage cells or other osteoblasts); and by odontoblasts and ameloblasts in developing teeth. Its production by osteoblasts was described by Thoma (1894). Except in the case of dental enamel, where the calcifiable matrix is laid down on a beta-protein and not on collagen fibrils the hydroxyapatite crystals deposited on it are small, rarely more than 70 Å to 200 Å across 10^8 Å = 1 cm: 10^4 Å = 1 micron). When sections of fixed material are viewed in the electron microscope the crystallites are not usually resolved, because of electron scatter by the surrounding calcifiable matrix, and do not give

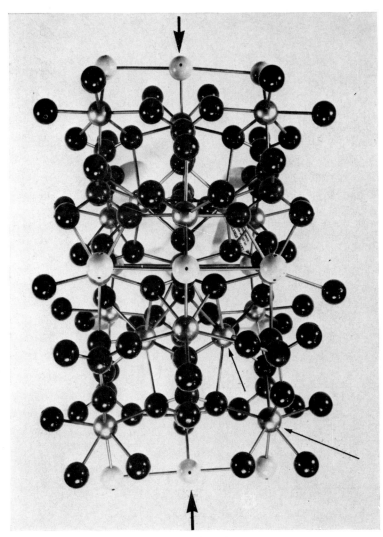

FIG. 1.44. Photograph of crystal structure model of hydroxyapatite. This shows the relative positions of atoms in the unit cell of a hydroxyapatite crystallite. Balls represent the centres of atoms, and lengths of the metal rods joining them are to scale, indicating the relative distances between these centres. Light coloured balls represent OH groups, while the metallic coloured calcium ions have two types of surrounding configuration (small arrows). Half the atoms in the unit cell are arranged in a single plane (arrowed).

Arrangement of adsorption sites on the matrix:

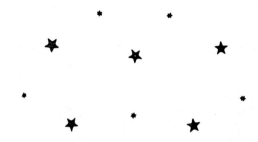

* Negative site for Ca^{++} ions

★ Positive site for PO$_4^=$ ions

I Å = 5 mm approx.

These Ca^{++} and PO$_4^=$ ions are in a single plane in the HA crystal lattice

Fig. 1.45. Arrangement of absorption sites on the underlying matrix which can act as a nucleation centre for hydroxyapatite.

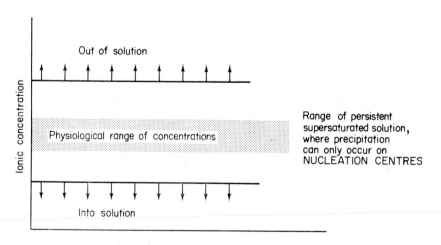

Fig. 1.46. Schematic representation of the relationship between the physiological range of ionic concentrations of calcium and phosphate and the range of persistent supersaturated solutions. Hydroxyapatite, $Ca_{10}(PO_4)_6(OH)_2$, has 18 ions. These ions must all move to the same place at the same time before precipitation can occur. When several are held in position on an underlying site it is easier for the others to move into place in an orderly manner.

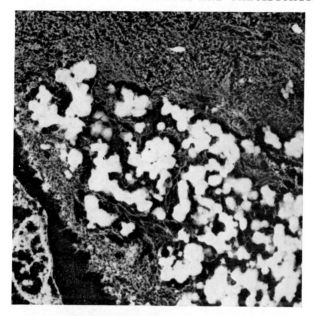

FIG. 1.47. Mineralization on material deposited in a blocked renal tubule. There are two types of mucopolysaccharide precipitate, only one of which has provided nucleation centres. E.M. 100kV. ×3500.

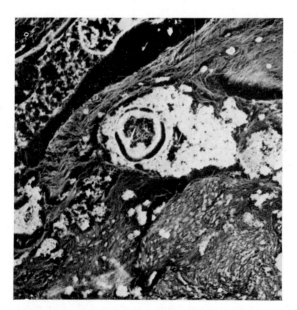

FIG. 1.48. Mineralization of cytoplasm of a cell trapped in the mucopolysaccharide in a blocked renal tubule. E.M. 100kV. ×3500.

F

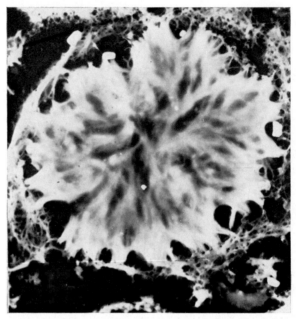

Fig. 1.49. Dendritic crystal formation blocking a renal tubule. The three photographs Figs 47–49) show diverse appearances in a single section of kidney, approximately 1 mm across, from a subject with multiple myeloma. E.M. 100kV. ×2000.

electron diffraction patterns. At 600 kV to 1000 kV the electron scatter from the non-crystalline organic compounds is reduced to a level at which the crystallites are resolved and diffraction effects may be observed. Figure 1.50 shows crystallites in primary calcification of bone, photographed at 600 kV and at ×250,000. Only those crystallites which are at a suitable orientation to deflect electrons give good contrast. To be certain that observed appearances are of crystals it is advisable to observe with dark ground illumination also. Only a small proportion will show up in dark ground illumination at any one time and angle, but as the angle of the specimen is altered different crystals appear bright. (Figure 1.51 is of a pathological calcification and Fig. 1.52 shows partial dark field illumination, so that both the crystallites which are bright and also those still dark can be observed. These crystallites are larger than the hydroxyapatite crystallites deposited on the calcifiable matrix.) In the type of hydroxyapatite deposited on calcifiable matrix there is an excess of phosphate present in the surface layers. In crystals as small as these about 17% of the ions are on the surface (Neuman and Neuman, 1953), available for the adsorption of other ions, and in Fig. 1.50 it may be observed that the surface layers show a different orientation to the main crystal, suggesting the presence of a different calcium phosphate,

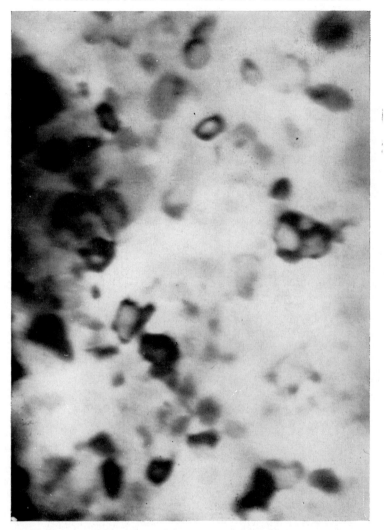

FIG. 1.50. Crystallites in primary mineralization of bone. Dimensions are in the range 70 Å–200 Å. The crystallites are plate-like, with a perimeter showing Bragg reflections at a different angle from the body of the crystal. This second crystalline phase prevents further crystal growth. E.M. 600kV. ×250,000. (This photograph is printed as a dark object on a light ground.)

Examination of the crystal structure models shows that hydroxyapatite and octacalcium phosphate have a crystal plane in common.

The resulting calcification when osteoblasts first produce bone is known as the primary calcification. As the bone matures the calcifiable matrix originally laid down is degraded and removed, and replaced by a

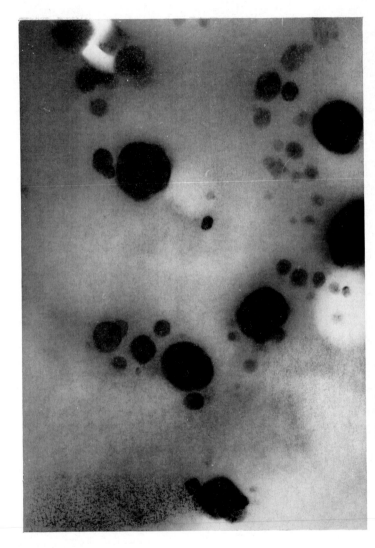

FIG. 1.51. Pathological calcification in aorta. Several crystal types are present. Bright field illumination. E.M. 600kV. ×80,000. (This photograph is printed as a dark object on a light ground.)

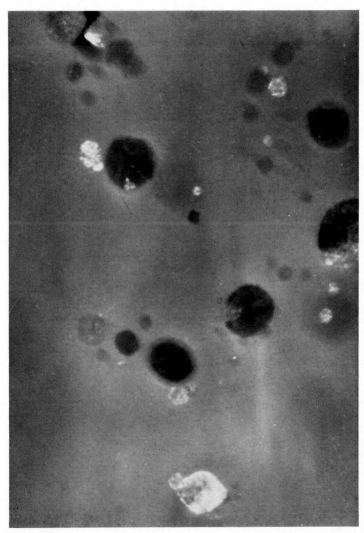

Fig. 1.52. Same area. Partial dark field illumination. Bragg reflections show as bright patches. Many particles are revealed as crystalline aggregates. E.M. 600kV. × 80,000. (This photograph is printed as a dark object on a light ground.)

secondary mineralization. Here the underlying matrix is the poly-saccharide-containing gel which surrounds the collagen fibrils. Since this is more coherent at the level of the bands in the collagen fibrils crystal growth is blocked and the secondary calcification contains crystallites of hydroxyapatite which are usually about 600 Å long (the spacing of the bands is 640 Å). Also, since they are in the spaces between bands, they are orientated in the direction of the underlying collagen fibrils. This is in contrast to the primary crystallization where orientation is limited. Typical crystallites orientated in relation to the collagen bands are shown arrowed in Fig. 1.53. The appearance in this and similar

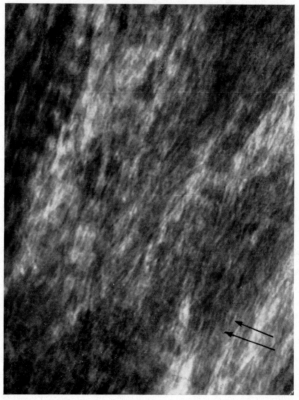

FIG. 1.53. Section through mature bone. Needle-shaped hydroxyapatite crystallites, about 600 Å long, are in parallel array between collagen fibrils, and between the 640 Å bands along these fibrils. Such a cluster, in the plane of the section, is shown arrowed. E.M. 600kV. × 64,000. (This photograph is printed as a dark object on a light ground.)

photographs of secondary mineralization in bone can be confusing be-cause of another type of diffraction effect. The deflected electrons shown in Figs 1.50, 1.52 are reflections from planes of atoms in the crystals and are known as Bragg reflections. There is another type of diffraction, caused by ordered structures being not quite aligned, known as Moire diffraction. It can be caused by planes of atoms in two adjacent crystals which are not perfectly lined up, or at the other end of the size range it can be caused by two sets of railings, with dark bands appearing at intervals usually several times longer than the distance between the posts. In the present example, bone, the underlying structure responsible for the Moire effects is the array of collagen fibrils. In the photograph shown in Fig. 1.54 only a few hydroxyapatite crystallites are

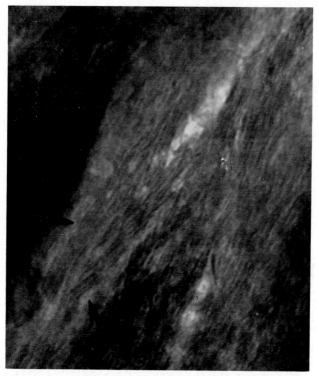

FIG. 1.54. Section through mature bone. The optical conditions here are such that long diffraction fringes are seen alongside the collagen fibrils. Some typical examples are arrowed. In the past such diffraction effects have been mistaken for hydroxyapatite crystals. A few crystals, similar to those shown in Fig. 53, can be discerned. E.M. 600kV. × 80,000.

discernable. Most of the detail is due to Moire diffraction effects. Some typical examples are arrowed.

Unlike the primary mineralization of bone, it is often possible to resolve crystallites of hydroxyapatite in the secondary calcification in the electron microscope at 100 kV, and electron diffraction patterns can then be obtained. This is because there is far less electron scatter from the underlying organic matrix. When a section through a junction of primary and secondary calcification is viewed using dark field illumination, with the image formed entirely from scattered electrons, it can be seen that there is less scatter from the denser area of secondary calcification (Fig. 1.55).

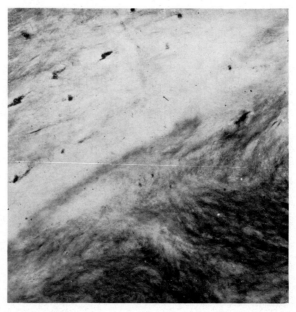

Fig. 1.55. Section of bone photographed using dark field illumination at 100kV. Using this dark field technique the image is provided entirely by scattered electrons. The area of primary calcification (top left) shows considerably more electron scatter than does the area of secondary calcification. ×3500.

Another crystal habit is found in dental enamel. Here with the underlying matrix involving a beta-protein and not collagen, the hydroxyapatite crystals grow bigger. Figure 1.56 is a thin section of dental enamel which shows the larger hydroxyapatite crystallites which have a mosaic structure. These crystallites again have adsorbed phosphate, while the proportion found on X-ray diffraction examination suggests that the crystallites have an internal composition corresponding to a higher phosphate ratio than the "ideal". There is probably water and phosphate adsorbed on inner surfaces of the mosaic crystallites (Bjerrum, 1958).

Pathological calcifications are of two main types. Changes in the applied forces may result in the metaplastic change of fibrocartilage or related tissues to the type of cartilage cell which produces calcifiable

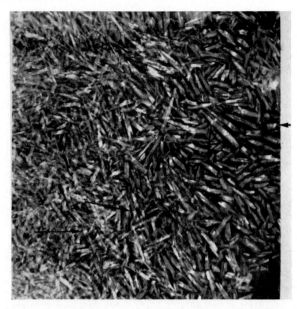

Fig. 1.56. Thin section of dental enamel, containing large crystallites. Some show regions of total internal reflection of the electrons. Variation of orientation within the crystallites so that only parts are at an angle to give the total internal reflection suggests that they are formed from subunits that are only partly aligned. A few examples of apparently mosaic crystals are indicated. E.M. 100kV. ×12,000.

matrix. Calcification of this is usually followed by enchondral ossification. The mineral is deposited as small phosphate-rich crystals. In the other case local tissue death results in degradative changes. The mineral crystals found on partially degraded tissue are hydroxyapatite of assorted sizes up to those of enamel crystallites, or magnesian whitlockite, or calcite (these are also present as large crystals), or mixtures of two or all three. Which type of crystallite is deposited depends on the composition of the underlying matrix and so may vary from one small patch to another. Figure 1.57 shows detail of an example of this type of calcification from the intervertebral disc, as seen in the electron microscope. Figure 1.58 is another example taken from a calcified aorta. The calcite crystals are so large that they can often be resolved in the light microscope. Figure 1.59 is from a patch of calcite in a section of necrotic intervertebral disc tissue taken at post-mortem. Each type of matrix, then, produces a different type of calcification. A common factor is the presence and partial breakdown of polysaccharides, while there is a gradually increasing amount of evidence that lipids may also play an important role. This aspect of the subject still requires further investigation.

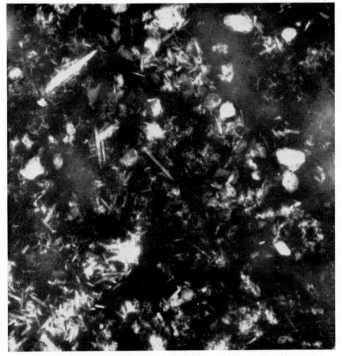

Fig. 1.57. Calcification on necrotic material in the intervertebral disc. Crystallites of hydroxy-apatite may be seen (elongated), of widely varying size, together with some crystallites of magnesian whitlockite. E.M. 100kV. × 10,000.

Calcium carbonate

The hydroxyapatite crystallites formed during secondary mineralization of bone have no adsorbed phosphate, but it is widely believed that they have carbonate adsorbed on their surfaces (e.g. Posner and Duychaerts, 1954). When treated with hydrochloric acid mature bone liberates carbon dioxide before the mineral goes into solution, while Carlström (1955) has gently heated bone to about 400°C to 500°C and caused calcite (one of the crystal modifications of calcium carbonate) to crystallize out as a separate phase. Very probably the carbonate is formed in air, after the bone is removed from the body, and before such experiments are performed.

The apparent deposition of calcite in the tissues has been the source of much confused thinking, and provides a good example of the care which needs to be taken in the interpretation of experimental results. Because carbonate could be obtained from calcified tissues which showed only hydroxyapatite diffraction patterns, one speculation, sometimes treated as a fact, was that carbonate was present as carbonate

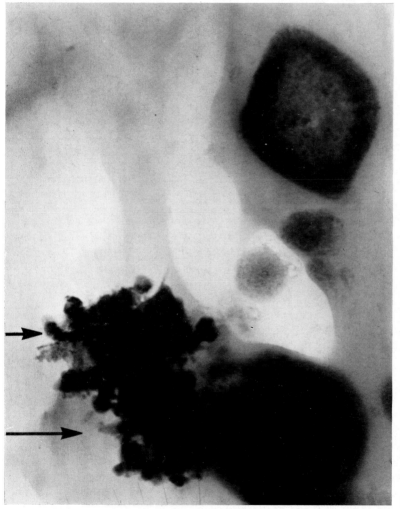

Fig. 1.58. Calcification on necrotic tissue in aorta. The two clusters of hydroxyapatite crystallites (arrowed) have each formed around a single nucleation centre. The large crystal shows a mosaic structure. E.M. 600kV. ×64,000.

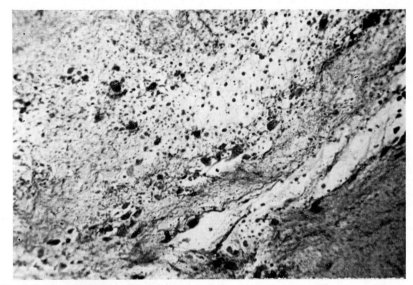

FIG. 1.59. Large calcite crystallites in a section of necrotic disc tissue. These crystallites have been formed, in all probability, by recrystallization from another compound with very small crystallites. ×200.

apatite (Gruner and McConnell, 1937; McConnell, 1938). But it was shown by Bredig (1933), Thewlis, Glock and Murray (1939) and Tovborg-Jensen and Møller (1944) that there would not be room in the hydroxy-apatite lattice for carbonate without a gross distortion which is not observed on the X-ray diffraction patterns; while later Trautz (1960) has attempted to make carbonate apatites, and produced amorphous mixtures rather than well-crystallized materials. Further, the size of those calcite crystallites actually found in dried samples of calcified aorta or intervertebral disc and other sites, makes it probable that on drying the specimens some recrystallization has occurred. This sup-position receives support from the complex appearance of the crystals when examined with the more penetrating electron beam of a high voltage microscope (Fig. 1.58). A possible explanation was provided by Taylor (1964; and Taylor and Little, 1963) who took samples of calcified lumbar disc tissue for X-ray diffraction immediately after removal at operation and found a different diffraction pattern, of a compound with small crystal size (Fig. 1.60), which after 1/2–3/4 h had recrystallized to calcite. In the intervening stages both diffraction patterns could be observed (Fig. 1.61). It thus became apparent that a labile compound was formed on the underlying matrix in these pathological calcifications, which was only converted to carbonate after removal from the body. This in turn suggests that the presence of carbonate in normal bone may also be a preparation artefact. The labile compound still awaits identification,

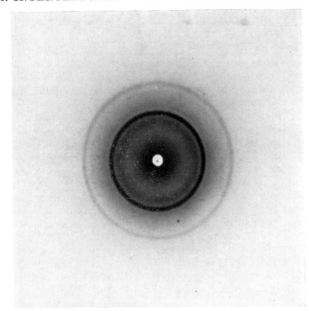

FIG. 1 60. X-ray fibre diffraction photograph. Pattern of compound with small crystal size, taken immediately after removal of disc at operation. The author thanks Prof. T. K. F. Taylor for this photograph.

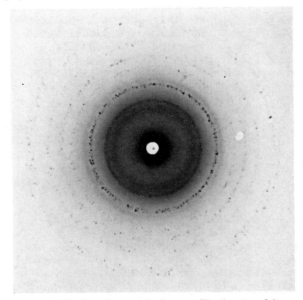

FIG. 1.61. X-ray fibre diffraction photograph. Recrystallization to calcite occurs 1/2–3/4 h after removal of disc. In this photograph there are rings due to the original compound with stronger rings of calcite. Speckling is an indication of the large size of the calcite crystals. The author thanks Prof. T. K. F. Taylor for this photograph.

Summary

1. Connective tissue cells produce intercellular matrices responsible for the mechanical properties of tissues. The majority of these cells are of the type which requires a substrate for movement. Others can exist and proliferate free in a liquid medium—some cartilage cells are of this type.

2. The main intercellular matrix components are the proteins and polysaccharides, which are polymeric compounds. The proteins are produced in the regions of the cells occupied by the endoplasmic reticulum, and extruded through segments of the cells surfaces which protrude and then retract.

3. The matrix components are extruded from the cells together, and in general each protein has its associated polysaccharide. The main groups of structural proteins are the collagens (immature in the foetus and infant), non-collagenous beta-proteins, and elastin. The non-collagenous beta-proteins, include an "immature" protein, a "mature" protein and a dense beta-protein which is often found associated with elastic tissue.

4. These main groups of proteins may be characterized by their X-ray diffraction patterns, their appearance in the electron microscope, their autofluorescence, and when information from these sources is used to assist interpretation, their appearance in histological sections.

5. In the body the intercellular matrices are present as gels or rubbers, each of which may vary from very loose and soft, to firm and resilient. In healthy tissues the physical state is that which best meets the needs of the cells in that tissue and the local mechanical requirements. The mature and dense beta-proteins and elastin are rubbers, and the other matrix components gels.

6. Another important type of intercellular matrix is the calcifiable matrix. This is laid down over the structural matrix components in cartilages prior to enchondral ossification, and in developing or remodelling bone tissues, and in teeth.

7. The main mineral component in the body is hydroxyapatite, $Ca_{10}(PO_4)_6$ $(OH)_2$. It is in direct equilibrium with the tissue fluids. Other compounds which are sometimes present include octacalcium phosphate, $Ca_4H(PO_4)_3.3H_2O$ and whitlockite, β-$Ca_3(PO_4)_2$. The relevant portion of the calcium–phosphate system is described.

8. The type of mineralization found is dependent upon the underlying organic matrix and not on the ionic content of the surrounding tissue fluids. The ionic concentrations in these fluids lie in the middle of the calcium phosphate supersaturation range, so that the presence of nucleation centres is necessary before minerals can be deposited. Even in pathological conditions the abnormal values still lie well within the supersaturation limits.

9. In normal tissues the deposited minerals are found:

(a) On calcifiable matrix in the epiphyseal growth cartilage and primary calcification of bone. Very small hydroxyapatite crystals, about 70 Å to 200 Å across, with excess phosphate present in the surface layers.

(b) During the secondary calcification of bone, on the polysaccharide-containing gel which surrounds the collagen fibrils. Hydroxyapatite crystallites about 600 Å long, with no excess phosphate, and orientated in the direction of the associated collagen fibrils.

(c) On the calcifiable matrix over the polysaccharide—beta-protein complex in dental enamel. Large plate-like mosaic hydroxyapatite crystals, up to 5–10,000 Å long and 600 Å wide, with excess phosphate present.

(d) On necrotic tissue. Hydroxyapatite crystals, without excess phosphate, of assorted sizes up to those of enamel crystallites; or magnesian whitlockite; or calcite, or mixtures of two or all three, depending on the nature of the underlying necrotic tissue.

10. Large calcite crystals are found on necrotic tissue, and carbonate has also been detected in normal bone after the material has been prepared for laboratory examination. In fresh material a labile compound, with small crystallites, is observed which rapidly changes to calcite when exposed in the laboratory. This suggests that the oft-recorded presence of carbonate may be a preparation artefact.

2. STAGES IN DEVELOPMENT

The account of the intercellular matrices given in the last chapter was a necessary introduction to an understanding of the changes which may occur in bone and cartilage over the years, for when considering ageing, some of the landmarks in development are marked by changes in the mode of production of the intercellular matrices. The underlying cause of these changes appears to be hormonal, and the stages of development are demarcated by the hormonal epochs. At the same time there is a more gradual process of ageing, with puberty as the only definite discontinuity. One indication of this discontinuity is the development of the thymus, stimulated by the polypeptide hormones, and in particular growth hormone. All steroid hormones, whether anabolic or catabolic, tend to cause it to atrophy, so that from puberty onwards as these become dominant there is a gradual involution of this gland. From adolescence onwards ageing may in this sense, the dominance of steroid over polypeptide hormones, be regarded as a continuous process. There is an interplay of the various hormones with certain tendencies overlaid on this which may cause partial discontinuities. Some of these are physiological, and some pathological.

In the early foetus cell division is the dominant feature in the development of the connective tissues. The time of the establishment of the foetal circulation is also the time at which formation of the intercellular matrices becomes noticeable. When a child starts walking or taking an active interest in its surroundings there is a change in the quality of the tissue components. In the early stages growth hormone dominates, then later intermittent variations in the level of cortisol production, influenced by the child's reaction to its surroundings, apparently play a part. After adolescence the steroid hormones dominate, and a balance is normally established between those with anabolic and those with catabolic activity. During the greater part of adult life their average level remains almost constant, with a rather higher proportion of anabolic in the male as compared with the female (Reifenstein, 1957). In men beyond the age of about 70–80 there commences a gradual decline in the total amount of both anabolic and catabolic hormones. In women there is a decrease in the proportion of the anabolic hormone for 5–10 years after the menopause; the two curves then become approximately parallel again, with a further decline of both beyond the age of 70–80. Throughout the time from adolescence onwards there is a gradual change in the quality of the intercellular matrices produced. They have a more ordered structure, with a corresponding decreased flexibility and water content, as age advances.

Overlaid on these normal ageing changes are a number of pathological changes, due to episodes of overproduction of catabolic steroids. These manifest themselves as osteoporosis, atherosclerosis, thrombus formation (with accompanying arterial lesions, brain damage and so on) and in various other ways. As hormone production decreases in the elderly, individuals become increasingly susceptible to the pathological changes caused by temporary hormone imbalance. Since few people remain unaffected there is a tendency to regard these pathological changes as the "ageing" process. Changes may, however, become apparent at an earlier age, and their appearance in the 5th and 6th decades or even sooner is unquestionably a pathological manifestation.

Foetus and Infant

Anlage cartilage and enchondral ossification

In the foetus bones develop as cartilage models, this cartilage being commonly referred to as anlage cartilage. At first it consists of a mass of

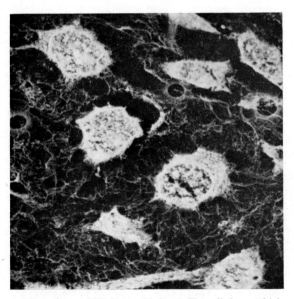

Fig. 2.1. Anlage cartilage from rabbit foetus (18 days). The cells have a high ratio of nucleus to cytoplasm and are surrounded by a very watery gel. Some intercellular matrix components have emerged from protruding cell processes. E.M. 100kV. ×2500.

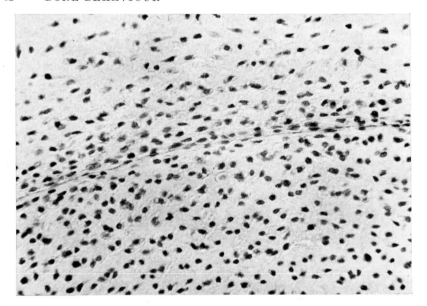

FIG. 2.2. Early stage of joint formation in human foetus (5 cm). A band of cells have flattened, but the two sides have not yet separated. ×200.

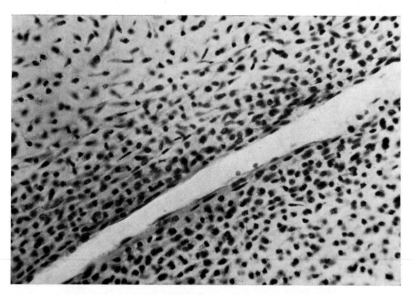

FIG. 2.3. Joint formation in human foetus (8 cm). Cells in the anlage cartilage tend to be elongated with a "tadpole-like" appearance. Cells close to the surface are more prolific and rounded, while surface cells are flattened. This is a very early stage in the development of articular cartilage. ×200.

immature cartilage cells with only a small proportion of cytoplasm to nucleus (Fig. 2.1). After the foetal circulation is established the proportions of both cytoplasm to nucleus within the cell, and matrix to cell within the tissue increases. The intercellular matrix consists of immature collagen and beta-protein, and their associated polysaccharides, as a very swollen gel. Figure 1.23 is a photograph of this gel after drying, with the polysaccharide clinging to its underlying protein.

At the time of joint formation a line of cells flattens (Fig. 2.2) and then separates. Near the separated surface a layer of more active rounded cells is the first indication of a distinction between articular and anlage cartilage (Fig. 2.3). Around the periphery cells differentiate to form a fibrous band (Fig. 2.4) which is the precursor of the synovial tissue and joint capsule.

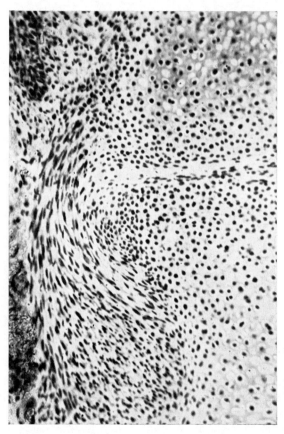

FIG. 2.4. Joint formation in a rabbit foetus. The band of fibrous tissue (left) is an early stage in the formation of the synovial membrane. Unlike the human, anlage cartilage cells in rabbits are rounded. ×100.

For growth of the anlage cartilage to take place an adequate blood supply is necessary. Examination of sections suggests that the cartilage cannot survive if more than approximately a millimetre away from the nearest vessel. The form of these vessels is characteristic. An artery and at least one vein occupy a vascular channel through the cartilage, and at the leading end these divide into a system of ramifying vessels. Figures 2.5, 2.6 show cross-sections in histological preparations of immature cartilage. Figure 2.5 shows an artery surrounded by four veins

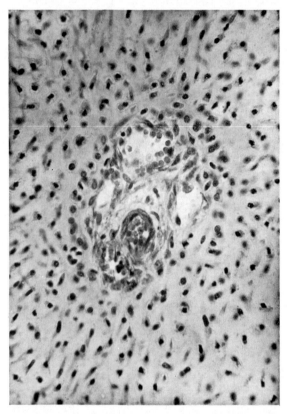

Fig. 2.5. Cross-section of vascular channel in anlage cartilage in the epiphyseal region. The anlage cartilage cells are asymmetrical. Newborn child. ×200.

in the vascular channel, while Fig. 2.6 shows a terminal vascular system. A similar vascular arrangement is seen in the ossifying front of the long bones in chickens, which do not have secondary bone nuclei. Figure 2.7 is of a perfused long bone in a chick, taken from a study by Beaumont (1965, 1967a), and Fig. 2.8 shows in more detail a vascular termination in the ossifying region. Behind the active vessels at the head of the

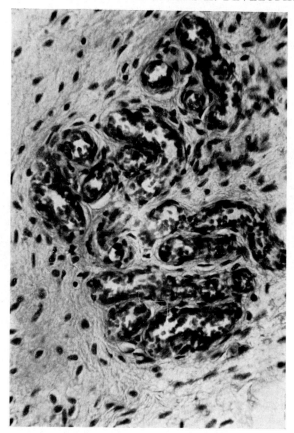

FIG. 2.6. Terminus of vascular channel in anlage cartilage between vertebral bodies, showing system of ramifying vessels. Three-month-old baby. ×200.

vascular channel in the chick ossification begins and the channel is lined with new bone. A similar vascular arrangement is also observed in fracture healing (Thoma, 1894) and during osteonal remodelling. In Fig. 2.9 two osteones in a region of active but irregular remodelling are seen side by side. One in longitudinal section shows the proliferation of vessels, while in its neighbour, seen in cross-section, the channel has almost filled with new bone.

Examination of histological sections of expanding anlage cartilage suggests that the main sites of cell division are close to vessels where cells are more numerous and active. Similarly the growth cartilage, before the development of the secondary bone nucleus, is served by a ceiling of vascular loops; and columns of cells in a mature growth cartilage are especially prolific under the vessels which penetrate the

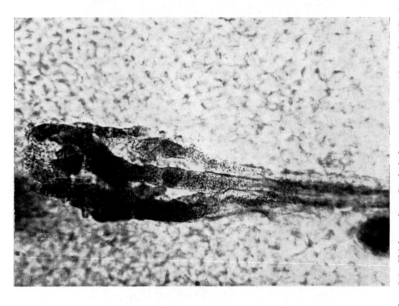

FIG. 2.8. Chicken ulna. Spalteholz preparation (cleared). "Basket-like", pattern of terminal vascular loops in ossifying region. ×200. The author thanks Dr. G. D. Beaumont for this photograph.

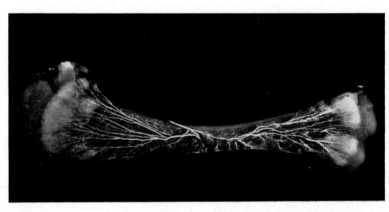

FIG. 2.7. Radiograph of humerus from 35 day old chick. Arterial perfusion with "Micropaque" (a colloidal suspension of barium sulphate). The author thanks Dr. G. D. Beaumont for this photograph.

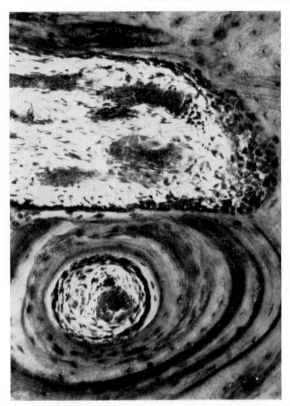

FIG. 2.9. Osteones in actively remodelling bone in arthritic head of femur. The osteone in longitudinal section shows proliferation of vessels and osteogenic cells; while in its neighbour, seen in cross-section, the channel is almost filled with new bone. The process was not continuous, and each phase is marked by a more heavily staining arrest line. In all probability there is more polysaccharide than protein laid down at the time of temporary cessation of activity (Johnson, 1964). ×100.

epiphyseal bone plate. The islands of cartilage which proliferate in the vicinity of the periosteum in an enchondroma also show cell proliferation near the vessels, and in regions of active proliferation in a chondrosarcoma the same is undoubtedly true. In many situations of this type the cell relationship with vessels is similar to that shown in Fig. 2.10, taken from a case of traumatic osteochondritis.

In a growing long bone the changes in the anlage cartilage which precede actual bone formation are first observed in the central regions of the bone. A cylinder of bone is laid down around the periosteum in this active region, and one of its functions appears to be to act as a support during the period when cell activity, with enlarged cells, early enchondral ossification and remodelling contribute to a lowering of

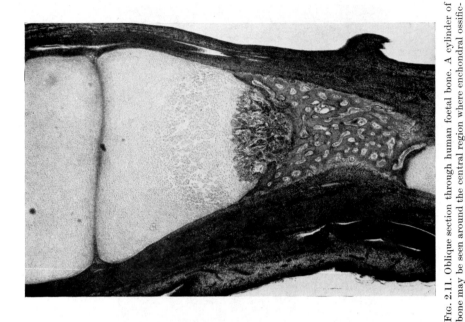

FIG. 2.11. Oblique section through human foetal bone. A cylinder of bone may be seen around the central region where enchondral ossification is taking place. There is a wide growth carti- lage containing proliferating and enlarging cells. × 35.

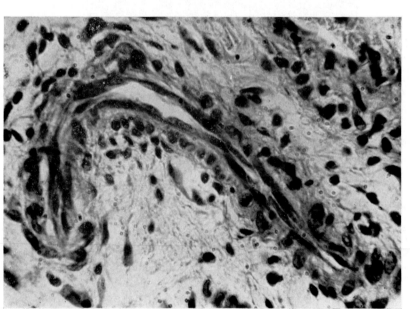

FIG. 2.10. Newly-formed cartilage from a case of traumatic osteochondritis. Active cell proliferation is close to the vessel. × 400.

mechanical strength (Fig. 2.11). As ossification proceeds along the shaft a regularly arranged cartilage develops (Fig. 2.12). Around its perimeter this continues to be protected by a bone collar extending to the region of accelerated cell proliferation. Figure 2.13 shows the extent of calcification in a foetus at the stage shortly before ossification of the shafts of the long bones is complete. The pattern of bone formation in the skull is somewhat different, allowing lateral expansion of the flattened bones.

Once the shaft has ossified, and the position of the growth cartilage has reached the epiphysis, this cartilage is no longer surrounded by an extension of the shaft of the bone, but by a band of firm cartilage, the perichondrial ring. At this stage the top part of the column of cell in the

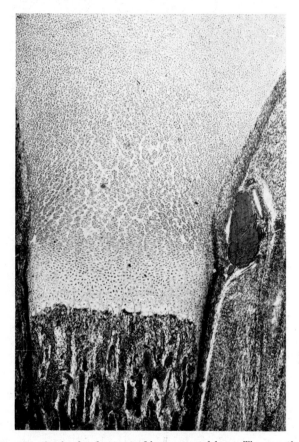

FIG. 2.12. Later stage in the development of human foetal bone. The growth cartilage and metaphysis are more regularly arranged with almost parallel vessels at the top of the metaphysis. The bone collar around the shaft extends to above the zone of enlarging cells in the cartilage. At the level of active cartilage cell proliferation is a blood vessel containing the perfusion mixture of Micropaque and Berlin blue. ×35.

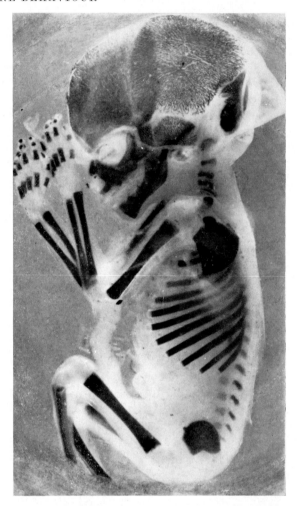

FIG. 2.13. Cleared preparation. Human foetus at the stage shortly before ossification of the long bones is complete. The back of the skull is detached, and it can be seen that the ossification pattern is different in skull and long bones. The author thanks Mrs. C. Robinson for providing this photograph.

growth cartilage is surrounded by anlage or articular cartilage and the top of the fibrous band of the perichondrial ring is level with the mid-part of the proliferative zone. Figure 2.14 shows this region of the femoral epiphysis in a 6-year-old child. Above the level of the growth cartilage the perichondrial ring merges into the perichondrium. Figure 2.15 shows the junction between the perichondrium and articular cartilage in more detail. Rigal (1962) has shown experimentally that an important func-

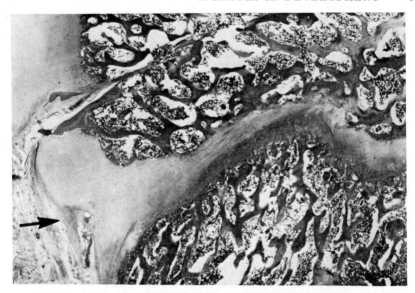

Fig. 2.14. Portions of epiphysis, growth cartilage and metaphysis of 6-year-old child. The region of the proliferative and enlarging zones is more heavily staining, while the residual anlage cartilage is lightly stained. The top of the fibrous band of the perichondral ring (arrowed) is level with the proliferative zone. An artery is seen to enter the epiphysis through the articular cartilage. ×35.

tion of the perichondrial ring is to hold the columns of cells in position. Slices of growth cartilage from the rabbit tibia, when placed in an *in vivo* culture chamber, maintain their shape in the region of the germinal zone (which may be regarded as a continuation of the anlage cartilage); but in the actively dividing proliferative zone the columnar arrangement is lost, and cells spread sideways as well as downwards. Figure 2.16 shows the irregular proliferation as seen after 10 days in an *in vivo* culture. *In vivo* culture means the placing of the piece of tissue under examination in a chamber which allows the passage of tissue fluids but not cells. This chamber is implanted in a suitable site in the animal. In an *in vitro* culture both the culture medium and the atmosphere over it are artificially controlled.

Immature bone

The bone tissue which is formed in early foetal bones is commonly called "woven bone". Unfortunately the nomenclature of bone is somewhat confused at present. This topic will be dealt with more fully in the chapter on bone formation and resorption, but will be mentioned briefly here. When bone is first laid down the mineral is deposited on the

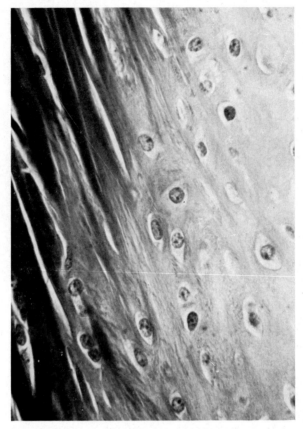

Fig. 2.15. Junction between perichondrium and articular cartilage. The more darkly staining fibrils of the fibrous tissue merge into the cartilage matrix. Cells with darkly stained nuclei are in the pre-division phase. ×400.

calcifiable matrix and is usually not very highly orientated. Later, and particularly when remodelling is taking place, the matrix is laid down by the osteoblasts in regular lamellae (Fig. 1.36) so that when secondary calcification takes place the mineral is highly orientated. In the foetus the somewhat irregularly arranged bone, with primary calcification and no secondary calcification, is that bone which is formed by proliferaton of cells from the vessel walls, and when histological sections are examined the line of osteocytes is nearly always seen to follow that of the vessels. Similarly in fracture callus, the irregularly arranged bone aligned with the ramifying vessels (Fig. 2.17) is frequently called "woven" bone.

But there is another sort of bone, also found in healing fractures and in Perthes disease, osteoarthritis and similar conditions, which is formed from a rather different type of cell, with different and less exacting

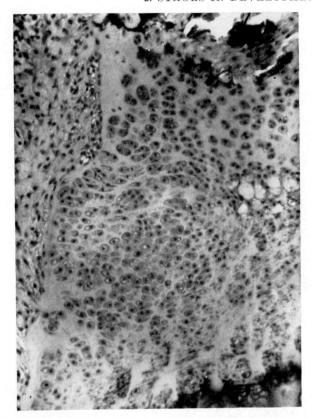

FIG. 2.16. The appearance of a block of growth cartilage after 10 days culture in an *in vivo* chamber. The cut edge of the germinal zone remains unchanged. Some cell division has occurred in the germinal zone, while there has been a considerable proliferation of cells of the proliferative zone. Without the constraining influence of the perichondral ring this zone of active proliferation bulges outwards and the columnar arrangement of flattened cells is lost. The whole explant is surrounded by proliferating fibrous tissue. × 100. The author thanks Dr. W. M. Rigal for this photograph.

nutritional requirements. This different type of bone is less directly dependent on vessels and does not mature and undergo secondary mineralization. Figure 2.18 shows the granulation tissue from which it is derived, in experimental Perthes disease at 48 h, and Fig. 2.19 shows the granulation tissue and bone derived from it at 5 weeks (Kemp, 1965). This is also called woven bone, and it would seem more logical for the term "woven bone" to be reserved for this special type of bone, rather than being applied to irregularly arranged ordinary bone in the stages before secondary mineralization has taken place. In this book, therefore, woven bone will be assumed to mean this special type of bone derived from granulation tissue.

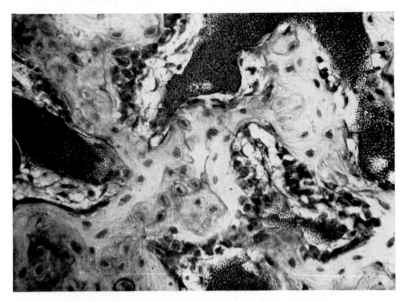

FIG. 2.17. Fracture callus. Vessels filled with perfusion medium. Irregular arrangement of vessels and bone, but cells in the bone are aligned with the vessels. ×200.

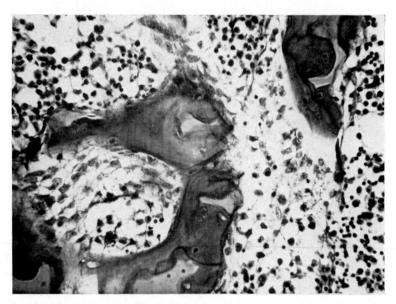

FIG. 2.18. Epiphyseal bone in experimental Perthes disease in puppy at 48 h. Granulation tissue is proliferating in the region where cell death had occurred. ×200.

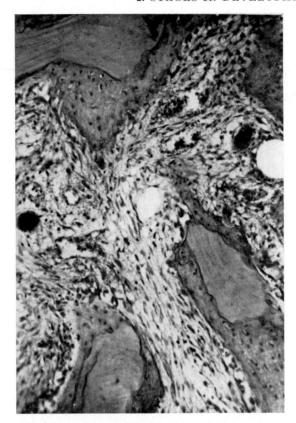

FIG. 2.19. Granulation tissue and woven bone derived from it cover dead trabeculae of the original bone. Experimental Perthes disease at 5 weeks. × 100.

Perthes disease, mentioned in the last paragraph, is a condition which sometimes develops in children after the formation of the secondary bone nucleus, in which some of the tissue within that nucleus is killed. The reason for this may be seen from a consideration of Fig. 2.14. One of the main arteries supplying the bone in this head of femur passes through the soft tissue outside the mineralized area. The vascular configuration varies from one individual to another, but in the children who are susceptible to Perthes disease an appreciable length of the artery is in the soft tissue close to the synovial fluid, and unprotected by any rigid structure. With a rise in fluid pressure from any cause the artery is temporarily closed, and some of the tissue supplied by it may die (Kemp, 1965, 1968). There is a transient pain which lasts for a day or two. Granulation tissue and woven bone are formed, while dead bone tissue present gradually degrades until a stage is reached when neither

the degraded bone tissue nor the new bone being formed by remodelling
have sufficient mechanical strength to support the weight of the body.
If weight-bearing is prevented at this time recovery takes place in 16
to 20 weeks. Otherwise crush fractures develop in the epiphysis which
may take 2 to 3 years to heal. Diagnosis during the initial stages is by a
slight displacement of the femoral head in the acetabulum as a result of
a temporary increase in size of the ligamentum teres (Boldero and Kemp,
1966).

In the foetus and infant osteoblasts are prolific and active, and it is
common to find bones covered with a mass of osteoblasts. There is a
species difference which may be observed here. In the human large
masses of osteoblasts are seen most often up to about 7 months, and by
birth their formation is already more restrained. In an animal such as

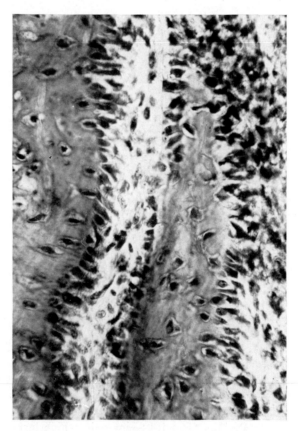

Fig. 2.20. Human foetal cortical bone at the level of zone of enlarging cells. The bone surface
is covered with active osteoblasts, about 1 in 6 of which survive to form osteocytes. They
tend to be elongated perpendicular to the surface. ×200.

the giraffe, the stage of bone development at birth is that of a human baby of about 12 months, and the baby giraffe is on its feet within hours of birth. In contrast, the new-born rat shows the very active stage of osteoblast activity.

Only a small proportion of the osteoblasts which cover a bone surface become surrounded by matrix to be buried as osteocytes. In the foetal bone shown in Fig. 2.20 it is about 1 in 6, with many of the remainder dying and disintegrating after they have made the required amount of matrix. Those that do become osteocytes retain their intercellular connections, with cell processes passing through canaliculi. These intercellular connections are present at all ages, and provide channels for the passage of the nutrients necessary for the maintenance of healthy osteocytes and bone. Most cell processes are found at the sides of cells (Fig. 2.21), but some are also present at the ends.

At the age when walking becomes possible there is a change in the

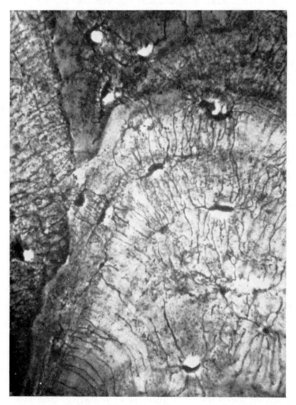

FIG. 2.21. Mature bone tissue. Silver stain to demonstrate the presence of canaliculi. In the osteone these link one osteocyte to another. The cells are elongated parallel to the surface at which they were formed, and most cell processes are found at their sides. ×400.

H

quality of the intercellular matrices, in fibrous tissue, cartilage and bone. The precise cause of this change is not yet known. The gel structure becomes firmer, while the individual components of the matrix are chemically more stable. In addition to gross species changes there are differences between one individual and another, so that one may find, say, the intervertebral disc tissue of a baby a few months old resembling that of another child at $2\frac{1}{2}$ years of age.

Childhood and Adolescence

During childhood, as growth continues, more mature components of the intercellular matrices are formed, collagen and the mature beta-proteins. The gels that form the greater part of the matrices increase in firmness, and their components are more stable. It is not till adolescence, however, that they approach the chemical stability of the adult tissues. This greater ease of solution or degradation in childhood facilitates resorption and tissue turnover. The matrix produced by cells which are being stimulated by the polypeptide hormones (including growth hormone) is always less chemically stable than the matrix produced by those same cells when stimulated by steroid hormones. Tissue turnover is an essential factor in growth. The long bones, for instance, as well as increasing in length by means of enchondral ossification at the growth cartilage also increase in diameter as new bone is laid down on the periosteal surface, resorption being preferentially from the endosteal surface. Modification of the shape of the bone, to correspond with external forces involves formation and removal of bone at both the endosteal and periosteal surfaces. An increase in diameter of the bones continues long after longitudinal growth has ceased.

One method of following this activity in experimental animals is by the administration of tetracycline, which is deposited in areas of new bone formation, so acting as a yellow fluorescent label when viewed in ultra-violet light. The administration of tetracycline to pregnant rabbits, for example, has shown that the rate of growth of the long bones in a baby rabbit is such that after three weeks none of the bone present at birth remains. In contrast to this, the skull grows by deposition near the suture lines and without removal of the bone already laid down. Figure 2.13 shows the contrast between skull and long bones in a human foetus. The very active growth in a young animal or child is accompanied by equally active wound healing. Fracture healing is also rapid, and in chidren leg-lengthening operations may be carried out by performing an osteotomy and gradually drawing the two halves of the bone apart. Once the adolescent changes have started this procedure is no longer practicable.

The beginning of adolescence is marked by the appearance of the sex hormones in substantial amounts in the circulating blood. They modify the behaviour of all cells of the connective tissue series. The tissues become less malleable (the reaction in the leg-lengthening operation is one example) and the changes in the cells of the epiphyseal growth plate mark the beginnings of plate closure. When this process is finally completed, and it may take several years, then longitudinal growth ceases. The interplay of hormones at this time is complex, but the mechanism of plate closure, which will be described in the next chapter, suggests that an alternation between a slight excess of first catabolic and then anabolic hormones is an integral part of the procedure. Behavioural disturbances due to these changes in hormone balance are, apart from a few rare cases, only slight. The adolescent behaviour in-

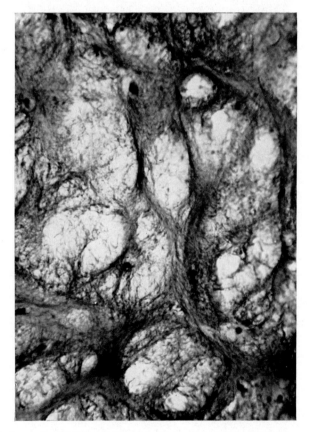

Fig. 2.22. Nucleus pulposus in baby. The section shows a dried gel (white spaces indicate the proportion of water lost during processing). Cells tend to remain in the more solid fibrous processes. ×200.

duced by exposure to pop music and similar external stimuli must be considered as abnormal, and is more closely related to the effects of habit-forming or hallucinatory drugs.

As well as bone, the matrices in cartilage, and particularly in the intervertebral disc, show changes at adolescence. In the early stages the fibro-cartilage of the nucleus pulposus consists of elongated cells in a uniform matrix (Fig. 2.6). Later the nucleus has the consistency of a very loose gel with the cells tending to cling to the more solid fibrous components (Fig. 2.22). Soon afterwards the spaces fill up with more matrix

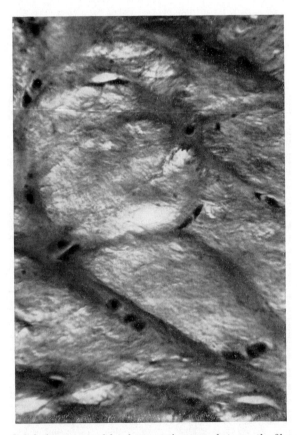

Fig. 2.23. At a slightly later stage of development the spaces between the fibrous processes in the nucleus pulposus are filled with more matrix. The cells on the processes are elongated. ×200.

(Fig. 2.23) in which a certain number of rounded cells are found (Fig. 2.24). The result is a tissue with a much higher proportion of matrix to cell than is the case with articular cartilage. Figures 2.25, 2.26, of adult

disc and articular cartilage, are comparable. At the time of adolescence
the cells produce a greater amount of the beta-protein, sufficiently polymerized to act as a stable rubber. As well as the hormonal changes
necessary for the more stable versions of the compound to be formed, the
cells must be stimulated by the correct physical forces, otherwise little
or none is produced. Another way of saying this is to say that during
adolescence adequate exercise is necessary for the correct maturation of
the spine. It is at this stage that lumbar disc lesions are initiated, which
may lead to prolapse from 5 to 15 years later. In a series of operations
for prolapse it has been observed that the normal parts of the disc
cartilage removed had very little of the mature beta-protein, in contrast
to the composition of the nucleus pulposus obtained at post-mortem
from subjects with healthy intervertebral discs (Taylor, 1964).

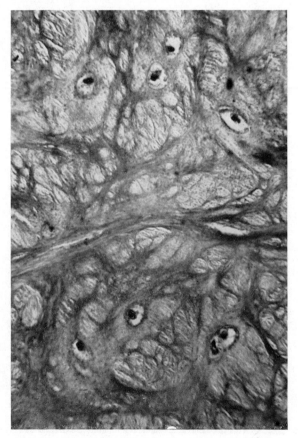

Fig. 2.24. Same baby as Fig. 2.22. Another part of the nucleus pulposus. Rounded cells are in
the matrix between the fibrous components. ×200.

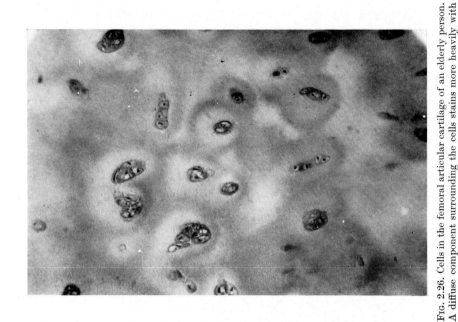

FIG. 2.26. Cells in the femoral articular cartilage of an elderly person. A diffuse component surrounding the cells stains more heavily with haematoxylin than does the rest of the matrix. There is a much lower proportion of matrix to cell than in the nucleus pulposus. ×200.

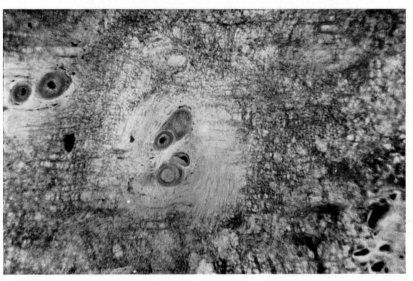

FIG. 2.25. Cells in the lumbar disc of an elderly individual. They have prominent "caps" and are surrounded by a large capsule. Between the widely separated groups of cells the matrix contains dense beta-protein which gives a dark brown colour with Hofmann's elastic stain. ×200.

The Adult

Tissue changes

In the adult, until the age of 35 to 40, changes in both cartilage and bone are towards greater stability of the intercellular matrices, with rather more bone tissue and stronger bones. Pathological changes may occur, in the intervertebral disc or in the arteries, but they are readily recognized as pathological. Beyond this age, the same trend in the composition of the matrices persists, and parallels the involution of the thymus and related phenomena, but the pathological changes affecting bones, blood vessels and connective tissues are at the present time becoming so common, particularly in urban populations, that in practice a susceptibility to these needs to be recognized as a dominant feature in the development of the middle-aged and elderly.

In the intervertebral disc in the adult the process of maturing is marked, in the normal individual, by an increasing firmness of both the gel and rubber-like components mixed with it, and by an increase in the degree of ordering of the beta-protein. At the age of about 40 the dense beta-protein starts to appear as a significant component of the nucleus pulposus, and by 50 or 60 years of age, it is a dominant component in some individuals. Beyond this same age of 40 the incidence of prolapse in the lumbar intervertebral discs shows a marked decrease (O'Connell, 1951). The "capsules" around the cells, which protect them from the quite considerable applied forces, become increasingly prominent (Figs 2.27, 2.28, 2.29).

In the bones, although longitudinal growth ceases after adolescence, there is a fairly steady increase in the amount of bone tissue, particularly in men, until the age of 35 or so. After this the proportion of bone tissue to marrow stays level for a time, then there is a gradual decline. Additionally, in pathological states such as those commonly known as post-menopausal osteoporosis and senile osteoporosis there may be an abnormal decrease in the amount of bone. A phenomenon similar to that observed in post-menopausal osteoporosis has been noted in some younger women taking the contraceptive pill. There are several causes for the gradual decrease in the quantity of bone once the peak has been passed. One is a direct hormonal action which leads to an abnormal rate of bone loss. The effects produced in the acute stage of post-menopausal osteoporosis have been simulated in animals by the alternate administration of cortisone and weakly anabolic steroids, to represent the increased blood cortisol levels present at times of stress and the surge of anabolic activity which follows after the stimulus to cortisol production has been removed (Storey, 1957). The alternation of steroids produces prominent

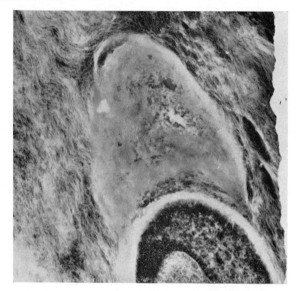

FIG. 2.27. Cap of altered matrix formed at end of cell in the intervertebral disc. E.M. 100kV. ×3500.

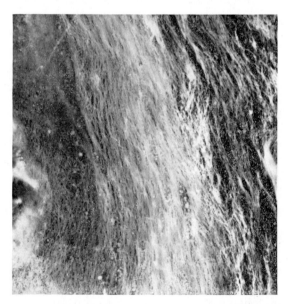

FIG. 2.28. Capsular material between edge of cell (extreme left) and the matrix of the nucleus pulposus. E.M. 100kV. ×3500.

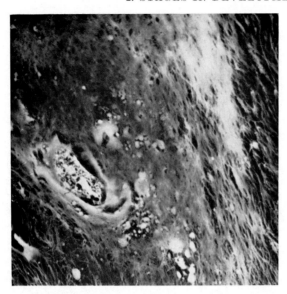

Fig. 2.29. Cell with "mummified" appearance and surrounded by capsule. Nucleus pulposus of elderly person. E.M. 100kV. ×3500.

arrest lines in bone and Fig. 2.30 shows 8 such lines corresponding to 8 alternations in the rabbit. Figure 2.31 shows the arrest lines in a trabecula from the human neck of femur taken during an active phase of the condition. Similarly Fig. 2.32 shows how bone removed from the end of a rabbit's cortex as the result of the alternation is replaced by haemopoietic tissue, while Fig. 2.33 shows the distribution of haemopoietic tissue at the junction of femoral neck and upper end of cortex in an active stage of the osteoporotic process in a woman. These mechanisms will be discussed in detail in a later chapter. Corticosteroids can also cause a decrease in the amount of intercellular matrix produced by each individual osteoblast.

Other mechanisms lead to a lowering of the flow of blood through the bone, and evidence will be described in detail in Chapter 5 which shows that a decreased blood flow through bone is accompanied by a decrease in the quantity of bone present. One important cause of decreased blood flow through bone is an indirect effect of hormonal action. Very frequently, and particularly in men, there is a narrowing of the lumen of the small blood vessels, not as a result of the type of fat deposition seen in the major arteries, but as a result of the deposition of thrombi and their subsequent organization. Such thrombus formation has been shown in animal experiments to be due to fluctuations in the ratio of anabolic to catabolic compounds, and the mechanisms involved will be

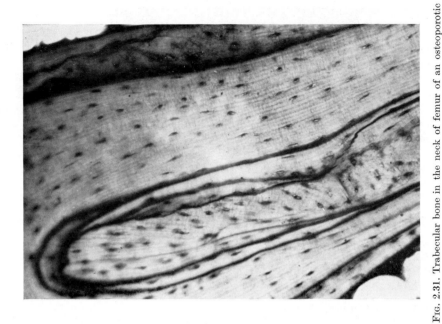

Fig. 2.31. Trabecular bone in the neck of femur of an osteoporotic subject, during an acute phase. The trabecular bone is surrounded by haemopoietic tissue. It contains very prominent arrest lines. ×300.

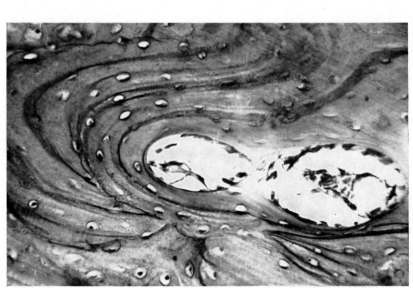

Fig. 2.30. Cortical bone from rabbit. Cortisone and lynoestrenol had been administered alternately for 8 cycles each of a week's duration (i.e. a total of 8 weeks). Each reversal of activity shows a prominent arrest line. ×300.

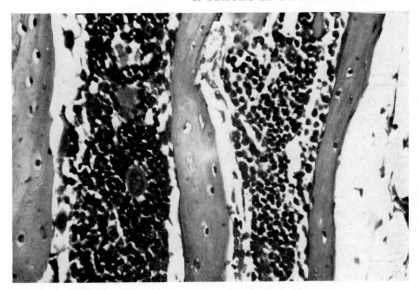

FIG. 2.32. Inner portion of cortex, towards metaphyseal side, of rabbit treated with cortisone for two weeks, followed by cortisone and methandienone. The resorbed bone has been replaced by haemopoietic tissue. × 200.

described in Chapter 6. Although the overall values of the anabolic and catabolic levels remain about the same during the greater part of adult life, there are fluctuations due to stress. This is a difficult term to define accurately, but in the present limited context is probably best regarded as any cause which can lead to a temporary increase in the plasma cortisol level. The effect is mediated by a change in pituitary output, and in other organs there may be different consequences of the pituitary changes. Recently formed thrombi can be found after episodes of preoperative stress, whether due to pain, discomfort or apprehension, and after severe terminal illness as well as in situations where histological confirmation is not so readily available. Figure 2.34 is a deposit in a synovial vessel removed at operation, while the tissues shown in Figs 2.35, 2.36 were taken at post-mortem from the lumbar region of an elderly man.

The flow of blood in a bone is partly regulated by the action of the heart pumping blood into the bone, and partly due to the action of the muscles pumping it out again. In the limbs these two mechanisms make approximately equal contributions. Stress reactions, whether by means of a generalized arteriosclerosis or the more local deposits such as those shown in Fig. 2.35 lower the contribution of the arterial blood supply. They also reduce the efficiency of the muscles, either by reducing their blood supply as in the case illustrated by Fig. 2.36, or by the weakening

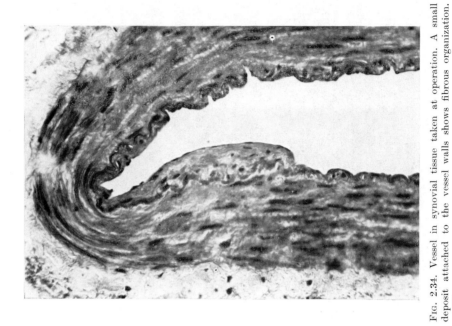

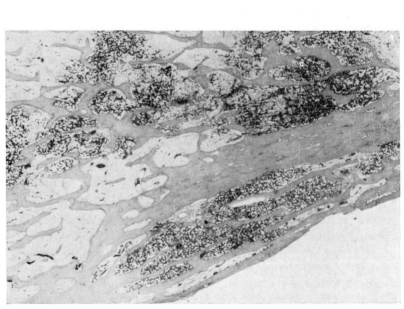

FIG. 2.34. Vessel in synovial tissue taken at operation. A small deposit attached to the vessel walls shows fibrous organization. ×200.

FIG. 2.33. Junction of the upper end of cortex and femoral neck at an active stage of the osteoporotic process. Haemopoietic tissue is present wherever bone resorption has taken place. ×35.

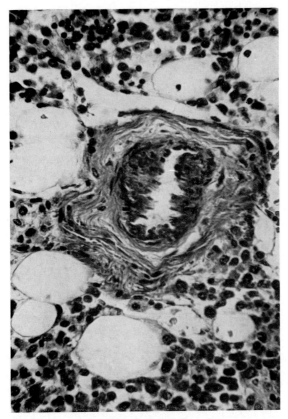

FIG. 2.35. Vessel in lumbar vertebra taken at post-mortem, after lengthy terminal illness. Granulation tissue has invaded a comparatively recent deposit so that there is a considerable reduction in the blood flow. $\times 200$.

of the muscle fibres that can be caused by the anti-anabolic action of the corticosteroids. There is another cause for reduced efficiency which may also operate in normal healthy individuals, and that is insufficient exercise. Frequently the cessation of the increase in the amount of bone tissue tends to coincide with a reduction in the amount of exercise taken by the individual. Too little exercise results in some atrophy of the muscles, and conversely increased exercise increases the muscle activity and efficiency, even of muscles whose function is slightly impaired, and so decreases bone loss. Exercise has other more indirect effects. It increases the partial pressure of oxygen in the circulating blood, as a result of more adequate ventilation of the lungs; it decreases the amount of unwanted fat; and it also suppresses the blood cortisol level (Cornil, de Coster, Copinshi and Franckson, 1965), so that one effect of adequate exercise is to diminish many of the consequences which might be

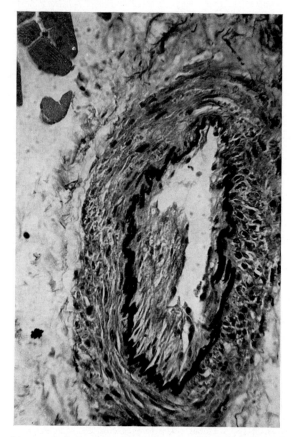

FIG. 2.36. Vessel in muscle in lumbar region of same patient. Stained to show the internal elastic lamina. An organized deposit more than half blocks the vessel. A few muscle fibres can be seen at the top left. ×200.

expected to follow exposure to stress-producing stimuli. In an earlier stage of society the physical running away from danger would diminish the undesirable side-effects of the hormonal response to fear, while not affecting the desirable ones.

Basic research methods as applied to vascular lesions

This is, perhaps, an appropriate place to mention the basic research methods which must be used whenever there is need to disentangle a complex set of phenomena. The first requirement is to make as many observations as possible of the phenomena under consideration. From these, speculation may result in the formulation of several possible hypotheses. But having formulated a hypothesis, it will suggest other observations which could either support it or eliminate it, or cause it to be modified. At this stage a not uncommon mistake is to choose a parameter involved in some particular hypothesis and to investigate it exclusively. Should the hypothesis be a mistaken one, further progress on the original problem is prevented. This has happened several times during the course of investigations on osteoporosis. It must always be remembered that any relevant facts which are not accounted for by a hypothesis must cause that hypothesis to be modified or abandoned. Further facts may lead to either a revised hypothesis or a new hypothesis.

Vascular lesions have appeared as an unexpected factor which modifies the behaviour of bone in the adult and the elderly, and so it will be useful to take the formation of these vascular lesions as an example of how the fundamental research methods may be applied.

The general pattern which has been observed is that in men there is the steady and continuous ageing process, but in middle age an increased susceptibility to the effects of vascular disease, and then after the age of 75 to 80 a further increased susceptibility to a number of degenerative processes, including vascular disease and osteoporosis. In women there is a discontinuity at the menopause, and after this an increased susceptibility to vascular disease, osteoporosis and other degenerative conditions. Osteoporosis is accompanied by an increased calcification of the aorta.

Over the course of years there have been various hypotheses to account for the observed vascular lesions. One of the most popular has been that an unsatisfactory diet might contribute to the vascular conditions. A striking observation was that clinical signs were accompanied by a raised blood cholesterol, while fat deposits on the artery walls are a dominant feature in many cases. One hypothesis was, therefore, that the cholesterol and other deposited fats were the only cause of the lesions, and another hypothesis was that since cholesterol and unsaturated fats are frequently present in the diet a diet containing these is the initial cause. Having formulated these two hypotheses, there is next the need to look for other related observations. A convincing one is that although on the basis of the hypothesis a modification of diet has been suggested to many patients, undoubtedly beneficial results are conspicuous by their absence. This, although a matter for simple observation, has also been the subject of carefully controlled tests. For example, a trial using soya-bean oil (Morris, 1968) has led to the conclusion that there was no evidence that the relapse rate in myocardial infarction was in any way affected by the unsaturated fat content of the diet used. Approaching the subject from another angle Friedman and Rosenman (1957) showed that the fat intake of American men and women was virtually the same, although there was a wide difference between the sexes in the incidence of clinical coronary disease.

As a result of many such observations the dietary hypothesis can be firmly eliminated. Insurance companies appear to have established a correlation between overweight and a liability to coronary heart disease, but this again is not simply a matter of either diet or cholesterol. Chapman *et al* (1966) have found that high cholesterol levels do not correlate with body weight. One hypothesis that might be considered again later is that exercise is a relevant factor. In the meantime the high cholesterol level remains to be considered. This was a fact and not a speculation.

As a result of observations on animals in the Philadelphia Zoological Gardens extending over 50 years information is available on a large number of species (Ratcliffe and Cronin, 1958). During the years 1901 to 1932 arteriosclerosis, defined in terms of lipid deposits, was found in less than 3% of autopsies on animals and birds in the zoo, but since then the frequency has risen to over 20%. Dietary changes were eliminated as a causative factor, but overcrowding and also quarrelling and loneliness, particularly when combined with inactivity, were found to cause an imbalance in adrenal secretion. These adrenal secretions were another factor to be considered, together with the idea that stressful situations are a primary cause, for over the years, rage, resentment and anger have been found likely to precede myocardial infarction and other incidents (Fisher, 1963). There is an abundance of evidence that such situations do result in rises in blood cholesterol. Chapman *et al.* (1966) reported high levels for men who are tense and nervous, living under a nervous strain, found their work trying and stressing, were exhausted at the end of the day. By contrast, living a hectic life did not itself raise the blood cholesterol. Another group of workers took as subjects for observation men in a profession which had periodic "dead-lines" to meet, and found the cholesterol levels closely related to the pattern of work (Friedman, Rosenman and Carrol, 1958). They also found as causes excessive drive, competition and economic frustration, and noted that the blood clotting time was halved at times of stress.

Advancing knowledge one stage further Wolf *et al.* (1962) showed that without any change in diet or exercise striking alterations in serum concentrations of cholesterol and triglycerides correlated with the occurrence of emotionally stressful situations. Such changes were brought about within 60 min. Similarly Peterson, Keith and Wolcox (1962) showed that the concentrations could vary widely during the course of a few hours in certain individuals. The changes could relate to anticipation of an event as well as to the event itself—apprehension is an emotion to be reckoned with.

A modified hypothesis could now be that stress causes a rise in the cholesterol and other fats in the blood, which are deposited in atheromatous plaques and are possibly directly responsible for conditions such as coronary heart disease. This hypothesis in turn, even on the evidence so far quoted, could not represent the entire story, since it does not include mention of the adrenal secretions or the reduced clotting time. So far the evidence for the more widely recognized rises in plasma cholesterol have been considered. But there is an abundance of evidence that stress also causes a rise in plasma cortisol.

In 1959 Mason considered a variety of anxiety states which caused temporary rises in adreno-cortical activity. He noted that novelty was a factor, so that people can become psychologically adapted to a situation, and also that the state which he described as "anxiety of a disintegrative nature" produced particularly high levels. In a review published in 1953 Dougherty and Dougherty recorded that stress of various types liberated cortisol. There are many reports that the severity of the stress reaction, in terms of raised cortisol levels, varies from one individual to another (Tesse, Friedman and Mason, 1965; Davis et al., 1962; Mason et al. 1965). Bursten and Russ (1965) showed that with a high level of preoperative apprehension the plasma cortisol levels dropped to that caused by the trauma of surgery, while with less apprehensive patients it rose to the level of surgical trauma. The same type of stimuli produced high cortisol levels as produced high cholesterol levels, and again it has been shown that the level follows the mood over a period of time (Bunney, Mason and Hamburg, 1965; Bliss, Mijeon, Branch and Samuels, 1956). The latter showed that the blood steroids may remain at a high level with chronic emotional tension. High levels are obtained with various types of stress; emotional, trauma, acute bacterial infection (Bassoe, Aarskoy, Thomsen and Stoe, 1965), acute illness (Sholiton, Werk and Marnell, 1961), genuine pain (Shenkin, 1964), terminal illness, and particularly high levels with advanced cancer (Werk, MacGee and Sholiton, 1964). The last three, like Bliss et al. (1956), noticed a disturbance in or a loss of the normal diurnal variations in cortisol levels. In contrast to all these varieties of stress, the cortisol levels are considerably reduced during hypnotic trance (Sachar, Cobb and Stor, 1966).

In recording the raised cortisol levels, plasma cortisol is sometimes measured, but at other times corticosteroids excreted in the urine are examined. These observations follow the plasma cortisol levels approximately, but not accurately. One instance in which this difference is significant is in the physiological rise of cortisol in pregnancy. Appleby and Norymberski (1957) have found that during pregnancy the average excretion rises to 40% above normal. There is an additional sharp increase following parturition, and one day later the urinary levels return to normal. But after labour ceases the plasma cortisol levels remain raised for several days.

Next there is a need to consider the relationship between the raised cholesterol and cortisol levels, and again the relevant information is available. When the adrenal is stimulated, corticosteroids are released by the cortex and adrenalin by the medulla. The adrenalin causes a rapid rise in the plasma concentrations of free fatty acids, cholesterol, phospholipids and triglycerides, but the presence of cortisol is needed for the mobilization of these in quantity (Peshef and Shapiro, 1960; Shapir and Steinberg, 1960). The changes in serum lipids are secondary to the increased mobilization of free fatty acids from adipose tissue (Forbes, Rudolph and Petterson, 1966). Jenkins, Lowe and Titterington (1964) have added another factor. Cortisol increased the release of free fatty acids from adipose tissue, while cortisone was inactive. In the human about a third of the cortisone administered experimentally or therapeutically would be metabolized to cortisol in an hour or two. The effect of the cortisol was completely overcome by the simultaneous infusion of insulin, which indicates that whenever there is any stimulus to increased insulin secretion the effect of the latter would predominate. This facet of the problem will not be considered further in the present discussion, although it is necessary for the complete elucidation of the mechanisms involved.

A further modification now of the cholesterol side of the hypothesis is that stress stimulates the adrenal glands, which in turn cause a rise of cholesterol and other lipids in the blood. For the deposition of cholesterol, the necessary conditions include a raised level in the blood, and the presence of a breakdown product of red cells (Gibbons, Alladine and Little, 1969). Some degree of haemolysis is often found in normal individuals (Roeser, Powell and O'Brien, 1968). In agreement with this Pierie, Hancock, Koorajian and Starr (1968) have found that when prosthetic heart valves in affected individuals are examined, cholesterol is usually deposited on the aortic valve, where the flow of blood is more turbulent. Figure 2.37 shows a deposit on the ball of an aortic prosthesis. In this case death had followed three weeks after its insertion. Once deposited, such crystals stimulate the propagation of granulation tissue. Hence the fat and fibrous tissue plaques found on the walls of the coronary arteries and the aorta.

One of the phospholipids produced by the combined action of adrenalin and cortisol can also help to account for the reduced clotting times which have been observed (Cannon and Mendenhal, 1914; Macht, 1952). Bolton, Hampton and Mitchell (1967) have elucidated the mechanism whereby an active phospholipid induces abnormal platelet sensitivity and rapid platelet aggregation. Here the platelets in the blood are

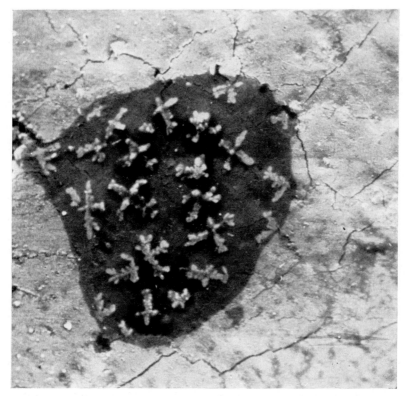

FIG. 2.37. Surface of silicone ball from a Starr-Edwards aortic heart valve. Death occurred three weeks after insertion. This is one of several patches of fat deposited on the surface of the ball. The specimen was metal coated, and the fine cracks are a preparation artefact. Stereoscan photograph. ×200.

introduced as yet another factor to be considered. As long ago as 1874 Osler had shown that platelets clump and fuse together into amorphous masses in the blood of some patients with febrile illnesses, and more recently Sharp (1961) has shown that in platelet clumping there are two separate stages, aggregation which may be reversible and fusion which is irreversible. The phospholipid affects clumping, while sticky platelets from abnormal megakaryocytes produced by the combined action of cortisol with certain other steroids fuse almost immediately to form thrombi (Little and White 1968; Little, 1970b).

Returning now to the portion of the hypothesis which states that stress stimulates the adrenal glands, some modification is necessary, because among the effects of the types of stress which have been described there are facts not covered by the simple theory dominated by a raised blood cortisol. Gastric ulcers are a common variant, and there are also rarer sequelae such as hyperthyroidism (Witte, 1966). The data required for a more comprehensive hypothesis is again available. One of the groups of cells that are affected by cortisol are the lymphocytes. Reduced mitosis, "budding" and loss of cytoplasm, and a failure to mature to macrophages are among the changes which have been observed (Dougherty, 1952). Dougherty and White (1944) have shown that these lymphocyte changes are under pituitary control and mediated by the adrenal cortex, which is now known to be responsible for the raised cortisol levels. It was also shown that these changes in the lymphatics and lymphocytes are produced by the various common forms of stress (Dougherty and Dougherty, 1953).

Since then the volume of evidence that stress causes the pituitary to release more ACTH which in turn stimulates the adrenal cortex to produce more corticosteroids has rapidly increased (Saffran, 1962). Saffran has pointed out that the activation of the pituitary-adrenal system by stress serves to provide metabolic reponses to help the organism to face altered circumstances. Prominent among these are additional supplies of carbohydrates which provide energy. A further interesting observation has been that fasting increases the plasma cortisol half-life (Mills, 1962), again facilitating extra mobility of carbohydrates to produce energy. Mills (1938) had earlier shown that the depression of glucose tolerance after exercise is connected with depleted carbohydrate stores. The form of the glucose tolerance curve was unconnected with the action of insulin. Jacobowitz, Marks and Vernikus-Danellis (1963) showed that the rise in ACTH was within a minute or two of the application of stress.

That the primary involvement is with the pituitary gland accounts satisfactorily for other effects following on from stress besides those initiated by the raised blood cortisol, because the pituitary controls several hormonal groups in the body. It also provides a possible line of contact between the emotions and their consequences, since there is a vascular connection between the hypothalmus and the pituitary. It is, however, possible for certain stimuli to act directly upon the adrenal cortex. One example is the action of low doses of radiation, of the order of 10 rad (Dougherty and White, 1946). It is not without interest that in some quarters low radiation doses are looked on as a method for "accelerating the ageing process".

Various pieces now seem to be fitting smoothly into the puzzle. Stress, as a matter of general observation, stimulates the clinical manifestations of vascular disease, and investigations have shown that stress acting through the hypothalmus stimulates the pituitary gland, which in turn releases ACTH that stimulates the adrenal gland. Cortisol is released, which can either have direct effects on its own, or assist the medullary hormones to release cholesterol, free fatty acids, phospholipids and triglycerides. The deposited cholesterol can account for the atheromatous plaques. Other manifestations of stress have also been fitted into the general pattern. *But the discovery of any awkward facts, as a result of observation, must cause hypotheses or theories at any stage of their development to be modified or abandoned.* Of the peripheral facts which should be fitted into any complete theory insulin has already been mentioned, while although hypotension and fluid balance are relevant, they are sufficiently peripheral to be omitted from the immediate discussion. Several other groups of facts are, however, directly relevant.

Exercise. This is concerned with the maintenance and development of the gels and rubbers of the intercellular matrices in cartilage and the connective tissues, and of the muscle fibres. It is also an important mechanism together with the pumping action of the heart, for pumping blood through the body, and in particular the bones, so maintaining a sufficient supply of oxygen for adequate tissue development. But it also seems to play a direct part in these stress conditions, and Morris *et al.* (1953) showed that men in physically active jobs have a lower incidence of coronary heart disease, and in milder form, than men of similar age in equivalent sedentary jobs. Cornil *et al.* (1965) provided a partial explanation of this by showing that muscular exercise by untrained normal men was accompanied by a significant fall in the plasma cortisol level. The mechanism of this decrease in the plasma cortisol still awaits elucidation.

Sex differences. It is the middle-aged men who are susceptible to serious vascular lesions but not middle-aged women. The interaction of the hormones is such that oestrogens lower the serum cholesterol and elevate the phospholipids, while androgens reverse the effects of the oestrogens. Then, when a vascular lesion is formed, the anabolic hormones in the men not only stimulate more granulation tissue formation as compared with the lower anabolic level of the female hormones, but the oestrogens prolong the half-life of the cortisol in the blood (Peterson *et al.*, 1962). Corticosteroids tend to inhibit granulation tissue proliferation. This question of anabolic and catabolic activity will be considered in a later chapter.

These two sets of facts tend to amplify the hypothesis, so that one might consider whether it could now be dignified by being referred to as a theory, but there is still a very big gap in knowledge, and that is the connection, if any, between these atheromatous lesions and clinical manifestations such as coronary heart disease. Ratcliffe and Cronin (1958), for example, in their survey of a wide range of species, were discussing the lesions in terms of post-mortem findings rather than of clinical symptoms. Mitchell, Schwartz and Zingler (1964) have examined in the human a large number of arteries and have observed the fatty lesions in most age groups, from children onwards, and come to the conclusion that they are benign. They found that lesions associated with clinical signs and symptoms had a somewhat different appearance and were rare before the age of 35 in men or 50 in women. There was a correlation between this second type of plaque and conditions such as cardiac infarction. Further, there was evidence of thrombus formation, with thrombi causing the lesions rather than *vice versa*. Complementary evidence has been obtained by Mason (1963). He found a considerable thickening of the intima of coronary arteries in a series of healthy young men in England, in the 20 to 30 age group. These men were killed as a result of either flying or car accidents. A closely similar degree of thickening of the intima of coronary arteries was observed in young men in the same age groups, killed in similar accidents, in the United States. But whereas in the English series the coronary artery disease was not accompanied by coronary heart disease, in a significant proportion of the American series it was. Clearly the factor of importance in the production of the cardiac ischaemia was not the underlying atherosclerosis.

Here one might interpolate several speculations as a basis for further investigations. It could be that exercise modifies the blood cortisol levels preferentially, without noticeable effect on the cholesterol levels, so that additional exercise was sufficient to prevent coronary heart disease being overlaid on the coronary artery disease in the men in the English series. There is also a probability that minor hormonal factors are partly responsible for the appearance of one result of stress in preference to another. It has been reported, for instance, that when stilboestrol (a synthetic compound with some actions similar to those of some natural hormones and of contraceptive agents) is given for the purpose of lowering the level of cholesterol in the blood the incidence of platelet thrombi is increased (Oliver and Boyd, 1961). Minor metabolic differences might also be considered as a possible means of accounting for the apparent correlation between being overweight and a liability to coronary heart disease. Again, although cholesterol is released into the blood almost immediately in a form which is available for deposition, it might be that megakaryocyte formation, and hence the production of the sticky platelets that form thrombi, is only disturbed if the diurnal rhythm of the cortisol is interfered with.

The situation now is that so far as both coronary heart disease and related conditions are concerned, and also the changes in vessels supplying bones and muscles, it is the second kind of lesion, involving a raised blood cortisol and thrombi, which is relevant. This puts bone into the picture in an active as well as a passive role, since the megakaryocytes which produce the platelets that coalesce to form thrombi are formed in the marrow. Accordingly, this topic will be pursued further in the sections of the book dealing with bone marrow. For the original problem hypotheses involving cholesterol are of only secondary importance. In the foregoing discussion only a small selection of references from among the large number available have been chosen. A comparison of some of the dates is of interest.

Such lines of reasoning, with observations, followed by hypotheses, followed by more observations, and consequent abandonment or modification of hypotheses, are the basis of all research methods. Technical manipulation of equipment in laboratories does not, of itself, constitute research. When the need for justification of the purchase of expensive equipment causes it to be applied to problems where its use is irrelevant, or when expensive and elaborate methods of assessing patients' conditions (e.g. a metabolic ward) are based on incorrect hypotheses, sophisticated experimental procedures become a positive hindrance. A point that must be emphasized, and remembered, is that among the invariable rules for genuine progress to be made are that awkward facts must not be swept under the carpet. And possibly even more important, *hypotheses are not facts.*

There are various difficulties and pitfalls in assessing observational evidence. Most common is to look at wholly irrelevant systems. For example, in investigating a condition such as osteoporosis, which has active phases, it is pointless to take bone samples from an inactive stage and use them to attempt to demonstrate the state of affairs in the active stages; or to make elaborate observations on the mineral, and expect to obtain information about cell activity. Again, there are some drug effects which depend on the simultaneous action of two or more compounds. To examine the effect of each separately gives no indication of what the joint action might be. Thrombus formation, depending on the joint action of corticosteroids with another type of steroid, comes into this category.

The Elderly

In the last section the period of life from adolescence to the mid-fifties was considered. In the next age group, from about 50 onwards, there is the same tendency towards connective tissue matrices with more stable components, having less resilience and a lower water content. It is also generally found that less matrix is formed per cell during the process of connective tissue or bone remodelling, which could account in part for the physiological decrease in the amount of bone tissue.

The main difficulty in describing the physiological changes in old age, *per se*, is that there are so few old people who do not show signs of the stress and degenerative diseases. Recently the problem has been quite clearly defined as a result of a survey of elderly people which was made in Holland (van Zonneveld, 1962). Over a quarter of the country's over 65 population (and their doctors) were interviewed. Among the results was the observation that whereas elderly women were frequently ill, elderly men tended to die. The same factor operates in England where the death-rate figures "rate for age" are lower in women because of a lower susceptibility to cardiovascular disease and chronic bronchitis. Another observation was that the age at which a general deterioration of the functions of the body frequently became apparent is about 85, except for those people who had lost interest in their activities or surroundings, and who had not enough to occupy their minds. In that sector of the population senile changes were observed even before the age of 70.

There is, then, a fairly definite change at the age of 80 to 85. Reifenstein (1957) recorded that beyond the age of 70 and 80 there is a gradual decline in the amount of both anabolic and catabolic hormones. The main consequence of this is that the balance between the two becomes more precarious, so that the individual becomes more susceptible to the effects of stress. This increased susceptibility to the effects of stress is such that there are only a comparatively small number of centenarians in the world. Most show some of the effects of the degenerative diseases, although a few are on record as still looking and behaving like "a well-preserved 80".

Many observations suggest that stress effects are the dominant causes of the degenerative conditions in old age. Loss of interest and loneliness are stressful, and would lead indirectly to thrombus formation. Working in the opposite direction is an as yet indeterminate factor which might be called "motivation". In several surveys of centenarians the common factor seems to be that they still retain an active interest and pride in what they are doing. In younger age groups a lack of motivation has been found to be a major contributory cause of mental disease and psychiatric breakdown—and 45% of the hospitals in Great Britain are for mental disease (Wright, Pincheri and Murray, 1968).

The degenerative diseases are, then, a dominant factor in a consideration of the elderly. Directly related to bone are osteoarthritis and osteoporosis, which will be discussed in detail in a later chapter. Indirectly related to bone, in that the marrow is closely concerned in their production, are the various consequences of thrombus formation. The changes start before this stage of life is reached. During the last few years there has been a very considerable increase in absence from work through causes such as chronic bronchitis, headaches and nervous debility. These are all early symptoms of the type of change which is being considered. In men cardiovascular disease and chronic bronchitis have tended to dominate and are responsible for most deaths in middle age and the following years. But the use of antibiotics during the present century has dramatically increased the average age of death, so that for the men who survive and most women there is a need to consider the more insidious effects of stress-induced thrombi.

Small thrombi, as well as the larger thrombi, contribute to the second type of arterial lesion described by Mitchell *et al.* (1964) and they also block small vessels. In arteriosclerosis there is the possibility of a portion of the plaque in the carotid arteries breaking away to form an embolus which can cause massive damage. There is also the possibility of the lumen of the artery being reduced to such an extent that an oxygen deficiency condition develops. In most parts of the body a colateral circulation is present or can develop, and the result is primarily the formation of a small amount of scar tissue or a benign pathological calcification. But the frontal lobes of the brain lack a colateral circulation, so that some neurones are irreversibly damaged. In elderly people there is often a progressive mental deterioration which histologically has atrophy and loss of neurones as the major feature. One might postulate as a basis for further study that a direct effect of steroids on cell membranes is a contributory cause. Perivascular zones of atrophy, which can vary from barely visible to massive, represent irreversible morphological changes, but there would seem to be at least a possibility that the physiological changes caused by the stimulus which has been termed motivation might retard the consequent mental deterioration. This suggestion is in the realms of speculation, but should form a worthwhile topic for research. The actual mechanisms of thrombus formation will be discussed in a later chapter.

Summary

1. There is a gradual process of ageing, with puberty as the only definite discontinuity. Before this the polypeptide hormones dominate, and afterwards the steroid hormones. There are partial discontinuities, marked by the changes in mode of production of the intercellular matrices, the underlying causes of which are hormonal. As age progresses the degenerative diseases become increasingly important.

2. Foetal bones develop as cartilage models, with the intercellular matrix a swollen gel. As age increases the gel becomes firmer. A vascular supply is required for its nourishment, the typical vascular arrangement during growth having associated artery and veins with a system of ramifying vessels at the end. The main sites of cell division are close to the vessels.

3. The development of foetal bone is by means of enchondral ossification,

starting at the central part of the shaft. Until after the position of the epiphyseal growth cartilage has been reached the bone and maturing cartilage are protected by a bone collar. Later the growth cartilage is held in position by a fibrous ring, the perichondrial ring.

4. Foetal bone is sometimes called woven bone, but it is in fact immature normal bone produced by cells from the vessel walls. Woven bone is produced from the granulation tissue present in bone, and does not develop a secondary calcification.

5. The lesions responsible for Perthes disease are briefly described.

6. During childhood more mature components of the intercellular matrices are found, but they do not approach the chemical stability of adult tissue until adolescence is reached. Before then there is a very active tissue turnover. At adolescence, as soon as steroid hormones are operative the tissues become less malleable.

7. During childhood the matrices in the intervertebral discs increase in firmness. At adolescence a combination of the action of steroid hormones and adequate exercise result in the formation of rubber-like beta-proteins. Intervertebral discs with an inadequate proportion of these are more susceptible to the pathological changes which lead to prolapse.

8. In the adult, intercellular matrices develop towards greater stability. Bones continue to show an increase in the amount of their bone tissue until the age of 35 or so, the quantity then remains stationary for a time and eventually falls off.

9. As age increases the degenerative diseases become increasingly important. Until the stage at which the dense beta-protein appears as a significant component of the nucleus pulposus prolapsed lumbar discs are the main degenerative condition, but only affect a small (but increasing) proportion of the population. After 40 there is a marked decrease in their incidence. Beyond 35 to 40 cardiovascular disease is increasingly common in men, while after the menopause women are susceptible to a pathological osteoporosis. Beyond the age of 70 to 80 an increasingly large proportion of both men and women suffer from a different type of osteoporosis, vascular lesions and senility. In old age those who remain healthy tend to retain the characteristics present at 80 to 85.

10. Exercise counteracts the tendencies which lead to degenerative conditions.

11. The method of research, whatever the problem, is to make as many observations as possible, formulate one or more hypotheses which cover these facts, seek other observational facts which may support or eliminate these hypotheses or cause them to be modified, formulate a modified hypothesis, seek more facts, and so on. Even at quite a late stage the hypothesis must be rejected if established facts oppose it. Vascular disease has been used to illustrate this approach to problems. Laboratory procedures or devised experiments do not come under the heading of research unless they make a positive contribution to the problem under consideration.

12. Stress, whether emotional, traumatic or caused by acute or chronic illness, stimulates the pituitary gland to produce excess ACTH. This in turn stimulates the adrenal gland. On occasion other hormonal pathways may be stimulated. The adrenal cortex releases corticosteroids so that there is a raised plasma cortisol. This assists adrenalin from the adrenal medulla to release cholesterol and other lipids into the blood. The cholesterol forms atheromatous plaques which have been found to be benign. The cortisol also assists in thrombus formation which is responsible for the cardiovascular diseases, some osteoporotic

changes and senile changes. Cholesterol is formed at all ages, but thrombi are usually formed in quantity only after the age of 35 to 40.

13. In the elderly stress diseases dominate, but have less effect on those who retain an interest in their activities and are "motivated".

14. Beyond the age of 70 to 80 there is a gradual decline in the amount of both anabolic and catabolic hormones and a corresponding increased susceptibility to the effects of stress. The effects of thrombi on brain tissue have the most important social consequences.

3. EPIPHYSEAL GROWTH CARTILAGE

A great deal may be discovered about the growth and behaviour of bone by a study of the growing epiphysis. In an experimental animal the system is a reproducible one, cells proliferate quickly, and there are present in a confined area cartilage cells, vessels, bone marrow, and also fibrous tissue and muscle, so that the effects of, say, vitamins and hormones on several cell types may be readily observed. There are quite considerable species differences, and the choice of experimental animals must be made with care. In general the smaller animals, once the secondary bone nucleus is developed, have a very narrow germinal zone, while in larger animals and in the human a half to two-thirds of the total width of the growth cartilage may be occupied by the germinal zone. Where this difference is not important the rabbit is one of the most satisfactory animals to use in a study involving the growth cartilage. When it is of importance the dog may be used. Figure 3.1 shows the growth cartilage in the tibia of a rabbit, and Fig. 3.2 the growth cartilage at the lower end of a rabbit's femur, while Fig. 3.3 is the growth cartilage from a puppy's femur. In the study of vitamins it is desirable to choose a species which does not produce its own supply of the vitamin in question. Consequently the guinea-pig is commonly used in the investigation of vitamin C deficiency and the rat for vitamin D deficiency. In all other respects the rat is the most unsuitable of the possible experimental animals for studies involving bone, cartilage or connective tissues. The cells behave differently to a great many stimuli, the matrix they form frequently has different properties, and perhaps most important of all there are hormones acting which are chemically different from those in man and most other species and have unusual properties. One consequence of this is that the growth cartilage does not mature towards plate closure but remains open indefinitely.

The Germinal Zone

The blood supply to the two sides of the growth cartilage is very different. Figure 3.4 is a section through a perfused rabbit tibia showing the distribution of vessels. At the epiphyseal side there are vessels penetrating through the bone plate at intervals to provide shallow loops at the top of

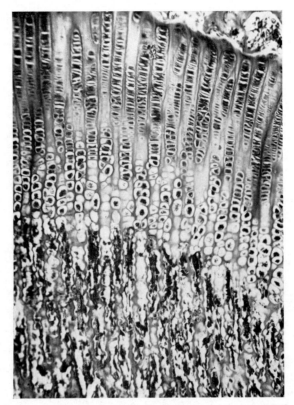

FIG. 3.1. The growth cartilage and upper end of metaphysis in tibia of rabbit at rapidly growing stage. There are: very narrow germinal zone, parallel columns of flat cells in the proliferative zone, rounded cells in the enlarging zone, and large cells with low density cytoplasm in the hypertrophic zone. A vessel (filled with perfusion medium) approaches each column, and between the vessels are bars of calcified cartilage. Rather lower in the metaphysis osteogenic activity may be seen. × 100.

the germinal zone, while at the metaphyseal side there are vessels approaching each column. Trueta and Amato (1960) have studied the function of these two sets of vessels by the simple expedient of implanting a polyethylene sheet either above or below the growth cartilage, so as to cut off the vessels, and then waiting for a week or two to see what happened. When the blood supply to the germinal zone was cut off the cells died after a time, both in the germinal zone and in the underlying proliferative zone. The tissues become necrotic, then calcified. This was followed by an invasion by other neighbouring vessels with the formation of a bone bridge across the growth cartilage. The effect of cutting off the blood supply to the metaphyseal side of the cartilage was quite different, and resulted in a build-up of hypertrophic cells.

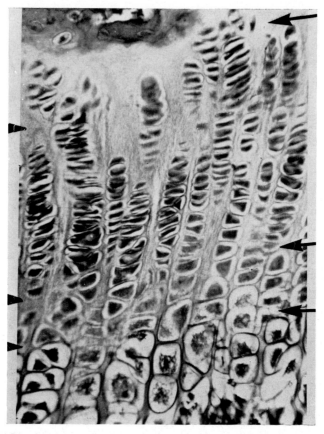

Fig. 3.2. The growth cartilage at the lower end of femur in a rabbit at the rapidly growing stage. The columnar arrangement is not quite so regular as in the tibia. In this photograph the enlarging and hypertrophic zones are clearly distinguished. Arrows indicate the boundaries of the various zones. ×200.

Where the defect on the epiphyseal side is smaller, an indentation in the growth cartilage, rather than a complete bone bridge is observed. This is very common in the growth cartilage of older children, particularly in the weight-bearing bones (Fig. 3.5).

The germinal zone is sometimes known as the resting zone. Cells have the characteristics of anlage cartilage cells. At infrequent intervals they divide to become the precursors of new columns of cells in the proliferative zone. Rigal (1962) has demonstrated the distribution of cells in their predivision stage by taking slices through the epiphyses of growing rabbits and placing them in a tissue culture medium, containing tritiated thymidine, for periods of up to 48 h. Cells which came into the predivision stage during the time in the tissue culture medium took up

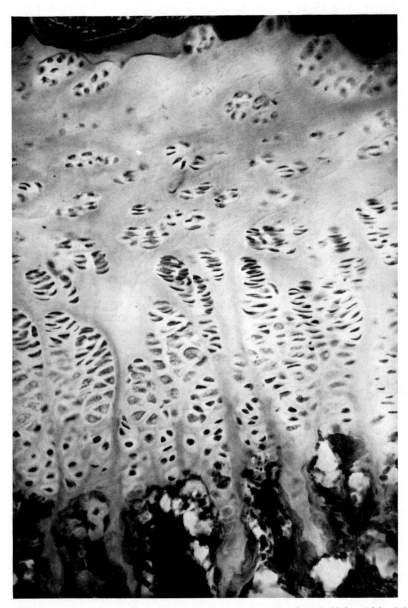

Fɪɢ. 3.3. Growth cartilage in puppy. The germinal zone occupies about half the width of the cartilage. Clusters of columns tend to be separated by bars of collagenous matrix, and in this slightly oblique section are seen to be arranged in cell nests. At the top of the metaphysis a vessel approaches each group of columns, and branches from this approach individual columns. Few cells have enlarged to the hypertrophic state. × 100.

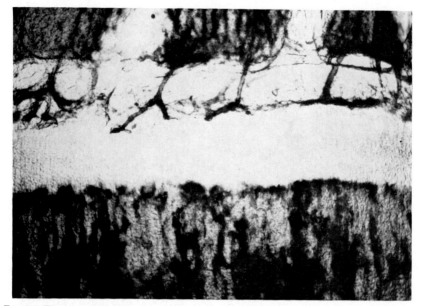

Fig. 3.4. Three hundred micron section through perfused rabbit tibia. Spatleholz preparation. At the epiphyseal side vessels penetrate the bone plate at intervals and spread in shallow loops at the top of the germinal zone. At the metaphyseal side vessels approach each column. In the tibia there is a region, about half the width of the growth cartilage above, where only calcified cartilage, vessels and newly formed bone are present. ×35.

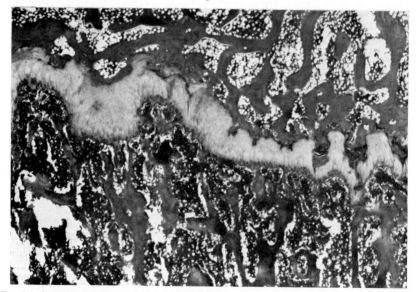

Fig. 3.5. Growth cartilage in boy's femoral epiphysis. There are indentations on the epiphyseal side of the cartilage, but no complete bone bridges. Such irregularities are common in the growth cartilage of older children, and particularly in weightbearing situations. ×35.

the thymidine, and were thus labelled with the radioactive isotope H³. Usually only one or two cells in the germinal zone in each histological section showed evidence of isotope uptake.

When growth hormone was administered to rabbits for a week or two before the slices of epiphysis were taken for labelling in the culture medium it was found that over 50% of the cells of the germinal zone became labelled (Rigal, 1964). It is thus apparent that an important action of growth hormone is the activation of such stem cells. Normally

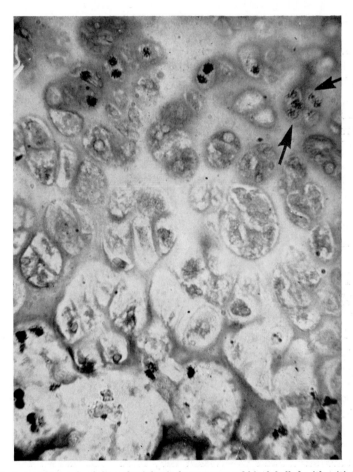

FIG. 3.6. Autoradiograph of slice of epiphysis from young rabbit, labelled with tritiated thymidine. The epiphyseal bone nucleus at this stage of growth is surrounded by a row of actively proliferating cells which act as a growth cartilage, so that the bone nucleus expands by a process of enchondral ossification. Proliferating cartilage cells and active cells in the bone are labelled. The group of cells (arrowed) at the top right of the photograph divided after the parent cells took up the labelled tritiated thymidine. ×100. The author thanks Dr. W. M. Rigal for this photograph.

K

growth hormone is only liberated into the blood stream at irregular intervals. It has a half-life in plasma of 20–30 min. There is an interaction between blood sugar, growth hormone and insulin, so that hormone secretion is related to meals, and the frequency of secretory episodes is increased during sleep (Rigal and Hunter, 1966).

The method which was used in the culture experiments, of labelling cells after removal from the body, rather than injecting the isotope labelled compound into the living animal has many advantages. In the case of the administration of tritiated thymidine to indicate the predivision stage in cartilage the information has been shown to be the same as that obtained by giving the labelled compounds to the whole animal. But when only small pieces of tissue are taken, a much higher level of labelling is possible, without the risk of radiation from the isotope altering the function of the adrenals or other organs in the body. Figure 3.6, of a row of dividing cells surrounding the secondary bone nucleus, shows the heavy positive labelling, which can be recognized at a low magnification. When a lower dose of isotope is spread throughout the body, it is necessary to count grains carefully to distinguish some of the labelled cells from the background. The labelling of tissue slices rather than the whole body means also that information can be obtained from human operation material which could not be sought by administration of the isotope to the patient—these have undesirable properties, including a carcinogenic action for which tolerance levels have not yet been determined.

The Proliferative Zone

Once cells from the germinal zone have entered into the state of active proliferation this proliferation continues for some time. As a result of the constricting band, of bone in the very young, and later of fibrous tissue in the perichondrial ring, the products of cell division are arranged in vertical columns, while the surrounding forces cause the cells in the columns to become flattened (Figs 3.1, 3.2, 3.3). Cell division within each column is usually synchronous (Rigal, 1962). When cartilage slices are placed in labelled culture media for short periods either all or none of the cells in a column take up the tritiated thymidine.

When cartilage cells which are not restrained by surrounding physical forces are stimulated to division they form "cell nests". Figure 2.16 showed what happened when the restraint was removed from growth cartilage, while cell nests are also found in regenerating articular and disc cartilage. When restrained and in their columnar arrangement growth cartilage cells are in elongated cell nests. This is more obvious in the cartilage of Fig. 3.3 than in the two preceding illustrations. Within these cell nests they are surrounded by the immature beta-protein. The texture of the immature beta-protein becomes firmer with age. Orientated collagen, also of the immature type, is found between the columns. The oblique section in Fig. 3.7 shows the border region between the intercellular matrix and the intercolumnar region.

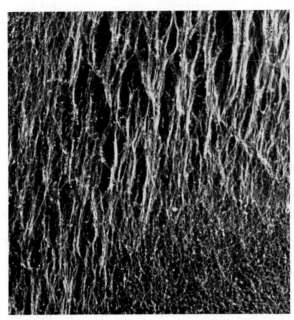

FIG. 3.7. Oblique section of the proliferative zone of the epiphyseal growth cartilage: to show the junction of the matrix between columns of cells which contains collagen fibrils, and the matrix containing immature beta-protein which surrounds cells in the columns. E.M. 100kV. ×5000.

Each column has only a limited life. After a time the repeated cell division stops, and the column grows out. When this happens cells at the level of the main proliferating zone begin to enlarge. Next the column is temporarily replaced by the intercellular matrix until a new column is formed by division of a cell in the germinal zone. While it lasts the stimulus to divide is a powerful one, and cell division will continue even in the absence of an adequate supporting matrix, as has been observed in scorbutic guinea-pigs.

Cell division is inhibited by an adequate dose of colchicine. The action of this drug is commonly said to be to arrest cell division at metaphase, but in cartilage cells of all types the effect is to isolate the cell nucleus from its surroundings, whether that cell nucleus be in the resting state, the predivision state or in the process of division. The cells in Fig. 3.8

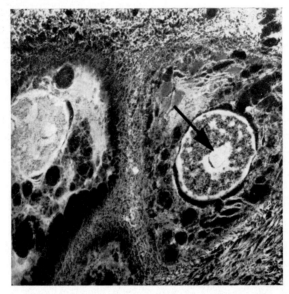

Fig. 3.8. Section from perichondrium of growing rabbit which had been given colchicine. The cell on the left, with denser nucleus, is in the early predivision stage, and the cell on the right in the resting phase. In both cells connections between the nucleus and its surroundings have been broken. There is also no connection between nucleus and nucleolus, and the latter (arrowed) is enlarged. E.M. 100 kV. ×3500.

have nuclei in the resting state and the early predivision state. The cell with the inactive nucleus should be producing matrix, but since the ribosomes have been hindered from leaving the nucleolus this has become considerably enlarged.

The Enlarging Zone

The next well-defined zone in the growth cartilage is the zone where the cells cease to proliferate and then expand. At the same time their production of the intercellular matrices based on the immature beta-protein and collagen ceases. Instead calcifiable matrix is produced, and is usually laid down on top of the collagenous matrix. The quality of this calcifiable matrix is readily modified by some of the chemicals which may be present in the surrounding tissue fluids.

Vitamin C has already been mentioned. An excess does not produce an effect beyond the normal, but when it is absent intercellular matrices are not synthesized properly. Although some of the calcifiable matrix is formed by the enlarged cells even in grossly scorbutic animals, the mode of calcification in scurvy is rather different from the normal. In the normal the sequence is for the calcifiable matrix to be first produced, and then to undergo modification to unmask nucleation centres for mineralization. There are usually a number of cells, producing the calcifiable matrix, present between the bottom of the proliferative zone and the level at which calcification is seen (Fig. 3.2). In the scorbutic animals an incomplete calcification is observed even at the bottom of the proliferative zone which partially hinders the process of cell enlargement (Poal-Manresa, Little and Trueta, 1970). This calcification tends to be uniform (Fig. 3.9) and without the discrete nucleation centres seen in the early stages of calcification in the normal growth cartilage (Fig. 3.10).

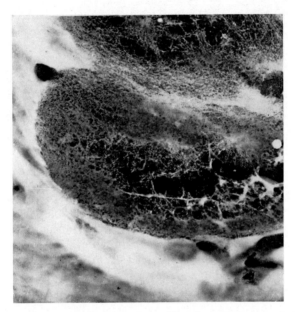

Fig. 3.9. Cell capsule immediately below the proliferative zone in a scorbutic guinea-pig. The calcification is of a uniform texture, with no visible indications of nucleation centres. This calcification of the surrounding matrix, although incomplete, prevents further enlargement of the cells. (The mineralized areas are the white or grey patches where there is an apparent loss of resolution.) E.M. 100kV. ×5000.

Vitamin D behaves quite differently. Both too little and too much cause abnormal matrix to be formed. With too little vitamin D (Rickets) the "calcifiable" matrix is produced in too large quantities and is too stable, and nucleation centres are not unmasked. This matrix is not only uncalcifiable, it is difficult to resorb. Consequently at the metaphyseal side of the growth cartilage vessels are unable to penetrate and there is a build-up of the enlarged cells, which accumulate more of the un-resorbable matrix. The experiment by Trueta and Amato (1960)

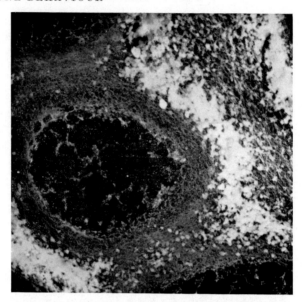

Fig. 3.10. Oblique section near the bottom of a normal rabbit growth cartilage. Calcification commences on discrete nucleation centres, and the calcified areas then expand and merge. Mineralized patches are white in this photograph. E.M. 100kV. ×3500.

already referred to, in which the blood supply to a portion of the metaphysis was cut off, also led to a build-up of enlarged hypertrophic cells. Mechanically preventing vessels reaching to the metaphyseal side of the cartilage prevents enchondral ossification, but does not affect the viability or activity of the cartilage cells. When the blood supply is restored, by the removal of the polyethylene sheet, vessels advance, one to each column (Fig. 3.11), and the process of enchondral ossification is resumed, at an accelerated rate, until the normal level of ossification is reached. But when the diet of a rachitic rat is restored to normal the blood vessels are unable to penetrate in the usual manner. They find weak points, penetrate through these to the base of the proliferative zone and only from there is more normal enchondral ossification resumed. Frequently a calcified zone, distinguishable on radiographs, is formed in the middle of the growth cartilage during the healing process, with the abnormal matrix remaining uncalcified.

In bone a deficiency of vitamin D leads to the deposition of the same abnormal matrix which is unable to calcify properly. In adult the condition is known as osteomalacia. When this condition is treated with an adequate quantity of vitamin D bone of normal quality and with normal calcification is laid down over the abnormal bone.

An excess of vitamin D leads to the production of a scanty and defec-

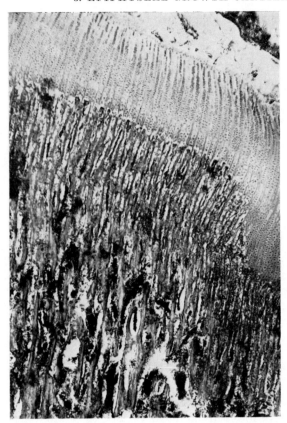

Fig. 3.11. Section through the metaphyseal region of a rabbit tibia which had had the meta-physeal vessels blocked by a polyethylene sheet which was subsequently removed. Newly proliferating vessels are advancing, one to each column, and enchondral ossification took about 4 days to complete. × 35.

tive matrix. The component most affected seems to be the polysacchar-ide. The gel structure is readily destroyed by minor trauma, and the vulnerable cells may then be killed. This is often followed by calcification of the necrotic tissue.

Fluoride affects the quality of the matrix, but with this compound it is seemingly the beta-protein which is most affected. As with vitamin D there is an optimum concentration for the formation of good quality intercellular matrix. With too little fluoride in the diet there is a lack of stability, and with too much a stable matrix is formed which does not easily calcify or remodel. This hindrance to bone remodelling shows radiologically when the fluoride content of the drinking water is greater than 25 parts per million (Johnson *et al.*, 1964). The tissue most sensitive to the effects of fluoride is dental enamel. When there is a fluoride deficiency the matrix within the enamel prisms is readily degraded by acid so allowing the crystallites to be lost. With a correct level of fluoride the matrix is stable, and is not lost from similarly treated enamel even after the lapse of over 1000 years. With rather too much fluoride the matrix is more irregularly formed. In one district in the Middle East there is 15 ppm in the drinking water. This level of fluoride causes irregularities in the tooth structure but has not harmed the local inhabitants. It is 10 ppm lower than the level at which the remodelling of the bones of sheep, cattle and other animals begins to be seriously affected. Fluoride metabolism in the rat is quite different, with a retention of the fluoride, so that results of rat experiments are irrelevant so far as humans are concerned.

The Hypertrophic Zone and Metaphyseal Bone

Some of the statements in the literature concerning the hypertrophic zone of the growth cartilage are confusing, because it is a region of the cartilage sensitive to both species differences and also age differences. In the study of this zone of the cartilage it is particularly important that those primarily interested in the human should not use a rat or a chicken as the experimental animal, since both have different hormones (also different from each other).

The true hypertrophic cells are those enlarged cells which have ceased all matrix production and whose cytoplasm contains a high proportion of fluid to solid. Their appearance is as shown in Figs 3.12, 3.13. Figure 3.12, with perfusion medium in the vessels which approach each column of cells in the rapidly growing stage in a rabbit, is from a paper by Morgan (1959). Figure 3.13 shows erythrocytes present in the last hypertrophic space under each column in a section of human bone. In the rabbit these conditions usually last until the stage of plate closure commences, but they are seen only until the age of about 2 to 4 years in the human. Figure 3.14 shows the manner in which the vessels approach the growth cartilage at this stage of growth. It is from a 300 micron section of a perfused rabbit bone. Figure 3.15 is a similar perfused section from a rabbit at a stage when the hormonal changes that cause the first stage of plate closure are in operation. During the stage of growth depicted in Figs 3.12, 3.13, 3.14 the vessel approaches the last hypertrophic cell in the column, and cell death takes place as a result of blood bursting into and filling the cell space. In each hypertrophic space there is a stage of the process when the blood is in direct contact with the intercellular matrix (Fig. 3.16). The resorption of the cartilage, other than the calcified portions, seems to be a direct chemical breakdown without the intervention of multinucleated cells. This direct resorption

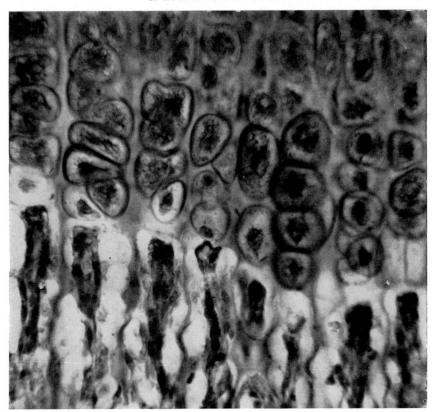

FIG. 3.12. Bottom of rabbit growth cartilage at the stage of rapid growth. A separate vessel approaches each column of cells. They are filled with perfusion medium, and it can be seen that they are present as vascular loops. ×600. The author thanks Mr. J. D. Morgan for this photograph.

is possible when the matrix components are not too stable. Later the influence of steroids confers a greater stability and the action of chondroclasts is then needed.

In the human, beyond the age of 2 to 4, and in the puppy at a somewhat later stage of development the cartilage columns are present in clusters. Vessels approach a cluster and divide towards their end, with a branch approaching each column. At this stage of development some cells at the bottom of the growth cartilage have proceeded to the full hypertrophic state while others are still in the enlarged state. Usually the former are seen to be removed by blood invading the cell space, while chondroclasts remove the latter. Particularly in the human, there is another factor to be taken into account at this stage of development, the result of stress. As has been indicated in the last chapter this

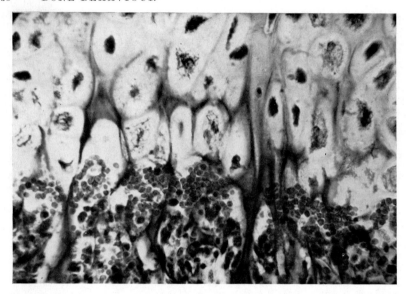

FIG. 3.13. Bottom of growth cartilage at the stage of rapid growth. Erythrocytes are present in the last hypertrophic space of each column of cells. ×400.

produces effects which are the same as the effects produced by the administration of cortisone or cortisol. Later at the time of puberty the combination and alternation of the anabolic steroid hormones and catabolic steroids lead to the sequence of events resulting in plate closure.

The mechanisms involved may be elucidated by observing the effects of catabolic and anabolic steroids on the rabbit, at the stage of rapid growth when there are no other complicating factors. When an anabolic compound is administered at this rapid stage of growth the production of matrix is enhanced, at the expense of cell division. Figure 3.17 shows the effect of 3 weeks administration of Stromba (androstano-pyrazole or stanozolol) at a dose level of 5 mg/kg. The production of excess matrix has caused the cells to elongate in the direction of the columns, while the extra stability of the matrix has hindered enlargement of cells to the hypertrophic state. Erythrocytes may be seen in one vascular space, but matrix removal is primarily by means of chondroclastic activity.

When corticosteroids are administered cell walls in the enlarging zone become more prominent. Matrix which is more stable than usual is produced, so hindering remodelling, and cells are prevented from proceeding to the hypertrophic state (Fig. 3.18). Corticosteroids also inhibit proliferation of the vessels that normally approach the hypertrophic zone from the metaphysis. When an anabolic compound is administered, or the animals's natural anabolic hormones take over

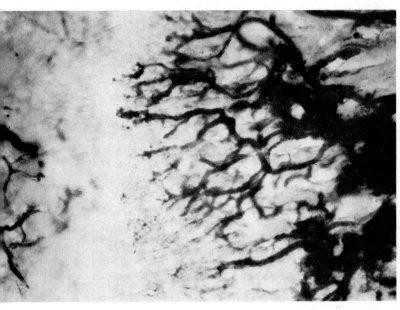

FIG. 3.15. Three hundred micron section of perfused bone in Spalteholz preparation. Rabbit metaphysis at the stage when the hormonal changes that initiate plate closure are in operation. The vascular arrangement is irregular, and branches from each vessel approach several columns. ×35.

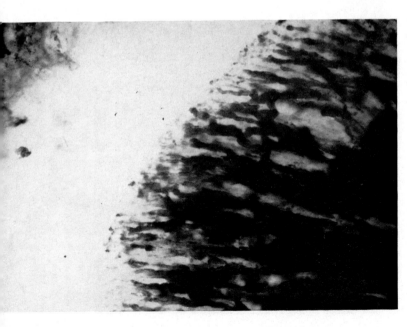

FIG. 3.14. Three hundred micron section of perfused bone in Spalteholz preparation. Rabbit metaphysis at the stage of rapid growth, with a vessel advancing to each column of cells. ×35.

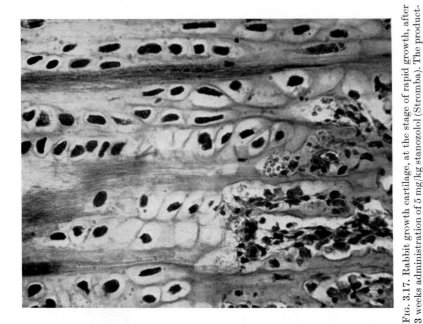

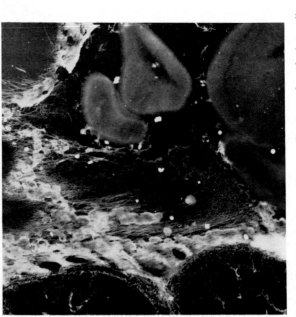

Fig. 3.17. Rabbit growth cartilage, at the stage of rapid growth, after 3 weeks administration of 5 mg/kg stanozolol (Stromba). The production of excess matrix has caused the cells to elongate in the direction of the columns, while the extra stability of the matrix has hindered enlargement of cells to the hypertrophic state. Erythrocytes may be seen in one vascular space, but matrix removal is primarily by means of chondroclastic activity. ×200.

Fig. 3.16. Rabbit growth cartilage at the stage when the intercellular matrix is removed directly by the blood, without the intervention of chondroclasts. Erythrocytes are seen in direct contact with the matrix. Patches of calcification around nucleation centres may also be seen. E.M. 100kV. ×4500.

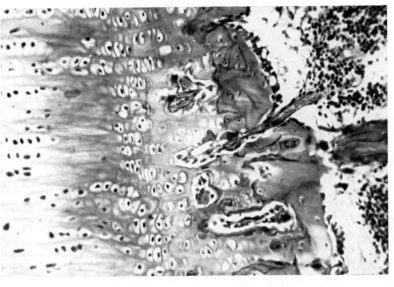

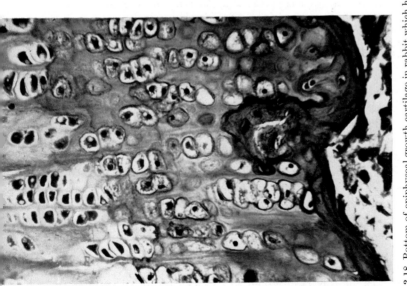

FIG. 3.19. Bottom of growth cartilage from a rabbit which had been maintained on cortisone for 2 weeks and then given stanozolol for 3 days. Blood vessels (filled with perfusion medium) penetrate through weak spots at the base. Matrix removal is by chondroclastic action. ×100.

FIG. 3.18. Bottom of epiphyseal growth cartilage in rabbit which had been given 10 mg/kg cortisone for 8 weeks. Cells in the enlarging zone have not proceeded to the hypertrophic state, their cell walls are very prominent, and the unusually stable matrix produced in this zone stains more heavily with haematoxylin than normal. The bottom of the growth cartilage is covered by a thin layer of bone. ×200.

then there is vascular proliferation. However, the stable matrix prevents normal resorption so that in a similar manner to the recovery from vitamin D deficiency, vessels penetrate weak spots and normal enchondral ossification resumes from the bottom of what had been the proliferative zone. Figures 3.19, 3.20, 3.21 show the effect of administration of stano-

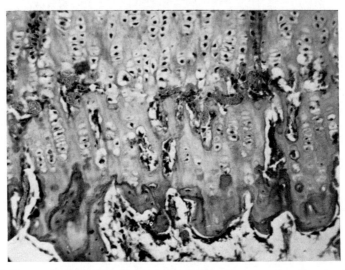

FIG. 3.20. The vessels penetrate to the base of the proliferative zone, where there is a tendency for them to spread horizontally. Normal enchondral ossification is resumed from this level. The altered growth cartilage remains behind in the metaphysis to be covered by bone or gradually resorbed. × 100.

zolol to an animal which had previously been given cortisone (Little and Munuera, 1970). The islands of altered cartilage left behind are gradually resorbed by chondroclasts (these are identical with osteoclasts, and the different name merely denotes a different tissue being removed), or they may become covered with a layer of bone. This bone is produced by the vessels which at the time of renewed proliferation form in a horizontal direction. The vascular distribution is as shown in Fig. 3.22. This was from a rabbit subjected to stress accidentally, as a result of a fractured leg. The leg was immobilized in plaster, then a week later the rabbit was killed and its vessels perfused with the Micropaque/Berlin blue mixture. In an intact epiphysis the line of horizontal vessels, with the subsequent more normal vascular proliferation, is clearly demonstrated, and shows a close resemblance to the effects produced experimentally by the administration of first cortisone and then stanozolol.

This appears to be the mechanism by which Harris lines are produced. "Harris lines" is the name given to the horizontal bars which are seen in the metaphysis on clinical X-rays of children who have recently

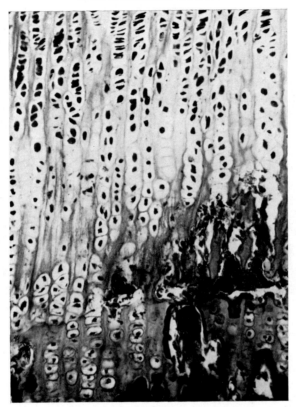

Fig. 3.21. In the initial stages the vascular penetration is uneven. In this area enchondral ossification has commenced in the region at the right of the photograph, but to the left vessels have not yet reached the base of the proliferative zone. × 100.

suffered an episode of acute illness or other form of stress. Usually cartilage in the horizontal bars is resorbed and replaced by bone, which is more gradually remodelled to form normal trabeculae. Such horizontal bars have been found in rabbits which were given alternating cortisone (C) and testosterone (T). When the timing was: 3 days C; 2 days T; 2 days rest (the animal's natural hormones, also anabolic); 2 days C; 3 days T; 2 days rest; and so on (Little, 1970a). The bars resulting from the 3 days cortisone administration remained, while those resulting from the 2 days cortisone administration were resorbed almost entirely, except for the very recent ones. Figures 3.23, 3.24 show the appearance of this zone in young boys; the cause of the stress in these two cases being acute illness. In Fig. 3.23 the appearance produced resembles that of the cortisone administration shown in Figure 3.17. Fig 3.24 is from a case where there had been a temporary remission. In a corresponding

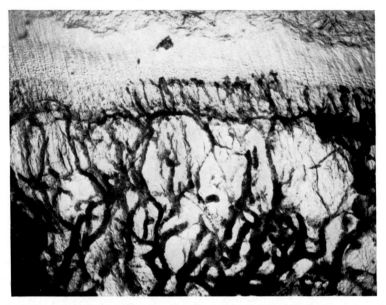

Fig. 3.22. Three hundred micron section through metaphysis and epiphyseal growth cartilage of a rabbit which had been subjected to traumatic stress. The limb was immobilized in plaster for a week. Spalteholz preparation of an unaffected perfused epiphysis. The vessels had spread horizontally along the base of the growth cartilage, then penetrated weak points, and enchondral ossification from the bottom of the proliferative zone is commencing. In one area the vessels have not yet reached the proliferative zone. × 35.

experimental situation where cortisone administration had been followed by the administration of testosterone there is also a gap between the altered cartilage and the bottom of the proliferative zone filled with haemopoietic tissue (Fig. 3.25). This reaction is rather different from that produced by stanozolol, when the gap is filled by new bone. Figure 3.26 shows the normal appearance in a boy at this stage of development. When the stress is very severe the cartilage may survive almost indefinitely. Figure 3.27 is from a puppy with the affected cartilage still remaining in mid-shaft after a year. Here the "stress" was caused by the action of plutonium on the adrenal glands. The isotope did not penetrate the cartilage.

At the time of plate closure both the anabolic steroids produced by developing sex organs and catabolic steroids are active, so that cell proliferation is hindered and more stable matrix formed, while in the anabolic phases vessels are enabled to penetrate more deeply into the cartilage. The levels of the catabolic and anabolic steroids tend to alternate, as shown by arrest lines in surrounding bone. When vessels, followed by bone bridges, have crossed the cartilage in a number of places growth is virtually at an end.

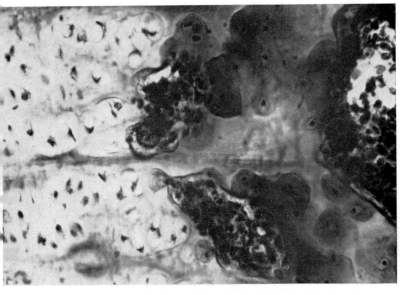

FIG. 3.24. Bottom of growth cartilage in boy. There had been a temporary remission of stress between injury and death, so that some vascular penetration has taken place through the altered zone at the base of the cartilage. Haemopoietic tissue has formed around the penetrating vessels. ×200.

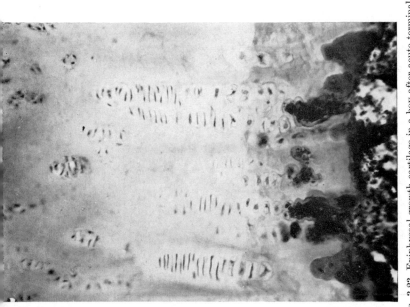

FIG. 3.23. Epiphyseal growth cartilage in a boy after acute terminal illness (tetanus). In the enlarging zone abnormal matrix, more heavily stained by haematoxylin than usual, has been formed, enlargement of cells has ceased, and there is a thin layer of bone along the bottom of the cartilage. This appearance may be compared with that shown in Fig. 18. ×100.

L

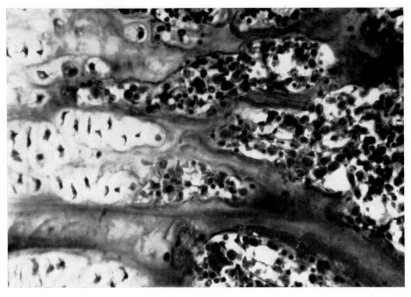

FIG. 3.26. The normal appearance of the junction of the epiphyseal growth cartilage and metaphyseal bone in a boy at the same stage of development as the one shown in Fig. 24. ×200.

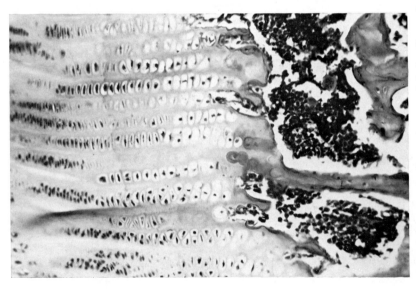

FIG. 3.25. Rabbit growth cartilage, where a period of cortisone administration has been followed by testosterone administration. Here also the gap between the altered cartilage and the bottom of the proliferative zone has filled with haemopoietic tissue. ×100.

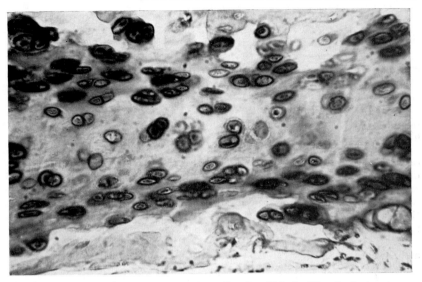

Fig. 3.27. Bone of unresorbed altered growth cartilage in midshaft of the rib of a beagle, seen a year after the severe stress caused by administration of plutonium. ×200.

Summary

1. There are considerable species differences. The germinal zone is narrow in small animals but occupies a half to two-thirds of the growth cartilage in larger animals and man. Where this fact is not of importance the rabbit is a suitable experimental animal to compare with the human. The rat is the most unsuitable animal to choose because cells and matrix differ and the hormones acting on the cartilage have unusual properties.

2. The germinal zone depends on a blood supply from the epiphysis for its nutrition. When this is blocked cells in the germinal and proliferative zones die.

3. At intervals cells in the germinal zone divide to become the precursors of new columns of cells in the proliferative zone. Their activity is controlled in part by growth hormone.

4. The secondary bone nucleus in the epiphysis expands by means of a less active "growth cartilage" which surrounds it.

5. Cells in columns are in elongated "cell nests". In the proliferative zone the cells are flattened. The columnar arrangement is maintained by the restraint provided by the perichondrial ring. Cell division is synchronous. While the stimulus lasts it is a powerful one, then repeated cell division stops and the column grows out.

6. In the enlarging zone calcifiable matrix is produced and laid down on top of the structural matrix. The production of this and the normal intercellular matrix is hindered by lack of vitamin C. Calcification in scorbutic conditions does not show the usual dependence on the unmasking of nucleation centres.

7. Both vitamin D and fluoride have an optiumum concentration. Vitamin D particularly affects the stability of the calcifiable matrix, and with a deficiency too much is produced in too stable a form, causing rickets or osteomalacia. With

an excess of vitamin D the gel structure of the matrix is readily destroyed and necrotic changes often result. Conversely, too little fluoride produces a lack of stability of the matrix and too much an unduly stable matrix.

8. A true hypertrophic zone is formed at the stage of rapid growth. Cells expand from the enlarged to the hypertrophic state and during enchondral ossification matrix is removed by blood. The period of growth occupied by this stage varies from one species to another.

9. In the presence of steroids expansion of cells to the hypertrophic state is hindered, and during enchondral ossification resorption of the matrix is by means of chondroclastic activity.

10. Stress, resulting in a raised cortisol level, affects the bottom of the growth cartilage. Cells in the enlarging zone form very stable matrix and the inhibition of resorption and vascular proliferation hinders enchondral ossification. When anabolic conditions are restored vessels penetrate through weak points to the base of the proliferative zone and normal enchondral ossification is resumed from that level. The altered cartilage is only gradually resorbed. Bone often forms on the surfaces. These horizontal bars in the metaphysis are the Harris lines.

11. Plate closure takes place as a result of the alternating action of catabolic and anabolic steroids.

4. BONE FORMATION AND REMOVAL

For many years certain phenomena, such as osteogenesis imperfecta, Paget's disease, osteosarcoma, and even the processes involved in more straightforward conditions such as osteoporosis and osteoarthritis have been regarded as mysteries. This has been because the mechanisms of bone formation and removal were not adequately described and understood. The literature on the subject of osteogenesis is by no means as clear as it might be. Most of the required information may be found, but in many papers there seems to have been little attempt to distinguish fact from vague hypotheses, and too often statements which were factually incorrect have been accepted without question. In this present chapter observations on the mechanisms of bone formation and removal will be described, together with an account of the circumstances under which each of the possible mechanisms operates.

Origin of Cells

Osteoblasts

Early work on the origin of osteoblasts was mostly concerned, not with normal bone, but with observations on pathological calcifications. In some sites, such as the lung, the vast majority were observed to be bone (Hasse, 1841). In other sites, such as the aorta, only a few of the calcified areas were bone. The first careful description of calcification in the aorta was by Andral in 1827. Other descriptions of the process followed, and it was realized that in the aorta calcification was predominantly on necrotic tissue (Thoma, 1894). It also became apparent that calcification was the usual prerequisite for subsequent ossification (Wells, 1910).

It is now known that the mineral is not the deciding factor, and also that there are situations in which osteoid is found but does not calcify. The significance of these facts will be considered further in the section on the stimulation of osteogenic activity.

Careful histological observations at the turn of the century (e.g. Thoma, 1894; Bunting, 1906) had indicated that there was a high probability that the bone cells were derived from the walls of vessels invading a calcified tissue. But in the early part of the twentieth century the technique of tissue culture was developed, and cells which could form bone were found free in culture media. It was not fully realized that the nature of surrounding proteins can modify the behaviour of cells (Berliner, 1965), and these cells observed in tissue culture media have sometimes been regarded as typical bone cells. More mechanical ideas of bone as an almost inert structural material also came to the fore, and for almost 50 years the vascular contribution to osteogenesis was ignored.

Trueta again drew attention to its importance in the 1950s, in a series of papers (1958, 1961, 1962 a, b, 1963) in which he considered various lines of evidence all of which pointed to the importance of the cells of the sinusoid vessel walls. By that time it was reasonably well agreed that there were often interconnected cells, the osteogenic precursor cells, which could differentiate to form osteoblasts. It was also established that the name given to a cell, i.e. osteoblast, osteoclast or osteocyte did not represent the name of the cell type, but rather the activity of the cell at the time when it was being observed. To avoid confusion, Pritchard (1956) has recommended that all cells actually on the bone surfaces should be called osteoblasts, whether in an active or resting phase. There was no knowledge, other than the earlier work that had been forgotten, of the origin of the precursor cells, although it was established that they could function as the precursors of either osteoblasts or osteoclasts, according to the local conditions (Ham, 1932).

The evidence produced by Trueta and his colleagues was of two main types, circumstantial and direct. The circumstantial evidence is that bone formation takes place in the vicinity of vessels. Observation of normal histological sections, or the tetracycline labelling of newly formed bone, or the location of new bone when ascorbic acid is given to scorbutic animals, shows that bone is laid down around sinusoid vessels. Similarly, when such vessels invade cartilage, as in fracture callus (Fig. 4.1) or in osteoarthritis (Fig. 4.2) the new bone is produced around the vessels. Experiments on growth cartilage reinforced the evidence. Trueta and Amato (1960) showed that when the vessels supplying the metaphysis are cut off enchondral ossification no longer occurs. Instead there is a build-up of the hypertrophic cells of the growth cartilage. When the vascular supply is re-established enchondral ossification is resumed, and the extra hypertrophic cartilage cells are replaced by metaphyseal bone up to the normal level (Fig. 3.11).

Direct evidence has depended on the fact that in certain sites bone formation takes place where there are no cells that could have acted as osteoblast precursors other than those of proliferating cells in the walls of the sinusoid vessels. One such site is the metaphyseal bone at the upper end of the rabbit's tibia, at the stage of most vigorous growth.

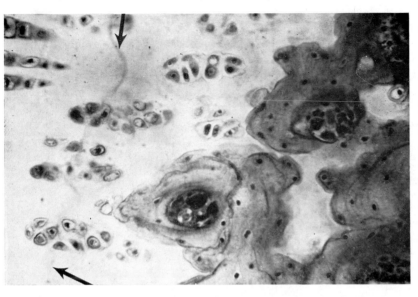

FIG. 4.2. Early osteoarthritic changes in adult articular cartilage. The texture of the cartilage matrix below the slightly more heavily stained line (arrowed) is altered. The change enables proliferating vessels to penetrate, and bone is formed around each. ×200.

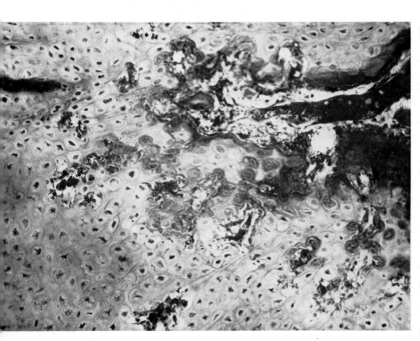

FIG. 4.1. Cartilage in experimental fracture in a rabbit. A proliferating vessel invades the fracture cartilage, and new bone is formed around the vessel and its branches. ×100.

Here Rigal (1961*b*) has demonstrated, both *in vivo* and *in vitro*, that the cells of the vessel walls, which are the only cells present between cartilage spicules at the upper end of the metaphysis, all divide during normal growth. This observation included not only the cells at the ends of the growing vessels, but cells along the walls, at a level where the calcified cartilage was not yet covered by bone, and along their length in the region of metaphyseal bone formation (Fig. 4.3). In this photograph

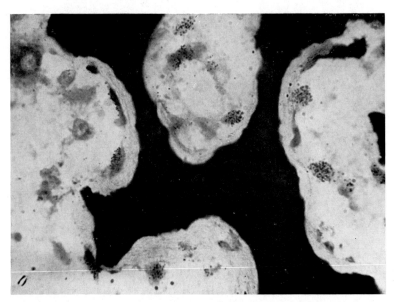

FIG. 4.3. Transverse section through upper metaphyseal region of rabbit tibia, at the stage of rapid growth. Mineralized areas are heavily stained, while the outer uncalcified matrix is only very lightly stained. The bone was placed in a tissue culture medium containing tritiated thymidine for 24 h, under conditions where the cells could enter the predivision stage, but not proliferate. Nearly all the cells in the vessel walls are labelled by the isotope, indicating that they had entered the predivision phase. ×400. The author thanks Dr. W. M. Rigal for this figure.

the mineralized part is heavily stained, while the uncalcified matrix covering it is only very lightly stained. Nearly all the cells in the vessel walls are labelled by tritiated thymidine, indicating that they are in the predivision phase. Figure 4.4 shows one of these cells in the process of division. Most convincing, perhaps, is the occasional appearance of a cell such as that shown in Fig. 4.5. This was from a perfused specimen, and a few patches of the perfusion medium can be seen in the lumen of the vessel. A part of the cell is acting as an endothelial cell attached to the basement membrane of the vessel wall (and a small portion of the membrane which has been torn away during sectioning shows a net-work

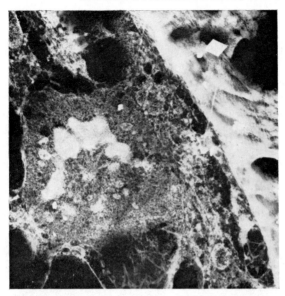

FIG. 4.4. Section through upper metaphyseal region of rabbit tibia, at a level where there was one layer of cells between the lumen of the vessel and the calcified cartilage. One of these cells is in the process of division, and the chromosome arrangement around a centriole can be seen. E.M. 100kV. ×3500.

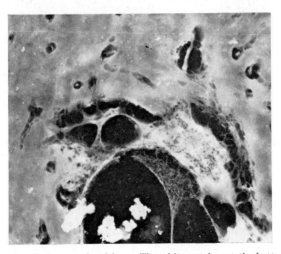

FIG. 4.5. Osteogenic cell, from perfused bone. The white patches at the bottom of the photograph are barium sulphate particles of the perfusion medium in the lumen of a small vessel. A part of the cell is acting as an endothelial cell attached to the basement membrane of the vessel wall; and a small portion of this membrane which was torn away during sectioning shows a network typical of reticulin. Another portion of the cell, towards the right of the photograph, is producing osteoid matrix, so fulfilling the function of an osteoblast, while the remainder of the cell and cell processes passing into canaliculi show the appearance of an osteocyte. E.M. 100kV. ×3500.

typical of reticulin). Another portion of the same cell has produced osteoid matrix, so fulfilling the function of an osteoblast, while the remainder of the cell and the cell processes passing into canaliculi show the appearance of an osteocyte. Parts of the same cell functioning as vessel wall, osteoblast and osteocyte leave no doubt about the potential roles of these cells of the vessel walls.

That cell processes link together, and that those from outside enter canaliculi to join processes from osteocytes was described as long ago as 1898 (Spuler). In all the sites mentioned in the last paragraph, suitable specimen preparation and staining can demonstrate that there are direct intercellular connections from the cells of the vessel walls, often through intermediate cells, to osteoblasts and osteocytes (Fig. 1.4). Figure 4.6 shows the connections to an intermediate cell at somewhat greater

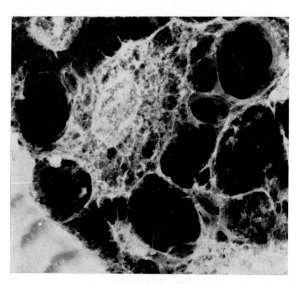

Fig. 4.6. Osteogenic cell in position intermediate between sinusoid wall and bone surface. There are intercellular connections with neighbouring cells, including the portion of an osteoblast (bottom right). E.M. 100kV. ×4500.

resolution. In an attempt to assess the relative importance of the various types of bone precursor which have been suggested, a variety of bone sections have been examined, including the upper end of the femur in all age groups from the foetus to over 90 years of age. The formation of bone from the differentiation of cells of the vessel walls, often through intermediate cells to osteoblasts has been seen as the normal method of bone formation in enchondral ossification, in osteonal remodelling, and in the majority of sites in bone at all ages. But the experiments in tissue culture media have suggested that osteoblasts can exist free in the culture media, and then lay down what appears to be bone. Pritchard (1956) in discussing such culture experiments has expressed the opinion that the same osteogenic cells can either join together or exist freely, according to the prevailing conditions.

The conditions in culture media and intact bone are very different, but there does seem to be at least one set of conditions in which the osteogenic cells can exist freely, and then join together before assuming an osteoblastic function. In some circumstances, and in particular in trabecular bone formation in the mature and elderly, bone formation from cells resembling the free type of osteoblast precursor described in the tissue culture experiments has been seen. These cells have been found around sinusoids and sometimes around larger vessels (Fig. 4.7), although in this latter case their origin could have been the

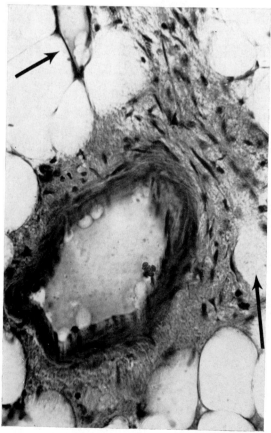

FIG. 4.7. Vessel in head of femur of elderly person. Connective tissue cells are proliferating in an effusion, around the vessel, which contains a high proportion of solids. Two neighbouring sinusoid vessels are arrowed. ×200.

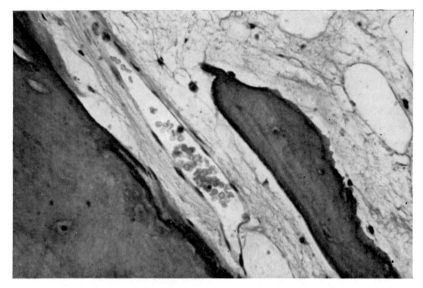

Fig. 4.8. Trabecular surfaces, somewhat eroded, in the head of femur of an elderly person. There has been an effusion from neighbouring vessels, but the solids and cells are sparse. × 200.

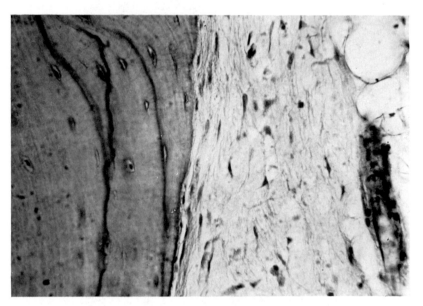

Fig. 4.9. Another region of the same head of femur. Prominent arrest lines in the trabecula are evidence that this bone is from an osteoporotic subject. Again there has been an effusion near the trabecula surface. With a rather higher protein content there is rather more cell activity, and a desultory osteoblast activity on the bone surface. × 200.

neighbouring sinusoids. The proportion of cells in a given volume varies (Figs 4.8, 4.9, 4.10). The accompanying observation in each case has been that these cells proliferate where the vessel is surrounded by an effusion, containing protein, which in the dried section contained a high proportion of solid. It may be as well to recall, at this point, that observation, especially in fracture healing, has shown that vascular and osteogenic cells require a solid or semi-solid substrate over which to move (Fig. 1.2). Before the precursor cells function as active osteoblasts they link up, so that at the bone surface they have the same appearance as ordinary bone (Fig. 4.10). If there were not an effective intercellular

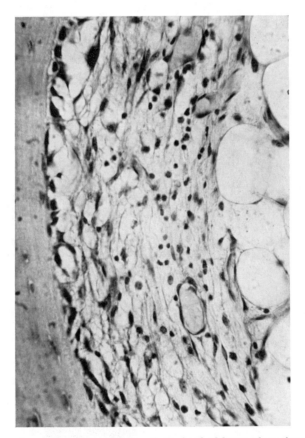

FIG. 4.10. A portion of an area in an osteoarthritic head of femur where there has been an extravascular effusion. In this bone there is abundant cell activity. The proliferating connective tissue cells, near the active osteoblasts on the bone surface, have formed intercellular connections. Small round cells in the region further away from the bone surface would seem to belong to the macrophage, or histiocyte, series. The presence of fat cells on the right of the photograph shows that the type of tissue breakdown product which favours haemopoietic activity is not present near this site. × 200.

link-up, then as soon as the bone matrix laid down by the cells had calcified they would die, since cell processes passing through the canaliculi are essential for osteocyte survival. Such acellular bone is known, particularly in fish, and it was the first type of bone to be formed. It has been called aspidin, and Tarlo (1963) has described its appearance and structure in the earliest bony fossils, the heterostracan ostracoderms which lived 400 million years ago.

Trabeculae

Trabeculae follow the lines of force, whether gravitational or caused by muscle pull. This phenomenon has been described by Ward (1838) and many others. The radiograph in Fig. 4.11, which is from the head of femur of a boy of 14, shows that in a child trabeculae commonly reach to all parts of the articular surface. In healthy people who

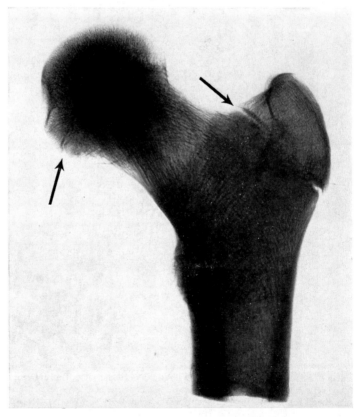

Fig. 4.11. Radiograph of head and neck of femur of boy of 14. In the head trabeculae reach to all parts of the articular surface. The epiphyseal growth plates are arrowed.

exercise their hips adequately this trabecular distribution remains. Figure 4.12 is from a 64-year-old individual. When hip movement is

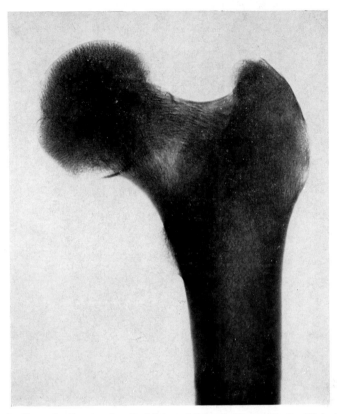

FIG. 4.12. Radiograph of head and neck of femur of 64-year-old man. During life he had taken adequate exercise, and bone trabeculae have continued to extend to all parts of the articular surface.

limited the trabeculae survive mainly in those portions of bone where there is active weight-bearing. Figure 4.13 is from a 37-year-old male. The angle of the head of femur is abnormal, and the portions of the bone to either side of the main group of trabeculae have not been subjected to adequate weight-bearing. What is probably more relevant, than that the trabeculae follow the lines of force, is that they follow the lines of open sinusoid vessels. These vessels have very thin flexible walls, so tend to be closed when they are transverse to the forces acting on them, but open when they are along the lines of applied forces. Sinusoids in cortical bone have equally thin walls (Fig. 4.14), but there they are protected by the surrounding bone. In Fig. 4.15 is illustrated the state of affairs arising after an osteotomy has altered the direction of the lines of

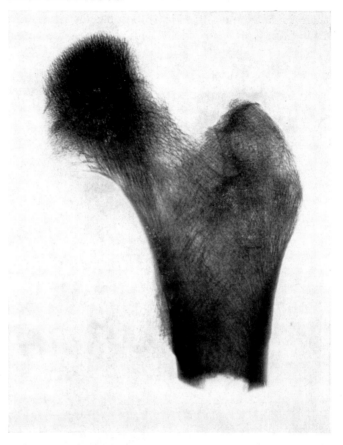

Fig. 4.13. Radiograph of head and neck of femur of 37-year-old man. The angle of the head and neck to the shaft of the bone is abnormal, and during life has limited the range of movement of the hip. The bone to either side of the main group of trabeculae has not been subject to adequate weight-bearing, and trabeculae are mostly missing from these regions. The bone formed at the time of closure of the epiphyseal plate remains, and has not been subject to remodelling processes.

force. The open vessels and new trabeculae are in one direction, while at an angle to this are the old and partially resorbed trabeculae. Figure 4.16 shows one stage in the process of trabecular resorption as a result of the changed mechanics of its surroundings. Here resorption has been preceded by the death of many of the osteocytes. It is possible that the effusion around some vessels, with a high content of solids, is due to a gradual build-up of pressure in areas of trabecular bone where the flow of blood has been temporarily hindered. When such oedema fluids are low in protein tissue growth does not occur, but when they are rich in protein they become a good cell culture medium (Drinker, Field

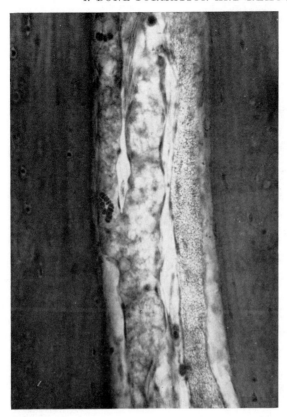

Fig. 4.14. Sinusoid vessels in a Haversian canal in the cortical bone of a dog. The vessel on the right is filled with perfusion medium. Vessel walls consist of a basement membrane on which are flattened widely spaced endothelial cells. ×200.

and Homans, 1934). Unsymmetrical trabeculae are often found associated with this type of osteogenic activity (Fig. 4.17).

A gradual remodelling of trabeculae continues through life, and there are indications that bone tissue in these sites does not survive intact for such long periods as bone in the cortex of long bones or in flat bones. One such indication was from an X-ray diffraction survey of the intercellular matrices in decalcified femurs. The collagen diffraction pattern together with a beta-protein pattern is seen in those specimens in which the calcifiable matrix is still present. Cortical bone in foetuses, infants and young children showed the beta-protein pattern in all specimens, but in the cortical bone from adults the beta-protein was rarely seen, and then only in small quantities. In trabecular bone the beta-protein pattern was observed at all ages.

M

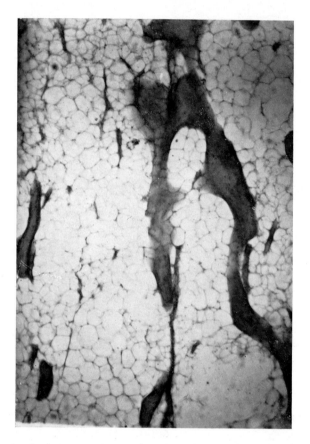

FIG. 4.15. Section through the head of femur a few months after an osteotomy, which altered the angle of the head relative to the shaft of the bone. In this figure the new direction of lines of force through the bone is vertical. Only sinusoid vessels along the lines of force are open. Some new trabeculae have formed along this direction. A previously formed trabecula remains at an angle to these new trabeculae (NNW to SSE). The surrounding marrow consists entirely of fat cells. The absence of haemopoietic tissue is an indication that in this field no active resorption is in progress. ×35.

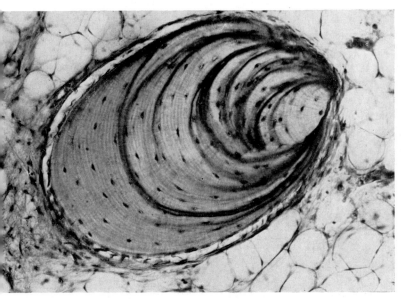

Fig. 4.17. Transverse, slightly oblique, section through trabecula in head of femur of an elderly person. The prominent arrest lines show that this bone is from an osteoporotic subject. The bone was obtained during an inactive phase. The trabecula is unsymmetrical, and bone in the process of being laid down on one side seems to be from cells in an extravascular effusion. ×100.

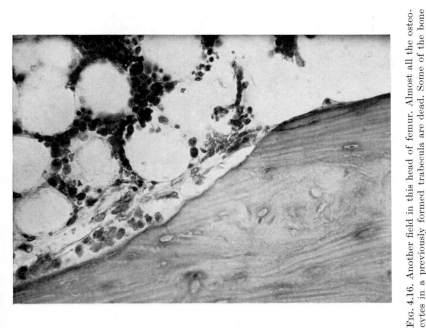

Fig. 4.16. Another field in this head of femur. Almost all the osteocytes in a previously formed trabecula are dead. Some of the bone matrix has started to degrade: it is less heavily stained than the intact matrix on the right. Resorption is in progress, and there is some haemopoietic activity in the vicinity. ×200.

Woven bone

A type of bone with somewhat different properties has been called woven
bone. In common usage the term "woven bone" is often applied to
foetal bone and to irregularly arranged bone in fracture callus (Fig. 2.17),
as well as to that type of bone which in this book is called woven bone.
Although foetal bone and some of the bone in fracture callus is irregularly
arranged, osteoblasts follow the lines of irregularly arranged vessels.
Woven bone is formed under quite different conditions, and looks and
behaves differently. The cell of origin again seems to be the vessel wall,
but where there has been cell death in the vicinity, from either trauma
or a loss of the blood supply, the cells which proliferate are granulation
tissue cells. W.M. Rigal (1963, pers. comm.) has grown short term

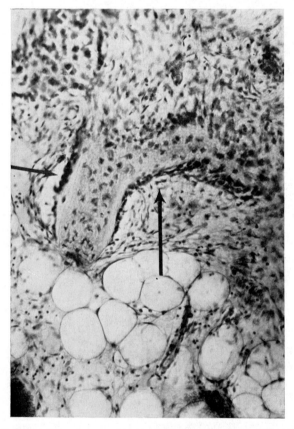

Fig. 4.18. Section through lumbar vertebra of an elderly man a short while after a small crush
fracture had occurred as a result of osteoporosis. Granulation tissue has proliferated from
damaged blood vessels and a patch of woven bone (arrowed) is in the pocess of formation.
×100.

cultures of rabbit metaphyseal bone using serum as the medium, and with tritiated thymidine added. After 6 h cells of the vessel walls alone had taken up the label, while after 48 h granulation tissue had proliferated.

In Fig. 2.18 granulation tissue cells are shown proliferating in the femoral epiphysis of a puppy 48 h after Perthes disease has been induced by temporarily constricting the artery leading to that part of the bone (Kemp, 1965). The cells are interconnected. In Fig. 4.18 is shown the early formation of woven bone from granulation tissue in the human. This illustration is taken from the lumbar vertebra of an elderly man where a small crush fracture had occurred as a result of osteoporosis. The woven bone is characterized by large irregularly shaped cells and irregularly arranged matrix and, unlike cells of the normal osteogenic type its cells do not readily coalesce to form osteoclasts. For comparison, Fig. 4.19

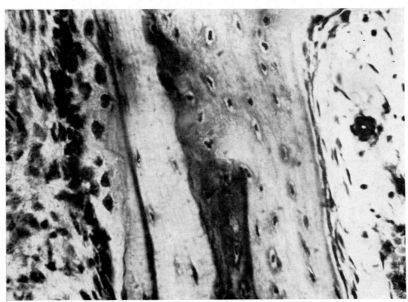

FIG. 4.19. The cells in woven bone are larger than those of normal bone formed under comparable conditions. The central part of this figure is occupied by the remains of one of the original trabeculae in an arthritic head of femur. A part of it has undergone additional calcification (more heavily stained). On the right ordinary bone has been laid down by osteogenic cells, and the osteocytes may be seen elongated in the direction of the trabecula and in a uniform row. On the left woven bone is being laid down by granulation tissue. These osteocytes and osteoblasts are larger, rounder, more heavily stained and less regularly arranged. × 200.

shows adjacent woven bone and ordinary bone on either side of a trabecula in an active area in osteoarthritis. This shows the difference in size and shape of the osteocytes formed in tissues at a similar level of activity. Woven bone is not a stable tissue, and remodelling takes place with the formation of ordinary bone (Fig.4.20).

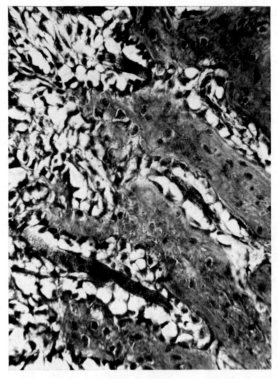

Fig. 4.20. Three almost parallel vessels have invaded the woven bone formed in a healing fracture. They are filled with perfusion medium. Osteogenic cells have proliferated from their walls and have begun to lay down ordinary bone. × 200.

Osteoclasts

The evidence that osteoclasts result from the fusion of pre-existing cells seems overwhelming, both from observation (Howell, 1890; Hancox, 1956) and by direct experiment. Hancox has observed that in embryonic tissues there is a tendency for the osteoclasts to contain other cells, which have presumably been trapped at the time of fusion. Baker (1939) and others have found that the formation of osteoclasts in response to a given stimulus is very rapid.

Fusion has been observed directly in culture media, both *in vivo* in rabbit ear chambers (Sandison, 1928) and *in vitro* (Tonna and Cronkite, 1961). By adding tritiated thymidine to a culture medium in which slices of rabbit tibia were placed, W.M. Rigal (1963, pers. comm.) has shown that whereas many of the surrounding cells took up tritiated thymidine as they went into the predivision phase, those which fused to form osteoclasts took up no thymidine. Very occasionally a cell which had entered the pre- division phase reversed its activity and coalesced with neighbouring cells. Both Sandison's *in vivo* and Rigal's *in vitro* experiments have given 48 h as the average life of an osteoclast.

Further evidence that osteoclasts are formed by fusion of osteogenic precursor cells has been obtained by administration of cortisone to rabbits. When it is administered regularly, osteoclasts are formed on all active bone surfaces (Fig. 4.21), and continue to be formed, remove

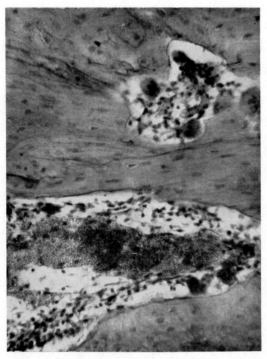

FIG. 4.21. Cortical bone from a rabbit to which cortisone had been administered. A distended sinusoid vessel may be seen filled with perfusion medium in the lower cavity. An abnormally large number of osteoclasts on the bone surfaces are enlarging the cavities. × 100.

bone and then die, until all the precursor cells are used up. But another way of causing bone removal is to prevent muscle activity. Experimentally, one method is to remove a portion of the Achilles tendon (Geizer and Trueta, 1958). This will be discussed in more detail later. When muscle action is prevented almost half of the bone served by those muscles is resorbed. When cortisone was given continuously to animals with a severed tendon, less bone was removed, apparently because all the available osteoclast precursors were used up before the final stage of the process had been reached (Little and de Valderrama, 1968).

Much of the confusion that has surrounded discussions on bone removal has been due to a failure to realize that the precursor cells can have more than one origin. The experiments mentioned in the last paragraph and many other observations are consistent with the hypothesis that osteogenic cells which have proliferated from sinusoid vessel walls are able to fuse together to form osteoclasts. In sections they may sometimes be found in the process of coalescing, and Fig. 4.22

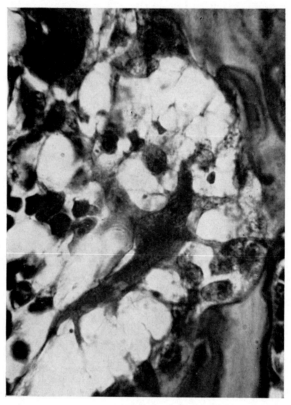

FIG. 4.22. Metaphyseal bone of rabbit. A group of osteogenic precursor cells between a vessel wall and the bone surface are in the process of coalescing to form an osteoclast. × 600.

shows a group of cells between the vessel wall and the bone surface which have joined together, while in Fig. 4.23 a cell of the vessel wall has been incorporated in the osteoclast. This vessel is filled with the Micropaque/Berlin blue perfusion medium.

That there is more than one cell type that can act as osteoclast precursors has been obvious at least since Gaillard (1955, 1959) took the first ciné pictures of bone in a culture medium where treatment with

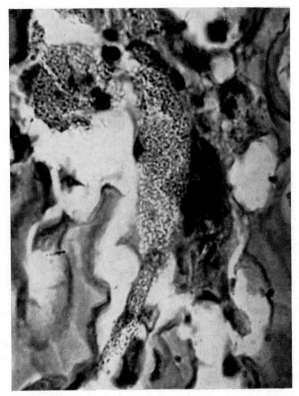

Fig. 4.23. An osteoclast (darkly stained) in the metaphyseal bone of a rabbit. A cell of the vessel wall has been incorporated into the multinucleated osteoclast. The vessel is filled with perfusion medium. ×400.

parathyroid hormone had produced vigorous bone resorption. In these pictures osteoclasts exhibited two types of behaviour. Some confined their activity to one spot, showing plenty of intracellular motion, but removing only the bone in their immediate neighbourhood, until the time came when all intracellular motion and activity suddenly ceased and the cell died. Others were able to move around freely. In osteonal remodelling Johnson (1964) has described them as "rolling" over the bone surface. It would seem logical to assume that the anchored osteoclasts were formed by coalescence of cells derived from the vessel walls, while the freely moving osteoclasts had some other precursor. The proportion probably did not represent the situation which exists in a normal animal or even in an animal treated with the parathyroid hormone, since the culture medium would itself exert an influence on the cell activity.

When reviewing the subject in 1956 Hancox considered the origin of many osteoclasts to be an open question. This was because of the frequent difficulty in identifying precursor cells in histological sections. As osteoclasts are formed their cytoplasm exhibits gross changes. Unlike osteoblasts, which have a gel-like structure, the osteoclast cytoplasm is fluid, with a corresponding low proportion of solids. Then as they progress to their active phase many organelles are found in the cytoplasm which produce the enzymes that degrade bone matrix. At this stage the cytoplasm stains heavily, while after resorptive activity ceases it loses its ability to take up stain. In Fig. 4.24 two osteoclasts

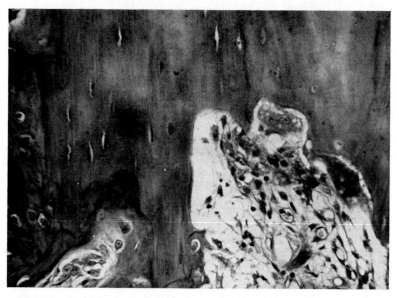

Fig. 4.24. Cortical bone in healing fracture in rabbit, with osteoclasts in the process of removing dead bone. An active osteoclast is heavily stained, while a lightly stained osteoclast is in the cavity that it has already produced. ×200.

can be seen, the active one heavily stained, while a lightly stained cell is in the cavity that it has already produced.

The situation has now been clarified as a result of observations by W. S. S. Jee and those working with him. In the first place Arnold and Jee (1957), using bone with plutonium deposited on the bone surfaces, showed that some resorbed matrix enters into the cytoplasm of some osteoclasts (Figs 4.25, 4.26), and later, after the death of these osteoclasts, is taken up into the cytoplasm of macrophages (Figs 4.27, 4.28). Then, in another series of experiments, Jee and Nolan (1963) introduced powdered charcoal into the long bones of rabbits by way of the nutrient artery. This powdered charcoal was removed from the sinusoids by

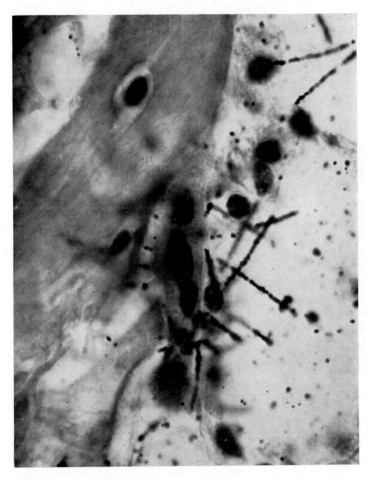

FIG. 4.25. The tissue level of a detailed autoradiogram of an osteoclast found to be a source of a concentration of activity on the surface of a trabecula in the vertebral body of a rat. 24 h after a ^{239}Pu injection. ×1560. Figure 10 from Arnold and Jee (1957).

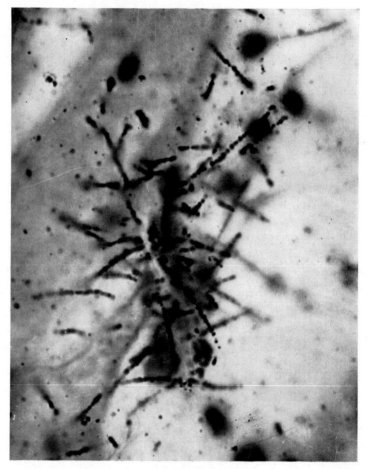

Fig. 4.26. The track level over the same osteoclast shown in Fig. 4.25. ×1560. Figure 11 from Arnold and Jee (1957).

macrophages (phagocytic reticular cells). The lowered blood flow caused by the charcoal initiated a phase of bone removal, and it was observed that macrophages "labelled" with charcoal coalesced to form a large proportion of the osteoclasts that were removing the bone.

A situation such as this appears to represent one extreme, with macrophages as the dominant source of osteoclasts, while the experiments in which bone removal is initiated by the action of cortisone or cortisol represents the other extreme. In that case one of the effects of cortisol is to inhibit the maturation of macrophages, so that the majority of osteoclasts must have been formed by coalescence of the osteogenic cells. In normal bone both mechanisms might be expected to play a part.

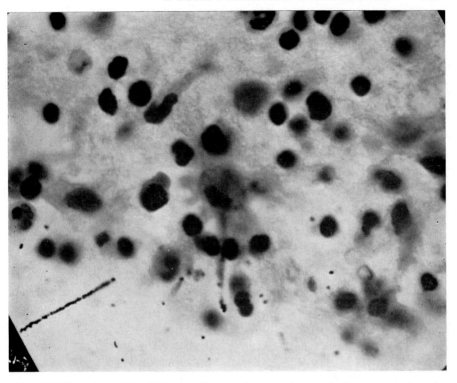

Fig. 4.27. Tissue level of detailed autoradiogram of a macrophage in the femoral metaphyseal marrow from a rat sacrificed 9 days after ^{239}Pu injection. $\times 1490$. Figure 14 from Arnold and Jee (1957).

The presence of parathyroid hormone is also needed before macrophages can coalesce, and Burkhart and Jowsey (1967) have found that immobilization osteoporosis is virtually eliminated when the thyroid and parathyroid glands are removed. Conversely, Faccini (1969) found, when fluoride was introduced into the drinking water of young rabbits and sheep that although the newly laid down bone became more resistant to resorption, the parathyroid glands were enlarged and became more active, and there was increased resorption of non-fluoride-containing bone. Thyroid hormone is also needed, and Adams and Jowsey (1967) showed that feeding dogs excess thyroxine resulted in an increased rate of activity.

These two mechanisms, with osteoclasts formed by coalescence of either osteogenic cells or macrophages, would seem to account for most of the observations on the subject recorded in the literature. Jacoby (1938) has pointed out that monocytes from the blood behave in exactly the same way as macrophages from other tissues. In the litera-

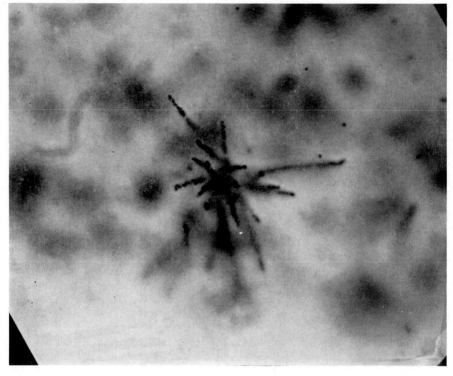

FIG. 4.28. The track level over the macrophage shown in Fig. 4.27. The convergence of the alpha tracks indicates that the ^{239}Pu was contained within the cytoplasm. × 1490. Figure 15 from Arnold and Jee (1957). The author thanks Prof. W. S. S. Jee for Figs. 4.25—4.28.

ture on bone the names given to the cells which are called macrophages in this book have varied. For instance, Lacoste (1923) and Hancox (1949) have used the term histiocytes, and Fischman and Hay (1962) mononuclear leucocytes, but it seems most probable that in each case the same cell type was observed. Observations on resorption by the osteogenic cells are more straightforward. The osteoblasts that have been implicated (Kolliker, 1873; Pommer, 1883) are part of the same cell network, and so are the osteocytes. Resorptive activity by osteocytes is shown not only by cells enlarging their lacunae (Fig. 4.29), but also by cell processes enlarging the canaliculi through which they pass (Fig. 4.30).

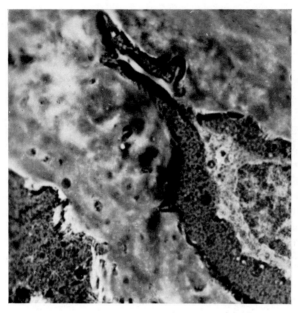

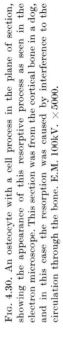

Fig. 4.30. An osteocyte with a cell process in the plane of section, showing the appearance of this resorptive process as seen in the electron microscope. This section was from the cortical bone in a dog, and in this case the resorption was caused by interference to the circulation through the bone. E.M. 100kV. ×5000.

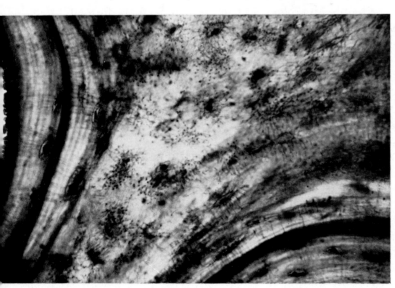

Fig. 4.29. A portion of a trabecula in the neck of femur of an osteo-porotic subject, during an active phase of post-menopausal osteo-porosis. Arrest lines are heavily stained. In the central part of the trabecula osteocytes have enlarged their lacunae, and also the canaliculi through which cell processes pass. In transverse section these can be seen as groups of dots. ×200.

Stimulation of Activity

There is thus ample evidence that bone is laid down by osteogenic precursor cells that are derived from the walls of proliferating vessels or sinusoid vessels; while it may be removed either by osteogenic cells coalescing to form osteoclasts, or by macrophages coalescing to form a different type of osteoclast. In either case the word osteoclast is used to denote a multinucleated cell which can resorb bone tissue, without regard to the origin of that multinucleated cell.

There remains to be considered in more detail those factors which make osteogenic and granulation tissue cells lay down bone tissue rather than fibrous tissue; and which determine whether bone is laid down or removed at any given time or place, the quality and quantity of bone tissue formed by osteoblasts, and which type of osteoclast is formed and how vigorously it acts. In each case it seems that the cell behaviour is influenced by the nature and concentration of the chemicals present in the surrounding fluids.

The osteogenic factor

In bone development the initial determining factor is a genetic one, which results in the formation of cartilage models (the anlage cartilage) of the appropriate shape and distribution. As the cartilage matures vessels proliferate and penetrate, and then bone is formed around them. Enchondral ossification, as it is called, is found as the anlage cartilage in the shaft is transformed to bone (Figs 2.11, 2.12), at the bottom of the growth cartilage (Fig. 3.1), around secondary epiphyseal bone nuclei where these are present, in fracture cartilage (Fig. 4.1), in cartilage formed by metaplastic changes in fibrous tissues (see next chapter), and also in an early stage of the osteoarthritic process, whether in young cartilage or more usually in mature adult articular cartilage (Fig. 4.2). In each of these examples of enchondral ossification a change in the cartilage has stimulated vascular proliferation. Similar vascular proliferation can occur in fibrous tissues, but only in the presence of cartilage or bone is the vascular proliferation followed by bone formation.

Many cartilage cells, as they approach the moribund stage, tend to enlarge and form the calcifiable matrix which was described in Chapter 1. A change in this matrix precedes the deposition of mineral. Irving (1960) has shown that a lipid is liberated. This was confirmed by Johnson (1964) who also showed that immediately preceding calcification an excess of phosphate is present. This is in accord with the observation that in this site the deposited mineral is mainly hydroxyapatite, but with the surface layers of the crystallites containing excess phosphate.

In bone vascular proliferation takes place where there is a breakdown of bone matrix. One example of this is in osteonal remodelling (Fig. 2.19). Johnson (1964) has shown that this is initiated at places in the bone where there are pressures capable of disrupting the membranes which cover bone surfaces. A breakdown product of the underlying bone matrix could then stimulate vessel and cell proliferation to give the characteristic vascular network that is seen immediately behind the cutting cone of osteoclasts. He has measured the rates of the various processes of this type in bone and recorded them in the chapter "Morphological Analysis in Pathology".

Vascular proliferation is also found in the vicinity of dead bone. Figure 4.31 is a typical example from an arthritic head of femur, where the vessel

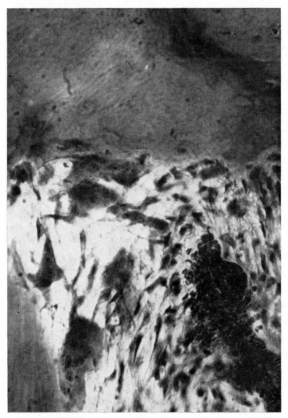

FIG. 4.31. Edge of a region of dead bone near the surface of an arthritic head of femur. To the left: a group of osteoclasts in the process of removing this bone. Bottom right: recently formed vessel containing packed red cells, and surrounded by mobile granulation tissue cells. ×200.

on the right has approached an area of dead bone, which is in the process of being removed by phagocytic osteoclasts. There is normally a time lag between osteocyte death and bone removal. When Irving and Handleman (1963) implanted dead rat bone there was a two week lag. In the adult femur the time lag between bone death after a fracture or other incident, and the vascular proliferation which is the first stage of resorption has been estimated as 5–8 weeks. When "Anorganic" bone (that is, bone with some of the organic constituents chemically extracted) is implanted it may stay 7 years or more with no sign of resorption. It would seem to be most probable that the time lag is due to a delay in the chemical decomposition of the tissue components to the products that stimulate cell proliferation. In the case of the "Anorganic" bone they had been extracted.

These observations, together with the fact that granulation tissue within bone is changed into woven bone, while elsewhere it is changed into fibrous tissue, can be explained if there is a chemical specifically responsible for stimulating osteogenic activity. All the available evidence is consistent with the hypothesis that the calcifiable matrix produced in enchondral ossification or by osteoblastic activity contains the substance which acts as a stimulant for osteogenic activity. There is an identical distribution and wherever the calcifiable matrix is present penetration of vessels into that tissue is followed by the production of bone.

The calcifiable matrix is produced *de novo* only by cartilage cells. Endothelial cells can only differentiate to ordinary or woven bone if there is some calcifiable matrix in their immediate neighbourhood, although once they have differentiated they can themselves produce calcifiable matrix. This matrix is complex, and known to contain protein, polysaccharides and lipids. There is as yet insufficient evidence as to whether or not the same components are responsible for both calcification and ossification—this is a field of investigation in which more observations are required. The few facts available would suggest that separate components are involved. Wherever the matrix change preceding calcification is observed suitable histological staining reveals the presence of a lipid, and calcification takes place in the altered matrix. It is a different lipid from the one which has been reported to be a normal component of collagenous tissue (Melcher, 1969). By contrast, there is evidence that the osteogenic factor can diffuse through the tissues. Thus, in the fracture repair process shown in Fig. 4.32, proliferating granulation tissue cells in the immediate vicinity of the fragment of dead bone are differentiating to woven bone, while those a little further away have differentiated to fibrous tissue. Similarly, in osteogenic osteosarcomas, in sites where cell proliferation outstrips bone

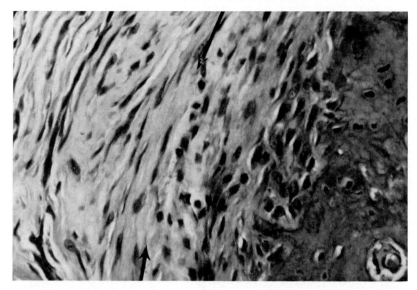

FIG. 4.32. Fracture callus in rabbit, near surface of callus. The woven bone (to the right) has formed on a chip of dead bone. The proliferating granulation tissue cells close to the fragment of dead bone are differentiating to woven bone, while those a little further away have differentiated to fibrous tissue. The boundary, which represents the limit of diffusion of the osteogenic factor, is arrowed. ×200.

formation patches of malignant fibrous tissue are found. In sarcoma derived from Paget's disease, where there is a particularly exhuberant cell proliferation, Price and Goldie (1969) have found a quarter of the lesions to be almost entirely fibrosarcomas.

Oxygen and carbon dioxide level

Cell activity is enhanced by a rapid flow of blood through the bone, whilst with a diminution of flow it becomes more sluggish. The flow of blood through bone is maintained by the action of the heart which pumps blood into the bone and the activity of surrounding muscles which pump it out of the bone (Trueta, 1968). The effect of a temporary build-up of pressure within a bone is to stimulate osteoclast formation and activity. This mechanism is demonstrated in Fig. 4.33. Here a defect was produced by cutting the cortex of a rabbit radius, across the main directional flow of the blood (Kemp, 1965). This blocked the flow in that part of the bone, and osteocytes deprived of their blood supply died. On the other side, where the blood flow was held up, osteoclasts are removing the bone.

Blood flow will be considered further in Chapter 5, but the aspect of

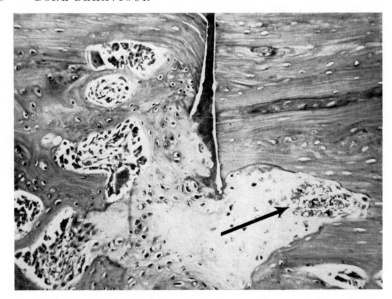

FIG. 4.33. A defect in the cortex of this rabbit radius contains clotted blood. The blood flow in the lamellar bone had been from left to right. The osteocytes on the right of the defect, having been deprived of their blood supply have died. On the left, where there was a build-up of pressure, osteoclasts are removing the bone. Towards the bottom is an area of fracture cartilage, and to the right of this newly proliferating vessels (arrowed) are stimulating osteoclastic removal of dead bone. ×100.

immediate interest is that with a high rate of blood flow there is a high partial pressure of oxygen in the tissues, and an increasing proportion of carbon dioxide as the rate of flow decreases. Oxygen is required to provide energy for cell activity, for proliferation and for the production of intercellular matrices or other secretions. With a low rate of flow less is available, while more is converted to carbon dioxide, which is less efficiently removed. In osteoporosis caused by immobilization Burkhart and Jowsey (1967) have shown that the blood in the affected limbs has an increased pCO_2 and decreased pH as compared with normal. Carbon dioxide tends to stimulate osteoclastic activity. A relevant observation is that an adequate oxygen supply favours the formation of cells whose contents are gelatinous (as are osteoblasts), while an increased partial pressure of carbon dioxide favours a change to a fluid cytoplasm (as have osteoclasts).

The effects of oxygen are somewhat complicated, and at first sight many reported observations would seem to be contradictory. There is an abundance of evidence that oxygen is one of the requirements for cell division (Bullough, 1952), but in some tissue culture media Goldhaber (1963) has shown that increasing partial pressures of oxygen caused increasing bone resorption. Goldhaber found that variations in the culture medium could vary the effects of the oxygen on resorption, and that possibly this was as a result of slight abnormalities in the cells. A the other end of the scale Bond, Matthews and Finney (1967) caused a local release of oxygen into the tissue of the jaw of a series of monkeys by injecting hydrogen peroxide and then irradiating. In this case there was prolific osteoblast activity subperiosteally, endosteally, and also within the dental pulp. These apparently contradictory effects of oxygen have been successfully employed in the treatment of a wide variety of neoplasms. Irradiation together with a high oxygen level in the tissues results in a more effective destruction of slightly or grossly abnormal cells, while the subsequent healing processes are accelerated (Mallams, Balla and Finney, 1965). The various effects of oxygen and carbon dioxide provide another topic which requires further elucidation.

Hormonal influences

In any consideration of osteoblastic and osteoclastic activity the action of the peptide and steroid hormones which may be present, together with related compounds that may be administered therapeutically or taken as drugs, are particularly important.

Growth hormone, as its name implies, dominates hormonal effects during the period of growth. It is a peptide hormone that has an anabolic action. That is, it stimulates the formation of intercellular matrices. These are less chemically stable than those whose formation is stimulated by the anabolic steroids (Davidson and Small, 1963), so facilitating the rapid tissue turnover that is necessary during growth. Growth hormone also stimulates stem cells to divide (Rigal, 1964). This action is probably responsible for the increase in total quantity of each tissue during growth. Some growth hormone continues to be produced in the adult. The adult Negro retains a greater capacity for growth hormone production than does the white adult, and there is a correspondingly higher proportion of osseous tissue present in any given bone in the Negro than in the white. This is particularly noticeable in the trabecular bone of the vertebrae.

The action of parathyroid hormone in bone is primarily on the macrophages. When these cells have enlarged, the presence of parathyroid hormone is needed for their coalescence to form osteoclasts. In the presence of an excessive amount of parathyroid hormone these osteoclasts display a correspondingly exhuberant activity, and selectively remove dead and moribund bone. The pattern of bone removal, from the cores of trabeculae as well as from the cortex is characteristic, and differs from other forms of osteoporosis. There are other accompanying symptoms of parathyroidism. The presence of thyroid hormone is necessary for parathyroid hormone to act.

In their effect on bone steroid hormones display three dominant types of behaviour, showing anabolic or anti-anabolic properties, catabolic or anti-catabolic properties, and modifying haemopoietic proliferation. Anabolic and catabolic are often thought of as opposites, but in fact anabolic properties relate to the quality and quantity of intercellular matrix produced by osteoblasts or other cells (and protein in muscle), while catabolic properties relate to vessel and cell proliferation (Little, 1970*a*). On the whole, but with minor variations, anabolic steroids are anti-catabolic, and catabolic steroids are anti-anabolic.

The most anabolic of the natural hormones is testosterone, with the female hormones showing a rather lower level of activity. Accordingly, a man has a greater proportion of osseous tissue in his bone than does a woman of similar height. Some synthetic steroids have a higher level of anabolic activity. Cortisol and other corticosteroids allow an osteoblast to produce only a small quantity of matrix, and that of an abnormal quality. They also cause muscle cells to lose protein from their fibres. In these activities they display an anti-catabolic characteristic.

The catabolic and anti-catabolic properties of steroids have an even more important effect on the properties of the bone. In this facet of their behaviour steroids influence the flexibility and mobility of cell membranes, and thus the rate and vigour of cell division. The catabolic compounds decrease this flexibility and mobility (Dougherty *et al.*, 1961), and the anti-catabolic compounds increase them (Bullough, 1952; Little, 1965–66). Of the natural steroids, testosterone has a greater effect on vessel and cell proliferation than do the female hormones, while some of the synthetic steroids promote still more vigorous proliferation. This does not mean that bone continues to be laid down indefinitely. Vessels and osteogenic cells are stimulated, but according to the other prevailing conditions, and in particular the rate of flow of blood, this vigorous activity may be either osteoblastic or osteoclastic.

At the other end of the scale are cortisol and other corticosteroids. They decrease the vigour and frequency of cell and vessel proliferation. There is an additional effect which provides a sharp line of demarcation between the weakly anti-catabolic and even the weakest of the catabolic compounds. The catabolic steroids hinder the differentiation of osteogenic precursor cells to osteoblasts, and instead stimulate their coalescence to osteoclasts. It is these steroids which are called corticosteroids. At the same time they inhibit the production of macrophages and prevent those already present from enlarging to the state where they can coalesce to form multinucleated phagocytic cells (Dougherty,

1952). Cortisol thus encourages the formation of one type of osteoclast, until the supply of osteogenic precursor cells runs out, whilst preventing the formation of the other type.

Cortisol is the most important of the corticosteroids because there is a raised level in the blood whenever an individual is under stress. By stress is meant in this context, the effects of such stimuli as pain, trauma, acute or terminal illness, or the unpleasant emotions such as anger, frustration, and jealousy. Fear and apprehension are very potent causes of a raised blood cortisol (see Chapters 2 and 7).

The steroids also affect the properties of marrow cells, and in particular the haemopoietic tissue. Acting separately or in combination they may alter the proportions and sometimes the properties of each of the components of the circulating blood which is formed in the bone. Thus, some steroids cause a considerable increase in erythropoiesis. One of the effects of cortisol is to increase the number of megakaryocytes in the marrow, and hence the number of circulating platelets. But when steroids with progestational properties are present abnormal megakaryocytes may develop. This is dependent upon the threshold level of excess cortisol needed to produce the abnormality, which varies for each steroid with which the cortisol interacts. For some it is above the toxic level of the cortisol itself, while for others it is very low. These abnormal megakaryocytes in turn produce abnormal platelets which quickly fuse to form platelet thrombi (Little and White, 1968).

The properties of hormones and steroids will be described in greater detail in Chapter 6 and thereafter.

Vitamins and trace elements

So far as bone is concerned, several dietary factors are of importance. Adequate amounts of vitamin C are required for normal healthy bone, while there are optimum levels for vitamin D and fluoride. In each case it is the quality of the intercellular matrix that is primarily influenced.

Vitamin C (ascorbic acid) affects the bone in two ways. In the first place a deficiency of vitamin C, while not directly affecting cell proliferation, causes a defective matrix to be formed by osteoblasts (Lind, 1753; Wolbach and Howe 1926; Boyle, Bessey and Howe, 1940). In a case of very serious deficiency matrix production may almost cease, so that this is the dominant cause of symptoms in children and in regions of rapid bone turnover. The effect on the walls of sinusoid vessels, particularly those which are formed during the course of normal tissue turnover, is more important in the adult. These vessel walls are defective, and so tend to dilate and rupture more easily than normal. Such weakened vessels lead to a larger proportion of the blood being held in the sinusoid system. Usually one tenth of the sinusoid vessels are open at any one time, but in scorbutic bone the proportion is increased. This in turn leads to a sluggish blood flow, and so to the type of bone removal due to phagocytic osteoclasts. The effect is enhanced by the easily degraded bone matrix formed during a lack of an adequate concentration of ascorbic acid. There are other accompanying symptoms of scurvy, particularly in the young.

Whereas vitamin C is water soluble, vitamins A and D are fat soluble, and tend to occur together. Vitamin D acts on the intercellular matrix, but while the effect of vitamin C is apparently on the whole matrix, vitamin D affects the non-collagenous parts of the intercellular matrices, and in cartilage and bone the calcifiable matrix. An excess of vitamin D weakens the gel structure, so that it breaks down with minimal trauma, and the matrix can then become calcified. With a deficiency of vitamin D the matrix is too stable, and this extra chemical and physical stability of the calcifiable matrix leads to pathological effects. The change in the matrix which precedes calcification is blocked, so that matrix laid down in the absence of an adequate amount of vitamin D fails to calcify. In the growing epiphysis it is more stable than normal, and requires chondroclasts for its removal. When enchondral ossification is blocked the condition is known as rickets; while when the result is an osteoid seam over trabeculi in place of normal calcified bone the condition is known as osteomalacia. Vitamin D deficiency may be caused by a straightforward deficiency in the diet, or alternatively by impaired absorption from the gut. A raised plasma cortisol level hinders this absorption (Caniggia, Gennari, Bianchi and Guideri, 1963); and so does phytic acid, the hexaphosphoric acid ester of inositol ($C_6H_6(O.H_2PO_3)_6$), which is present in many cereals (Mellanby, 1950). In Indians it is thought that a biochemical effect may also be present, which would account for their vitamin-resistant late rickets and osteomalacia.

Because of the failure of the osteoid seams to calcify in osteomalacia and rickets, it is sometimes thought that a deficiency of calcium is involved. Mellanby's work has shown that this is not the case, but that the controlling effects of vitamin D and phytic acid are more important. When there is an actual calcium deficiency, the pathological consequences are quite different. Scott, Greaves and Scott (1961) and Scott (1968) have shown that the effects are mediated through the thyroid gland, while the histological changes eventually produced in bone (Kayanja, Scott and Scott 1965) resemble those produced by cortisone.

The effects of vitamin A are different, and deficiency results in a distortion of the shape of the bones. A series of meticulous experiments was performed by Mellanby (1950). He worked at a time before the importance of the blood flow, hormone effects, and the presence of two types of osteoclast with different controlling mechanisms were recognized. His results showed that it was not the intercellular matrix, but the abnormal distribution of osteoblastic and osteoclastic activity in the absence of vitamin A which can result in sufficient bone distortion to compress nerves contained within the bone. His descriptions are consistent with the suppression of osteoclast formation from macrophages, leaving normal osteoblast mechanisms, and only those osteoclasts from osteogenic precursor cells formed. Photomicrographs he shows are typical of this type of osteoclast. It would thus appear possible that vitamin A acts on the thyroid or parathyroid glands.

Fluoride is included with this group of vitamins because it has a closely related mode of action. It affects the intercellular matrices, but this time observations are consistent with it being the non-collagenous protein moiety that is affected. With too little fluoride the compound is unstable. Effects on bone are minimal, since their mechanical stability is primarily dependent upon the collagen and gel components of the matrix. The tissue that shows most clearly the effect of a fluoride deficiency is dental enamel, because the protein component of enamel matrix is predominantly non-collagenous protein. In areas of fluoride deficiency the spread of dental caries is facilitated. It is possible that fluoride deficiency might also affect the properties of the intervertebral disc, as a result of defective beta-protein production, but this possibility has not as yet been investigated. An excess of fluoride causes the beta-protein to become too stable, and the production of "mottled" teeth suggests that it is laid down in a rather more condensed form than the normal protein. This mottling shows at concentrations above about 3 ppm, but hindrance to normal bone remodelling as a result of resistance to resorption does not become noticeable till about 25 ppm.

As was stated at the beginning of this chapter, the subject of bone formation and removal has been more than usually confused because of various incorrect statements often naïvely accepted as facts. This has partly been due to a tendency, as different facets of the basic mechanisms of bone formation and removal came to the fore, to attempt to explain all properties in terms of too few mechanisms. In considering the various theories and hypotheses two not unimportant criteria to apply are: "Is the hypothesis understandable?" and "Is it in accord with common sense?". Additionally, valid hypotheses should advance knowledge of the mechanism of obscure conditions. In the next section, therefore, osteogenesis imperfecta will be discussed in terms of the available information which has been outlined at the beginning of this chapter, while the mechanisms of osteoporosis, osteoarthritis, Paget's disease and osteosarcomas will be discussed in Chapters 8 and 9.

Osteogenesis Imperfecta

This is a condition, fortunately rare, in which the bone tissues fail to form and calcify normally, with consequent multiple fractures and deformity. Most probably it is a generalized condition of the connective tissues. The sclera are often thin and blue, the skin may be thin with its collagen showing staining characteristics reminiscent of reticulin, mechanical weaknesses may be found in the aorta, and cartilage often stains abnormally. Dominant clinical characteristics, however, are associated with the bones. The severity of the condition varies, so that all stages may be found, in different individuals, between normal and grossly abnormal.

The pattern of defects is seen most clearly when sections of bones are examined after autopsy of a very severe case. In the long bones the growth cartilage develops almost normally, and the secondary bone nucleus enlarges, but instead of the expected enchondral ossification cells form a material which has a low mechanical strength, does not calcify, and gives an X-ray diffraction pattern showing no rings attributable to collagen, but only to a beta-protein. In the metaphysis the calcified cartilage is resorbed by osteoclasts at the expected level, and the abnormal material is between and below the calcified cartilage spicules. An observation which might seem to be unexpected is that this material is formed not only by the osteoblasts but also by their precursors and by cells of the vessel walls. Figure 4.34 shows an area of active proliferation in the metaphysis with this abnormal intercellular material both within and without vessels. In Fig. 4.35 is an area which should contain trabecular bone. Again there are fat cells interspersed with areas of the abnormal matrix and here the vessels containing it are viewed in cross-section. That this grossly abnormal bone matrix is found inside vessels as well as between them is easily understood if the cells of the vessel walls are, as postulated, the precursors of the cells which differentiate to form osteoblasts.

For such a material to be formed in these sites there would seem to be two abnormalities in the cell behaviour. In the first place only partial differentiation has taken place before matrix production, while the abnormal and chemically unstable matrix is itself formed prematurely. The abnormal matrix formed in very severe cases, such as that illustrated in Figs 4.34, 4.35, is replaced by normal looking marrow quite soon. In less severe cases it is generally seen that the more normal the differentiation of osteogenic cells the more normal is the matrix they produce, until a stage is reached when it calcifies. That the two abnormalities are parallel in their degree of severity would point to one underlying defect.

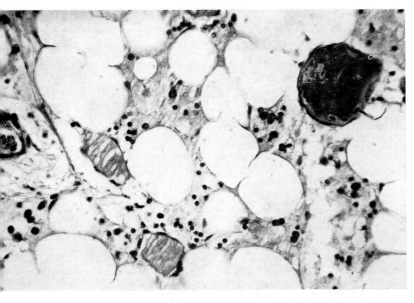

Fig. 4.35. Osteogenesis imperfecta. Same case as Fig. 4.34. Cross-section of metaphysis. Fat cells are interspersed with areas of the abnormal matrix. Several sinusoid vessels contain this same matrix. The parallel cracks are a sectioning artefact. ×200.

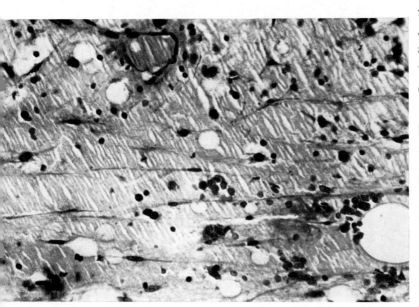

Fig. 4.34. Osteogenesis imperfecta. Age 2½ years. Longitudinal section of metaphysis, in an area of active proliferation. An abnormal intercellular material has been formed which is both inside and outside sinusoid vessels. ×200.

In the very severe cases periosteal bone is not produced, but a fairly common observation is the presence of multinucleated cells that look like osteoclasts in the vicinity of the periosteum, on the "bone" side and not on the periosteal side of the border. These cells are invariably on the vessel walls (Fig. 4.36), and could well have resulted from an attempt at differentiation.

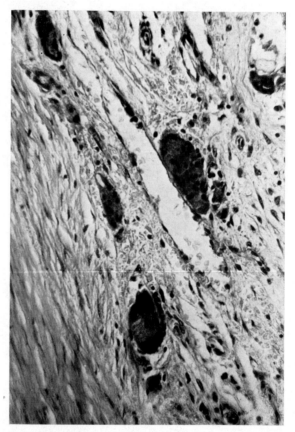

FIG. 4.36. Osteogenesis imperfecta. Same case as Fig. 4.34. Periosteal border. Multi-nucleated cells that look like osteoclasts are on the "bone" side of the border. There is one on a sinusoid vessel near the centre. Top right shows granulation tissue cells and blood vessels in place of cortical bone. ×200.

When cell death as a result of blocked vessels or fractures occurs, then granulation tissue proliferates and woven bone is formed from it in the normal manner. In the femur from which Fig. 4.37 was taken all the bone present in the cortex was woven bone formed from granulation tissue. An interesting observation, suggesting that genetic factors must

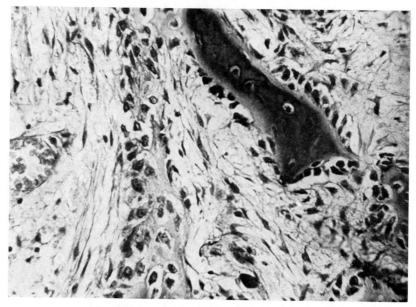

FIG. 4.37. Osteogenesis imperfecta. Same case as Fig. 4.34. In the cortical region granulation tissue cells have proliferated and woven bone is being laid down. ×200.

not be overlooked, was that the tissue was present as a grossly abnormal cortex surrounding a fatty marrow. Even though, as a result of multiple fractures, normal forces were not acting on the bone, the area occupied by the granulation tissue and woven bone was, very approximately, the right thickness.

In the last section, evidence was discussed which leads to the conclusion that there is a chemical "osteogenic factor" which stimulates osteogenic activity. Examination of bone from cases of osteogenesis imperfecta has provided confirmatory evidence. One method of treating the weight-bearing bones in this condition, so as to prevent gross deformity, is to cut the bone into segments and string them along a Kuntschner wire. As healing takes place granulation tissue is formed around the wire. It is found that this granulation tissue differentiates in two directions. Close to the wire fibrous tissue is formed, while the part of the tissue near the bone and marrow develops into woven bone (Fig. 4.38). Since originally it was all derived from cells which proliferated from vessels in bone into the blood clot around the inserted wire, it is reasonable to assume that the border between woven bone and fibrous tissue represents the depth to which the "osteogenic factor" had penetrated.

The influence of hormones on connective tissue and bone has also been

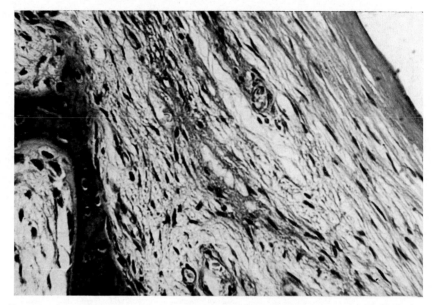

Fig. 4.38. Osteogenesis imperfecta. Same case as Fig. 4.34. A Kuntschner wire had been placed in the centre of the bone, to hold it in place and prevent gross deformity, three months previously. Granulation tissue formed around this wire, and its surface can be seen top right. Close to the wire it differentiated to fibrous tissue, while the part nearest the marrow and bone has developed into woven bone. ×200.

mentioned, the polypeptide hormones being responsible for less chemically stable intercellular matrices than those which are produced in the presence of steroid hormones. In osteogenesis imperfecta, when individuals reach adolescence and the proportion of steroid hormones increases, the bone formed becomes almost completely normal. The site in the cell where the defect resides must therefore be one subject to hormonal control.

Summary

1. Osteogenic cells and osteoblasts are derived from cells of sinusoid vessel walls. The term osteoblast covers all cells on the bone surface whether active or resting. The terms osteoblast, osteocyte, and osteoclast refer to different activities of osteogenic cells and not to different cell types. In most types of bone formation there are intercellular connections from vessel walls, through intermediate cells to osteoblasts and osteocytes.

2. In some sites, where there is tissue fluid containing protein around the vessels, osteogenic cells are separate and exist as in a tissue culture. They join together before forming bone. Cell processes passing through canaliculi are essential for osteocyte survival.

3. Trabeculae follow the lines of force, whether gravitational or caused by

muscle pull, because they follow the lines of open sinusoid vessels which have very thin flexible walls and so tend to be closed when transverse to the forces acting on them. When the lines of force are altered, as after an osteotomy, the direction of open vessels alters and as remodelling proceeds so does the direction of the trabeculae.

4. When granulation tissue proliferates from vessel walls it differentiates into a calcifiable tissue if in the vicinity of bone. This altered calcified granulation tissue is known as woven bone. Osteocytes are arranged irregularly and are larger than osteocytes in normal bone formed under comparable conditions. Woven bone is not a stable tissue and remodelling takes place with the formation of ordinary bone.

5. Osteoclasts arise from the fusion of pre-existing cells, and nuclear division does not take place within these cells. Their average life is probably of the order of 48 h. During that time they develop organelles in their cytoplasm that produces enzymes to remove bone tissue. The cytoplasm then tends to clear again before the cells disintegrate.

6. There are two types of osteoclast. One is formed by the coalescence of osteogenic cells. These confine thier activity to one spot and remove bone in their immediate vicinity. The other type of osteoclast is formed by the fusion of macrophages. These osteoclasts are able to move around freely. The proportion of the two types varies. Osteoclastic activity as a result of the action of corticosteroids is primarily due to the coalescence of osteogenic cells, while when there is a hindered blood flow those formed from macrophages dominate. After the death of osteoclasts debris is taken up into the cytoplasm of macrophages.

7. Osteogenic cells are formed only in the presence of a material known as the osteogenic factor. This is present in the calcifiable matrix which is formed by maturing cartilage cells, and by active osteoblasts which have been stimulated either during the process of enchondral ossification or by other osteoblasts. This osteogenic factor can diffuse for a short distance through the tissue.

8. Cell activity is influenced by the partial pressures of oxygen and carbon dioxide in the blood. Oxygen provides energy for cell activity, both for proliferation and for the production of intercellular matrices, and so a plentiful supply of oxygen favours osteoblast activity. The presence of excess carbon dioxide in the vicinity favours the change of cell contents from a gel consistency, as in osteoblasts, to a fluid consistency, as in osteoclasts.

9. The peptide and steroid anabolic hormones favour cell proliferation and osteoblast activity. Catabolic hormones cause osteogenic precursor cells to coalesce to form osteoclasts, and at the same time prevent the formation of osteoclasts from macrophages. The presence of parathyroid hormone is needed for macrophages to coalesce to form osteoclasts, and this parathyroid hormone action itself requires the presence of thyroid hormone.

10. Steroids show anabolic or anti-anabolic properties, according to whether or not they favour the production of intercellular matrices; catabolic or anti-catabolic properties according to their effect on the flexibility and mobility of cell membranes, and thus the rate and vigour of cell division, with catabolic decreasing and anti-catabolic increasing the mobility; and they also affect the properties of marrow cells so that, acting separately or in combination, they may alter the properties of each of the components of the circulating blood.

11. Vitamin C deficiency hinders the production of intercellular matrices, and also causes a laxity of the walls of sinusoid vessels.

12. Vitamin D excess weakens the gel structure of intercellular matrices, so

that they readily break down and calcify. A deficiency of vitamin D leads to too stable a matrix, particularly of the calcifiable matrix. As a result it fails to calcify and is more difficult to resorb than normal. Both a raised plasma cortisol level and the presence of phytic acid in the diet cause impaired absorption of vitamin D by the gut.

13. Vitamin A deficiency causes a distortion of the shapes of bones. Descriptions of the histological appearance of bones given by Sir Edward Mellanby are consistent with the hypothesis that vitamin A is necessary for the formation of osteoclasts from macrophages, but does not affect the formation of osteoclasts from osteogenic precursor cells.

14. Fluoride is another trace material for which there is an optimum concentration. It affects the formation of non-collagenous proteins. These are rather unstable in the absence of fluoride, and in the presence of increasing quantities of fluoride become increasingly stable. At a concentration of 25 ppm bone remodelling is hindered.

15. The underlying defect in osteogenesis imperfecta, which is partly under hormonal control, causes two abnormalities in osteogenic cell behaviour. Only partial cell differentiation takes place before matrix production, while the abnormal and chemically unstable matrix is itself formed prematurely. Granulation tissue and woven bone appear to be normal, and the ordinary bone approaches normal after adolescence.

5. MECHANICAL INFLUENCES

Mention has already been made of some of the effects that mechanical forces can have on bone and connective tissues. There are forces such as gravity to which the body is always subject, and it is a well-known fact that a person cannot be completely healthy without taking sufficient exercise. The dominant effects of exercise on the fibrous and connective tissues are on individual cells. Applied pressure can modify the behaviour of these cells, and consequently the intercellular matrices they produce. Inadequate or incorrect forces can lead to lesions such as prolapse of the intervertebral discs and osteoarthritis. In bone the mechanical effects are more concerned with blood flow and pressure, and the influence these have on bone function and removal. Exercise also reduces the level of cortisol in the blood during times of stress.

Other phenomena which come under this heading are the effects of those abnormal mechanical forces which result in trauma, so that this would seem to be the logical place to deal with some aspects of the behaviour of cells in wound healing and fracture healing.

Cartilage and Fibrous Tissue Metaplasia

In Chapter 1 evidence was mentioned which shows that cells of the cartilage and fibrous tissue series have flexible and mobile surfaces, and that this mobility enables an essential stage in the production of intercellular matrix to take place. Briefly, this sequence is:

(a) The formation within the cell of membranes commonly known as the endoplasmic reticulum. In the resting state of the cell such membranes are not found, but as soon as matrix production is imminent they are formed.

(b) These membranes of the endoplasmic reticulum are sometimes called "rough" membranes, whereas membranes of the cell surface and certain other membranes within the cell are "smooth" membranes. The rough membranes are concerned with protein production and the formation of the intercellular matrices, whereas smooth membranes are more concerned with ion transport within the cell and biotransformations affecting cell behaviour. The roughness is caused by small ribonucleic acid particles, the ribosomes, adhering to the membranes. These ribosomes are formed in the nucleolus, which is an extension of the cytoplasm located within the nucleus and joined to the remainder of the cytoplasm by a narrow channel. When formed the ribosomes migrate and attach themselves in regular sequence to the membranes of the endoplasmic reticulum. In cases when there has been a hindrance to the formation of these membranes, as in vitamin C deficiency and in some areas of tumours, prominent nucleoli are seen, packed with ribonucleic acid, while the matrix that is formed is of abnormal quality.

(c) Polymerization of the protein components of the intercellular matrix takes place in the vicinity of the ribosome-covered endoplasmic reticulum. These products then pass through that region of the cell known as the Golgi apparatus, it being here that there is evidence to suggest that the polysaccharide components of the matrix are added. Collagenous matrices also contain some lipid, but no evidence seems to be available yet about the stage at which this is added to the matrix. When all the components have been added the matrix proceeds towards the cell surface.

(d) Sectors of the surface of these connective tissue cells are normally in a state of motion, protruding and retracting. Ciné pictures have been taken of fibroblasts and cartilage cells in culture showing this process. At the time of protrusion the matrix is extruded from small openings in the surfaces. As was shown in Fig. 1.13 it is possible for the matrix to trap these cell processes in the extended position. When excess corticosteroids are present movement becomes more sluggish (Dougherty et al., 1961), and at the same time the properties of the extruded matrix show changes, which include altered staining properties (Fig. 3.18), and which are generally in the direction of greater chemical stability. The stability results in a greater difficulty of resorption, as was illustrated in Figs 3.19, 3.20, 3.21.

(e) After matrix production has ceased the endoplasmic reticulum disperses, and is not found in resting cells. The Golgi apparatus, however, has been reported as remaining intact. Possibly linked with this statement is evidence, not so well documented, but compatible with other available evidence, that cells maintain the quality of the matrix by a frequent renewal of the polysaccharides. When for any reason the gel structure of the matrix is broken down, it takes several days, and possibly 2 to 3 weeks, for the cells to renew the quality of the matrix, apparently by selective polysaccharide production.

(f) Where the matrix is extruded from the end of elongated cells the dominant product is an orientated collagen, and the fibrils originate at the cell surface. When the matrix is extruded from the sides of the cells, a cartilage type of matrix, or sometimes cell "capsules" are found. Here the evidence is in favour of the matrix being precipitated after it has been extruded.

Tensional forces acting on cells

With a mechanism of this type it is apparent that applied forces could affect cell behaviour by an action on either the outer cell membranes, or the intracytoplasmic membranes, or both. The result of tensional forces acting on flexible cells would be to elongate them, so that in regions of the body where such forces are operating, as in tendons or the annulus fibrosus of the intervertebral disc, orientated fibrous tissue is found. Movement along a substrate such as occurs in the invasion of a blood clot (Fig 1.2) also results in elongated cells. Figure 5.1 shows a

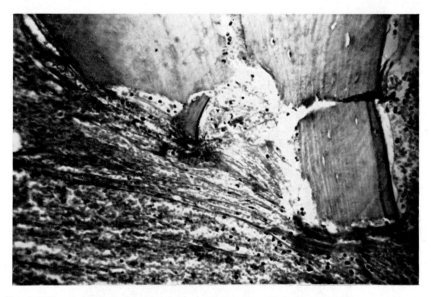

FIG. 5.1. Fractured head of femur removed at operation. Fibrin is arranged in strands in the recently formed clot near fragments of broken bone. × 100.

newly formed blood clot near fragments of broken bone in a fracture. The fibrin is organized in strands, and Fig. 5.2 is a later stage of a similar fracture with orientated fibrous tissue along what had been the fibrin direction in the clot. Figure 5.3 shows a cell migrating through loose tissue with a damaged gel structure. An active cell in such sites leaves behind a band of firm fibrous tissue which helps to provide a framework of greater mechanical strength in the tissue under repair.

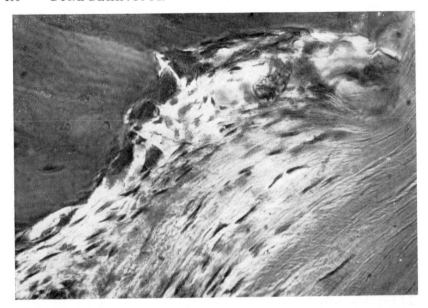

Fig. 5.2. A similar fractured head of femur removed at a later stage. Orientated fibrous tissue covers the bone fragments; it is arranged in a similar manner to the fibrin illustrated in Fig. 5.1. Multinucleated phagocytic cells are in the process of removing the dead bone. ×200.

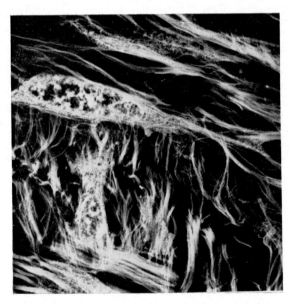

Fig. 5.3. Loose tissue near surface in an arthritic head of femur. A fibroblast is migrating through the tissue. E.M. 100kV. ×3000.

Compressive and rotational forces acting on cells

Where the forces are of a compressive and rotational nature, then rounded cells would be expected to result. These cells produce the cartilaginous type of matrix, containing unorientated collagen in a more or less tangled array. That a change in the shape of a cell is sufficient to cause a change in the type of intercellular matrix it produces is the reason that changes in applied physical forces can cause metaplastic changes in tissue structure and behaviour (Scapinelli and Little, 1970). Often this happens during the natural process of development. Tendons and ligaments, for example, have a cartilaginous appearance at their points of attachment to bone. Frequently also metaplastic changes occur during the course of processes that may be regarded as pathological, or as a part of the reaction of surrounding tissues to a pathological process. Figure 5.4 shows a change in the border of the annulus fibrosus of the

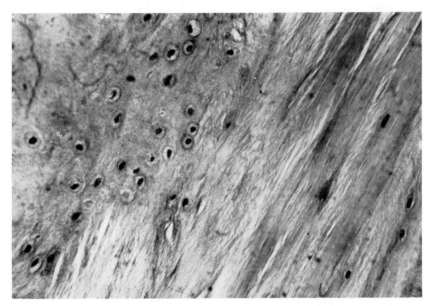

Fig. 5.4. Annulus fibrosus of intervertebral disc, near border with a partly degenerated nucleus pulposus. Towards the left of this area there are a group of cells more numerous than in the surrounding tissue, suggesting that some cell division has taken place. They show the characteristics of cartilage cells rather than of fibrous tissue cells. × 200.

intervertebral disc, apparently in response to a change in the mechanical stability of a neighbouring portion of the nucleus pulposus. Cells are closer together, suggesting that cell division has occurred, while they have surrounded themselves with a cartilaginous matrix, instead of the orientated collagenous matrix of the remainder of the annulus.

Another example, also from the lumbar spine, is a change which may take place in the interspinous ligaments. Starting at the opposite apophyseal insertions they may be partially changed to the more flexible fibrocartilage, and in some elderly subjects the whole inter-spinous space may be involved (Scapinelli, 1960a). In the cervical region, at the C5-C6 level, where the mobility of the neck is greatest, Scapinelli (1960b, 1963) has demonstrated in different subjects all the stages from a change from fibrous tissue to cartilage on the posterior border of the ligamentum flavum, through enchondral ossification to the formation of pathological bones with cortex and marrow cavity.

In the aorta there may be changes in the intima from fibrous tissue to cartilage. It is where this has happened that enchondral bone formation is found instead of the more usual pathological calcifications of necrotic tissue. There is at least one case on record where this cartilage, formed in the aorta of a young woman, proceeded on to the formation of a chondrosarcoma, which grew as a sausage down the lumen of the artery, and in due course interfered with the circulation to the legs (T. Edgington, 1963, pers. comm.).

Plastic implants in loose tissue can cause local trauma, and so become surrounded by fibrous scar tissue. Particularly near corners the motion may be such that patches of cartilage are formed, with the possibility of enchondral ossification. In rats, awkwardly shaped implants have caused repeated trauma with the eventual formation, not only of fibrosarcoma (Oppenheimer et al., 1958), but also of osteosarcoma (Alexander and Horning 1959), apparently derived from such patches.

Metaplastic change plays an important part in many repair mechanisms. For example, damaged articular cartilage is frequently covered or replaced by fibrous repair tissue (Fig. 5.5). With the resumption of normal cell nutrition this changes to fibrous tissue (Fig. 5.6), and if the forces acting on the joint are sufficiently normal it may then be converted to cartilage (Figs 5.7, 5.8). By the time the stage of Fig. 5.8 has been reached, even though the change to a true cartilage is not quite complete, the joint can function reasonably normally. This last example was from a joint where the defect was localized. The appearance of the section suggested a small area of healed avascular necrosis rather than osteoarthritis due to the general mechanics of the joint. Figure 5.9 is the final state, after 5 years, of repaired articular cartilage from a damaged elbow joint described by Jellinek (1955). Here an electrical injury had completely removed part of the cartilage from the underlying bone, which was exposed at the base of the wound. Joint function was restored after a little over a year and the smooth join between old and new cartilage allowed a complete range of movement. Figures 5.8, 5.9 represent two extremes in the range of appearances observed in healed

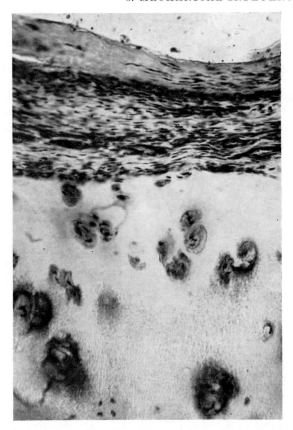

FIG. 5.5. The surface of damaged articular cartilage in a femoral head. It is covered by a layer of fibrous repair tissue which had spread from a defect. Cells in the cartilage have reacted to abnormal pressures, and are surrounded by heavily staining new matrix (haematoxylin). Some have divided to form small cell nests. × 100.

articular cartilage, the one having no cell nests and the other having very large cell nests. Appearances are usually somewhere between the two. Isolated cells are formed from fibrous repair tissue, and the cell nests by repeated division of cartilage cells. Figures 5.10, 5.11, 5.12 show in more detail stages in the transition of cell type caused by the application of compressional and rotational forces, from the fibrous tissue resulting from granulation tissue, and cells such as that shown in Fig. 5.3 to cells resembling those seen in the nucleus pulposus. These were taken from different areas in a partly formed pathological joint.

In addition to changes in the cell shape, with a transition from one mechanism of matrix production to another, the applied forces may also affect the performance of the membranes responsible for these two main

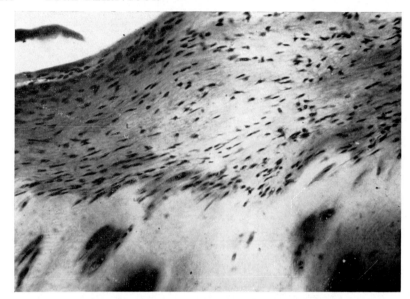

FIG. 5.6. A similar area of damaged articular cartilage. The surface layer of granulation tissue has matured to fibrous tissue. Surviving cells in the original cartilage are surrounded by new heavily staining inter-cellular matrix. × 100.

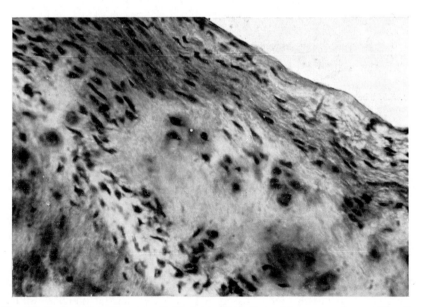

FIG. 5.7. Surface of cartilage in arthritic joint. Tissue formed from a previous proliferation of granulation tissue has been transformed to cartilage, and later abnormal pressures have caused these cartilage cells to extrude extra heavily staining matrix. A more recent proliferation of granulation tissue has matured to fibrous tissue. × 100.

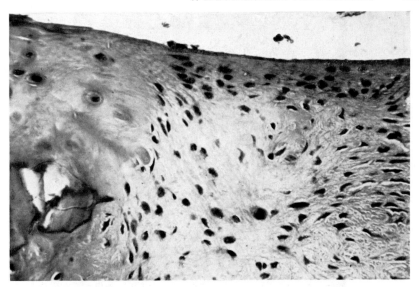

Fig. 5.8. Surface of articular cartilage. Edge of a healed localized defect. The surface level and texture have been restored, and the joint was functioning normally. Cells have the appearance of fibrocartilage, and this would appear to be a stage in the transition between fibrous tissue and true hyaline cartilage. Some of the original cartilage is seen on the left. ×100.

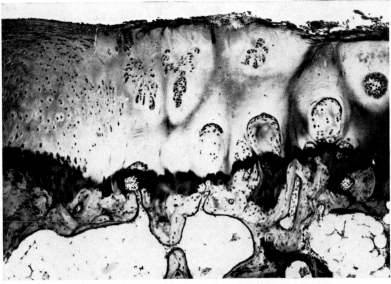

Fig. 5.9. Surface of healed articular cartilage. Cartilage had been stripped off the bone on the right as a result of an electrical injury. Comparatively little granulation tissue was formed, and cartilage thickness was restored by the formation of very large cell nests. Joint function was normal after a little over a year, and the figure shows the appearance of the cartilage at death 5 years later (diptheria). ×40. The author thanks the late Professor S. Jellinek for this photograph.

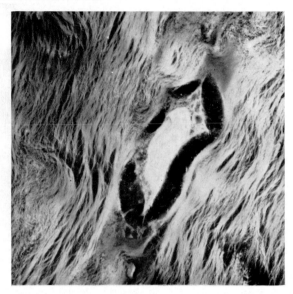

FIG. 5.10. Tissue from partly formed pathological joint. The intercellular matrix is that of fibrous tissue or fibrocartilage, while the cell has characteristics of fibrocartilage cells. The nucleus has a high electron density (and thus appears white in the photograph) indicating that it is in the predivision phase. E.M. 100kV. ×2600.

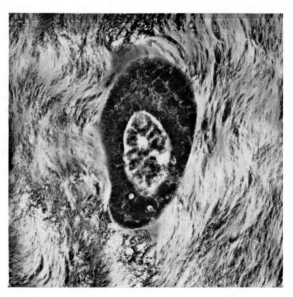

FIG. 5.11. An area a little nearer to the central part of the pathological joint. This cell is rounded, and has all the characteristics of a cartilage cell. E.M. 100kV. ×2600.

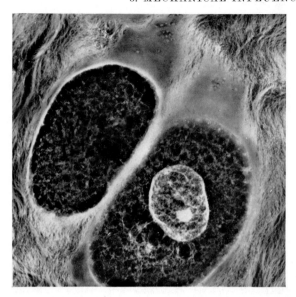

FIG. 5.12. An area in the part of the pathological joint with maximum rotary forces. Some small cell nests were present, and these cells show caps of non-collagenous material similar to those that are frequently found in cartilage cells in the intervertebral discs. E.M. 100kV. ×2600.

types of matrix. The membranes of the endoplasmic reticulum in a cell process such as that shown in Fig. 1.6, could not possibly remain undisturbed during the transition to a rounded state of the cell. What appears to happen in this situation is that as the previously elongated cells are gradually compressed attempts at matrix production from the ends become steadily more inefficient, until a "cap" containing grossly abnormal matrix forms at the ends of the cell. Figure 5.12 was an early example. Such cells are very commonly seen in the nucleus pulposus of the intervertebral disc (Fig. 2.27). The abnormal matrix, formed when comparatively large pressures have been operating, often contains small dense particles, whose nature has not yet been established (Fig. 5.13) although there is reason to think they are lipids which have been prevented from being incorporated in the normal manner.

The segments which extrude matrix from rounded cells do not protrude so far as the segments at the ends of cells, but their movement may also be harrassed by higher pressures. When this happens there is a change in the quality of the extruded matrix, and instead of collagen fibrils beta-proteins are produced. In the young these also have a gel structure, cell nests in the epiphyseal growth cartilage being one example, but once adolescence has been reached they normally have a rubber-like texture. In areas of lesser pressure the rubber-like protein

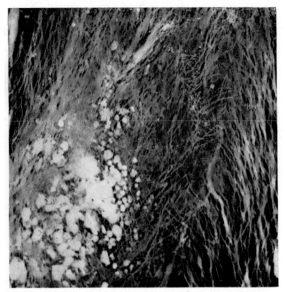

Fig. 5.13. Section through the non-collagenous cap adjacent to a cartilage cell in the inter-vertebral disc of an elderly subject. Particularly in the elderly, this material frequently contains small dense granules. E.M. 100kV. ×3500.

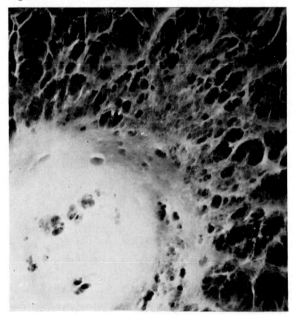

Fig. 5.14. Section through intercellular matrix in prolapsed lumbar disc tissue, closely adjacent to a cell. The rubber-like beta-protein has been extruded by the cell, together with a few collagen fibrils. The latter give the appearance of having been formed in the early stages. E.M. 100kV. ×3500.

may be mixed with collagen (Fig. 1.27) but where the pressure is greatest almost the whole of the extruded matrix may be in the form of the rubber-like beta-protein (Fig. 5.14). Being rubber-like, it can protect the cells from damage far more efficiently than do the gels in ordinary collagenous tissue, which are themselves subject to mechanical breakdown. Figure 5.15 shows undamaged cells, surrounded by the rubber-like beta-protein, at the edge of a necrotic area in the nucleus pulposus.

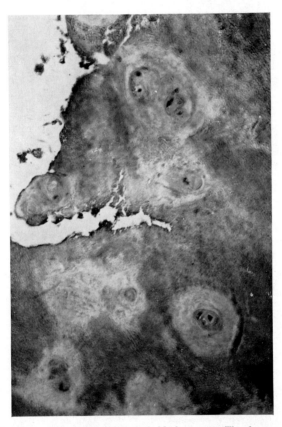

FIG. 5.15. Section through nucleus pulposus of elderly person. The dense rubber-like beta-protein is a dominant component of the matrix between cell nests. In this figure it is more darkly stained with silver than the mature beta-protein of the cell nests. Top left: the edge of a necrotic area. Cells protected by the beta-protein, even though close to the edge, remain undamaged. × 100.

When the change of force has been fairly abrupt, previously resting cells are stimulated to matrix production, cell division, or both. This is most probably mediated by a breakdown of the gel in their immediate vicinity releasing chemicals which activate the process. Figure 5.16 is

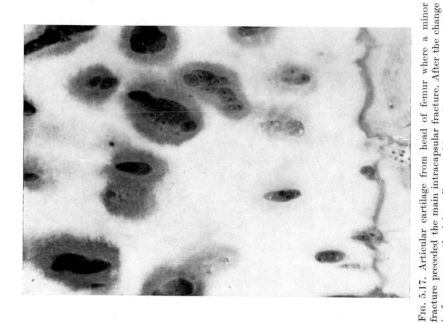

Fig. 5.17. Articular cartilage from head of femur where a minor fracture preceded the main intracapsular fracture. After the change in forces across the joint cells reacted by producing new intercellular matrix, which is heavily stained. ×200.

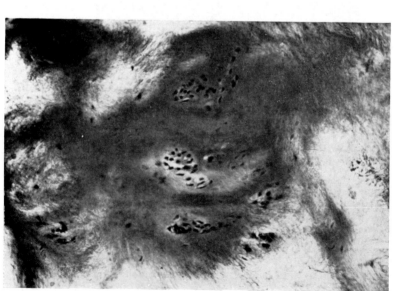

Fig. 5.16. Section through tissue of lumbar prolapse. Cell nests are surrounded by newly formed mature beta-protein, which during the period immediately after extrusion takes up haematoxylin. ×100.

taken from prolapsed intervertebral disc tissue, and shows both cell nests and an expanse of the rubber-like matrix surrounding them. Heavier staining here indicates the presence of comparatively new matrix. Its identity as a matrix containing a very high proportion of the rubber-like beta-protein was established by X-ray diffraction. A survey using X-ray fibre diffraction has shown that prolapsed lumbar disc tissue is the best source of the mature beta-protein; the presence of some collagen is almost inevitable, but it is virtually unmixed with the other beta-proteins (Taylor and Little, 1965). Figure 5.17 is another example of pressure-stimulated matrix production, this time taken from articular cartilage. A histological examination of the whole section suggested that changes in applied forces were the result of a minor fracture preceding an

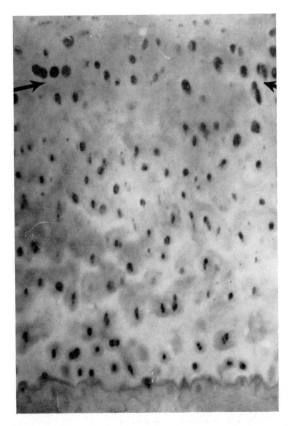

FIG. 5.18. A similar head of femur from a case of post-menopausal osteoporosis. High cortisol levels over an extended period had resulted in the formation of more stable cartilage matrix than usual. In this section only a single row of cells (arrowed) a little below the articulating surface have reacted to form additional beta-protein. × 100.

intracapsular fracture in the head of the femur. Where the new matrix is rubber-like, cells may well survive additional compressive forces. When this new matrix formation occurs at a time when there is an episode involving a high level of catabolic steroids, the hormonal background also contributes to the stability of the matrix. Early stages of the process have been followed in cartilage of the head of the femur where this has been removed following an intra-capsular fracture, and also in cases of Paget's disease with bone involvement fairly close to the joint. Figure 2.26 showed well established stable protein whereas Fig. 5.17 shows it heavily staining when newly laid down. The stain in these instances was haematoxylin, which combines mainly with phosphate or sulphate groups that may be attached to either protein molecules or their accompanying polysaccharides. Again, the use of X-ray fibre

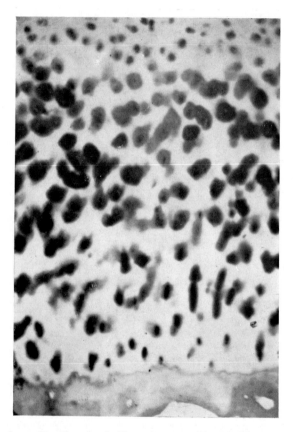

FIG. 5.19. Articular cartilage from head of femur in a case of Paget's disease, after bone changes close to the joint had altered the forces across the joint. Cells in almost the whole thickness of the cartilage have reacted to produce new more resilient matrix. ×100.

diffraction helps to clarify the situation. Alternatively, the blue auto-fluorescence of unstained sections may be observed.

The result of further compression and rotary pressure on a stable cartilage is shown in Fig. 5.18, where only a row of cells a little below the surface of the cartilage have produced additional matrix, although some cell division may be seen near the base of the cartilage. In a cartilage, previously of gel type, new matrix may be formed all through the cartilage (Fig. 5.19). Where the forces are not suitable, as at the edge of the weight-bearing zones, the new matrix may be formed through only a part of the thickness of the cartilage (Fig. 5.20). A further abrupt force,

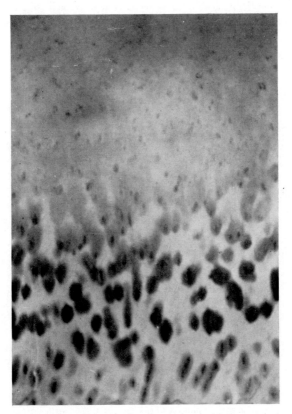

FIG. 5.20. Articular cartilage from new weight-bearing zone in arthritic head of femur. The cells in the inner part of this cartilage have reacted to form the resilient matrix component, but forces on cells in the outer part of the cartilage were unsuitable. This matrix has partially lost its gel structure, so that the cells in the outer cartilage are vulnerable to even minor trauma. × 100.

of traumatic type, would then result in the death of the unprotected cells. It is usually observed that the inner cells are better protected than those near the surface of the cartilage. Figure 5.18 showed that only a zone fairly near the surface required extra protection, and in the early stages of osteoarthritis this is frequently the level at which cell death is first observed.

In the young, there is a definite zone containing stem cells which acts as a "germinal zone" for the articular cartilage. It is at first well separated from the germinal zone of the secondary bone nucleus but at a later stage of development the two bands of cells merge (Rigal, 1961b). In the adult cell proliferation and renewal of the articular cartilage continues as required, but there is no evidence of any zone of stem cells remaining. Instead cell proliferation occurs as a result of stimulation of cells by breakdown products of the intercellular matrix. This means, in practice, that it occurs when and where it is most required, which may be at any depth in the cartilage. Sometimes it is in the inner zone, while Fig. 5.21

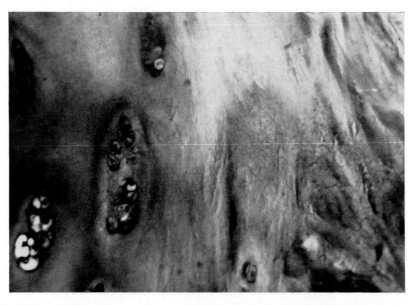

Fig. 5.21. Articular cartilage at edge of arthritic lesion. To the right is the arthritic cartilage, containing dead cells, and with collagen fibrils orientated in the direction of the prevailing dominant applied forces, almost normal to the surface of the cartilage. The edge of the more normal cartilage is seen to the left. Cells have proliferated to form cell nests, and new polysaccharide-containing matrix has formed around them. This area was half way through the cartilage. ×200.

is an example taken almost exactly at the mid-point of the cartilage at the end of an arthritic region. Fig. 5.22 shows vigorous cell proliferation with cell nest formation near the surface of the cartilage.

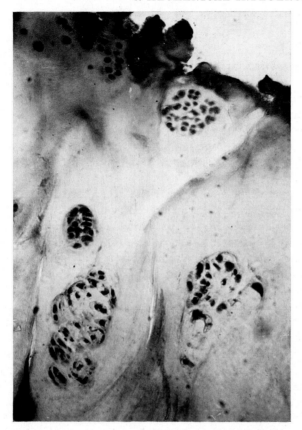

FIG. 5.22. Damaged surface of articular cartilage. A proportion of the cells have died, while the remaining cartilage cells have proliferated to form cell nests. ×200.

Sheer forces

So far the effect of tensional forces, and then of compressional and rotary forces has been considered. There is a further modification of tissue behaviour when a sheer force is applied to cartilage, in addition to the compressive and rotary forces. The cartilage then tends to separate into two, with flattened cells first forming and then separating as new surface layers, and the result is a synovial joint. Such joint formation is fairly common in non-union of fractures, and may also be found between the spinous processes of the lumbar vertebrae with increasing lordosis. The sequence of events is similar to that seen in joints in the developing foetus (Figs 2.2, 2.3, 2.4). The stimulus for the formation of the synovial membrane, with secretion of synovial fluid, is not yet known.

Blood Flow

In cartilage, with flexible cells and matrix, the influence of applied forces is felt directly by the cells. For bone, with a considerably more rigid intercellular matrix, the dominant influence of applied forces is indirect, and changes are mediated by alterations in the blood flow and pressure. One way that this can happen was described in the last chapter—the influence of pressure on the extremely flexible sinusoid vessel walls helps to determine the direction of the main weight-bearing trabeculae.

Trueta and others have shown that there are two main pumping mechanisms which propel the blood through the bones. If one considers the long bones, then the first part of the circulation depends upon the systolic blood pressure and the calibre of the arteries. The main artery is the nutrient artery, which has a muscular layer, so that its diameter is under nervous control. Other arteries enter the epiphyseal regions. These vessels break up into smaller branches, and the blood passes into the sinusoid network. Here at any one time when the flow is normal only about a tenth of the vessels are open (Johnson, 1964). Changes occur rhythmically ever one or two minutes. The pressure in the diaphysis is slightly higher than in the metaphysis. Blood passes back to a central collecting vein, but then disperses again, with many small branches passing into the cortex from the inner side. Outside the cortex the blood collects into larger veins. In the human the action of the muscles in pumping blood out through these veins is of almost equal importance with the arterial action in maintaining adequate circulation. The situation is in some ways analogous to the manner in which movement of the diaphragm helps to maintain flow upwards through the vena cava. de Valderrama and Trueta (1965) have measured the pressure within the bone in the dog's tibia, and Shaw (1966) has carried out similar measurements in the cat's femur. When the muscles contract the pressure within the bone builds-up, then at the end of the contraction there is a sudden fall of marrow pressure to near zero values. This lasts only a fraction of a second, and suggests that the muscles have exerted a suction effect on the marrow bed, which is of great assistance in ensuring a refill by newly oxygenated blood. The main effect of the muscles, then, is that contraction blocks the venous outflow, and next, following the sudden short-lived drop of pressure, vascular engorgement ceases as the muscles become inactive.

Two situations require further consideration, the effect when muscle activity is grossly diminished or ceases, and the effect of very vigorous muscle activity. In the first there is for a time a gradual build-up of

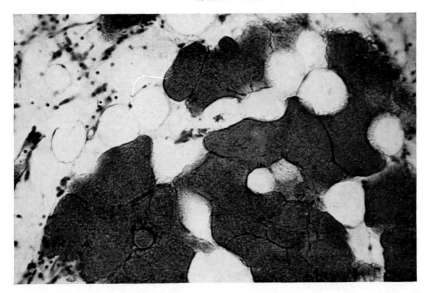

Fig. 5.23. Open sinusoids in marrow of osteoporotic bone. These sinusoids are filled with Micropaque/Berlin blue perfusion medium. The appearance of the section suggests that in this type of situation the blood is stagnant. This would allow a build-up of carbon dioxide, which causes sinusoid vessel walls to relax. $\times 200$.

marrow pressure, with many open sinusoids (Fig. 5.23). In this Figure the open sinusoids are filled with Micropaque/Berlin blue perfusion medium. Appearances suggest that in this type of situation the blood becomes stagnant so that there is no new bone formation analogous to the remodelling of the weight-bearing trabeculae (e.g. Fig. 4.15). Neither is there the type of cell proliferation and activity seen when there is a vigorous flow of blood, as in the large number of vessels sometimes seen in an active response in osteoarthritis. (In Fig. 5.24, taken from an arthritic head of femur, there are many open vessels, but with a different appearance from the sinusoids of the bone marrow, and surrounded by actively proliferating cells and new bone formation.) The period, after muscle activity ceases, during which there is an elevated marrow pressure, lasts about three weeks. During this time some of the vascular channels through the cortex become enlarged, as a result of osteoclast activity. As in normal osteonal remodelling, there is a proliferation of vessels with ahead of them a "cutting-cone" of osteoclasts (Fig. 5.25). Unlike osteonal remodelling, the channels through the cortex remain wide. When these enlarged channels reach the outer surface (Fig. 5.26 shows the boring process almost completed) then the pressure is released and the bone settles down to normal activity, but with a smaller quantity of bone.

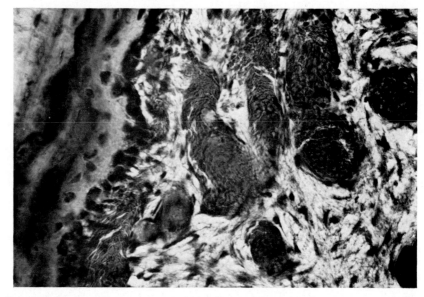

FIG. 5.24. Section through arthritic head of femur. In the areas of bone activity there are many open blood vessels, surrounded by active proliferating cells and new bone formation (left). ×200.

Disuse osteoporosis, then, is the result of bone resorption which removes obstacles and so releases the pressure caused by a lower rate of flow, together with a failure to lay down new bone, as a result of diminution in flow rate. In contrast to this, where there is a vigorous muscle action, there follows a vigorous osteogenic activity, with frequent remodelling and usually a fairly vascular bone. Figures 5.27, 5.28 show two extremes in the spine. Figure 5.27 is from the lumbar spine of an old man, with the typical ballooned disc of osteoporosis, accompanied by very little bone in the walls of the vertebrae. Figure 5.28 is a portion of the wall of the vertebra from one of the most muscular of all animals, a dinosaur. It is healthy compact bone, but noticeably more vascular than any normal human bone.

A raised blood flow stimulates osteonal remodelling. This remodelling is essential for the formation of healthy bone with adequate mechanical strength. Normally it is found that in the cortex of the main weight-bearing bones remodelling of the original lamellar bone is completed soon after adolescence. In the child the cortical bone is all lamellar bone. Then as development takes place there is osteonal remodelling, starting at those sites where there is greatest muscular activity. The last part of the tibia to be involved in remodelling is at the upper end of the bone where there is little muscular cover, and just beyond the last of the internal

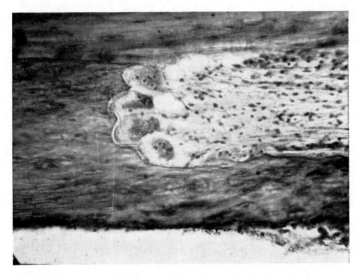

FIG. 5.26. A cutting cone of osteoclasts in a channel almost parallel to the periosteal surface (left). From another rabbit in the same experiment as illustrated in Fig. 5.25. ×100.

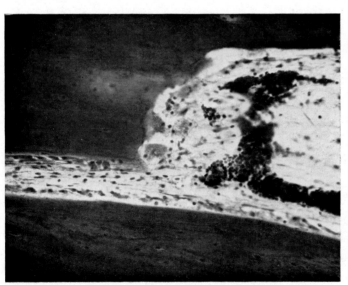

FIG. 5.25. Cortical bone in experimental animal. Surrounding muscles were inactivated by removing a section of the Achilles tendon. A vascular channel is being widened by a "cutting-cone" of osteoclasts. Behind these are proliferating vessels. ×100.

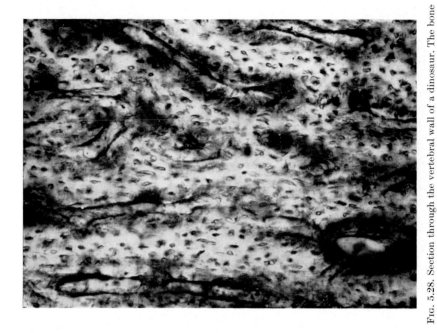

Fig. 5.28. Section through the vertebral wall of a dinosaur. The bone contains a higher proportion of vascular channels than is normal in compact bone of smaller less muscular vertebrates. ×100.

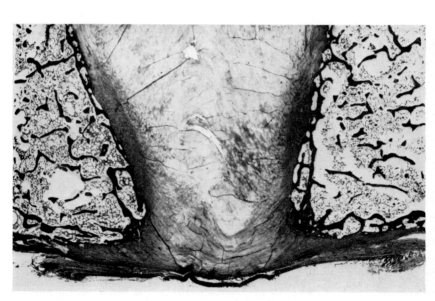

Fig. 5.27. Section through the lumbar spine of an old man, with the typical ballooned disc of osteoporosis. The walls of the two vertebrae (top left and bottom left) contain very little of the bone tissue (darkly

bracing trabeculae of the metaphyseal cancellous bone. Certain Marines have provided an object lesson on the mechanisms involved when bone is subjected to a sudden increase of muscular activity and consequently blood flow (Johnson *et al.*, 1963). It so happened that before these Marines started their period of intensive training they had had little exercise for several years, so that remodelling of the last portion of the tibia to osteonal bone had not yet taken place. It will be remembered, too, that osteones usually develop at places in bone where there are pressures that could disrupt the membrane covering the bone surfaces. The sudden increase of violent exercise therefore stimulated osteone formation in the region of lamellar bone. The timing, however, is such that whereas it takes about a week to produce resorption cavities during osteone formation, it takes about three months to fill them in (Johnson, 1964). These Marines therefore developed a localized osteoporosis. But the pressures involved were sufficient also to disrupt some of the thin-walled vessels emerging from the bone. The sequence of periosteal events were then the same as those which will be described in the next section for fracture healing, with ruptured vessels, clot formation, granulation tissue proliferation and callus formation. Symptoms were apparent in the second week, and reached a maximum at six weeks. At about three weeks the cortex became sufficiently porotic for pathological fractures to develop—that is, after there was already an abundance of "fracture callus". At one stage an epidemic of osteosarcoma was suspected!

This was not the most usual site for "march" fractures. Bones in the feet are more commonly affected. Which bone shows the changes is mainly dependent on the type of drill. "Let me hear the left on every 4th" has produced stress fractures of the left metatarsal, while with "Let me hear those heels dig in" the oscalcis was the site of fracture (Gilbert and Johnson, 1966). In these bones also the onset of symptoms was during the second and third weeks of training, with a few in the fourth and fifth weeks and none afterwards. As with the tibia a previous lack of exercise had prevented normal bone remodelling and development. Those who had failed to take part in normal school athletics or any other form of physical activity were the individuals affected. It is thus apparent that without adequate exercise in childhood and adolescence bone remodelling is hindered. Such bone defects could provide a substantial contribution to osteoporotic and osteoarthritic processes later in life.

Trauma

Some of the effects of trauma, and the reactions of cartilage and bone during the healing process have been mentioned in the last two sections.

In bone, trauma may be either extensive with displacement, bleeding and clot formation, or may affect only a small number of trabeculae and without any spectacular displacement. Minor breaks and cracks occur chiefly in weight-bearing bones, in sites such as the lumbar spine and the head of femur, when the total quantity of bone has been diminished during the osteoporotic process, and when death of cells and subsequent embrittlement of their surroundings takes place in the remaining bone. Sometimes only a single trabecula may be involved. Figure 5.29 shows fracture callus on the surface of an isolated trabecula in the head of femur from an elderly woman. Occasional healed trabecular fractures may also be seen near "ballooned" intervertebral discs. Rather more drastic is the production of a crush fracture of the type shown in Fig. 5.30. Here the recently formed fracture callus and the original very rarified

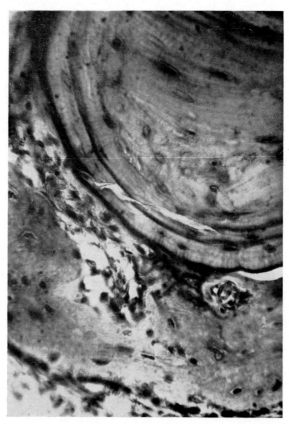

Fig. 5.29. Fracture callus on the surface of a trabecula in the head of femur from an elderly woman. Surrounding trabeculae were undamaged. Another more recent crack may be seen in the bone. × 200.

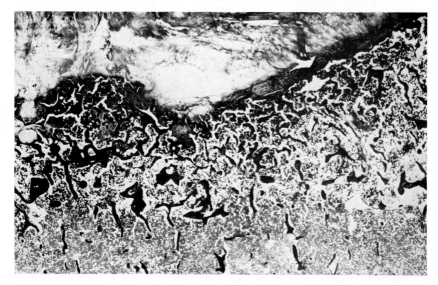

Fɪɢ. 5.30. A fairly recent crush fracture in the osteoporotic vertebra of an old man. The junction between the partly healed bone containing fracture callus and new trabeculae, and the original bone with very few trabeculae is an almost horizontal line. The border of the disc tissue has also been damaged. ×35.

bone are separated by an almost horizontal line. Much of the new disc tissue has the appearance shown in Fig. 5.31 and contains an abundance of beta-protein. It is basically of the "fracture cartilage" type (see Figs 1.1, 1.3) although the pressures operating through the spinal column result in first beta-protein formation and later the dense beta-protein and elastin.

Major fractures, however, are invariably accompanied by bleeding, and organization of the clot (as illustrated in Figs 5.1, 5.2) is an integral part of the healing process. The healing mechanisms in an ordinary fracture are complex, but a general rule is that where there has been adequate clot formation there is an invasion of vessels and granulation tissue with direct formation of bone, but that where a space has been filled with fluid fracture cartilage is found (Fig. 1.1) which is later converted to bone by enchondral ossification (Fig. 4.1). Fracture healing is thus dependent on the time when the bone is immobilized, and on the distribution of the remaining intact blood supply. Experimental bone defects, without displacement, have been used by Kemp (1965–66) to elucidate details of the early part of the process, and of the effect of anticoagulants at this stage. In the early stages of clot formation, the direction of precipitated fibrin tends to be along the "lines of force" in the gel, apparently produced as a result of shrinkage. The subsequent

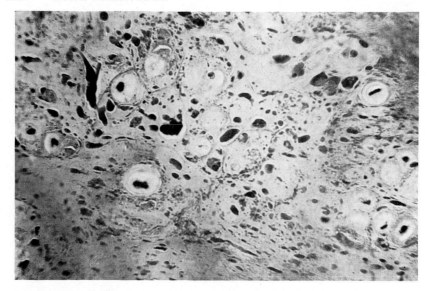

Fig. 5.31. Repair tissue in a ballooned intervertebral disc. The dominant beta-protein is elastin, which can be seen spread through the tissue. × 100.

vascular invasion from the periphery follows these same lines, so that with a symmetrical defect there is a symmetrical arrangement of the vessels. In the defect shown in Fig. 5.32 the clot had adhered to the periosteal surface of the bone in the area illustrated, so that the row of vessels which has penetrated the clot is shown in parallel array on the right. On the left, where the raised periosteum still remains, the vascular array is somewhat less regular. Shortly afterwards a suitable plane of section reveals a very regular arrangement of new bone around the parallel array of vessels (Fig. 5.33).

For the invasion of the clot by vessels and granulation tissue, the texture needs to be that of a loose gel. In Fig. 5.34 such a gel is shown, of necessity after having been dried. Penetrating vessels are filled with perfusion medium. In haemophilia, or after the administration of an anticoagulant the blood settles out into a dense non-fibrous solid separated from the fluid. Vessels then have difficulty in penetrating. Figure 5.35 shows success only around the periphery of a clot in a fracture produced while the animal was on anticoagulants. When anticoagulants are given to patients for any reason, wound healing as well as fracture healing is affected, the extent being partly dependent upon the dose. Figures 5.36, 5.37, 5.38 show appearances in a section of scar tissue, taken after three weeks on anticoagulant therapy. The development of fibrous tissue shown in Fig. 5.36 is comparatively normal, but

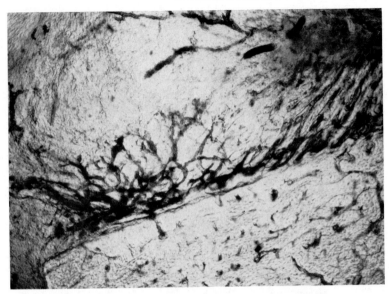

Fig. 5.32. The edge of a defect cut in bone (bottom left), cortical bone (bottom third). At the time the defect was cut a blood clot formed between the periosteal surface of the bone and the overlying tissue. New vessels have followed the direction of fibrin strands in the clot. On the right they are in parallel array. ×100. The author thanks Mr. H. B. S. Kemp for this photograph.

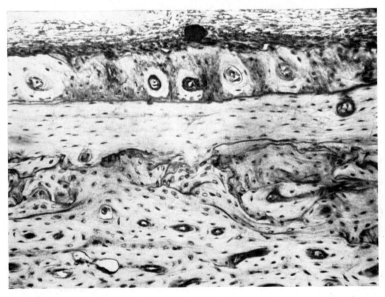

Fig. 5.33. A later stage of repair. The new periosteal bone, near the top, is uniformly arranged around a series of parallel vessels. ×100. The author thanks Mr H. B. S. Kemp for this photograph.

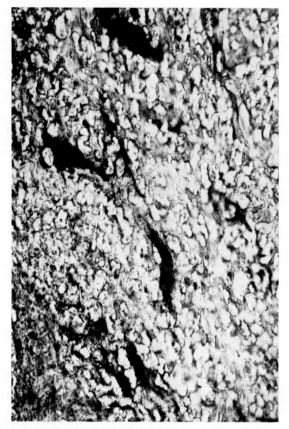

Fig. 5.34. A normal blood clot is in the form of a loose gel, and the first stage of repair is the penetration of blood vessels through this gel. Here these vessels are filled with perfusion medium. ×200. The author thanks Mr. H. B. S. Kemp for this photograph.

Fig. 5.37 5.38 each show an area containing fragments of clot too dense for adequate cell penetration.

In brief, the main sequence of events in normal fracture healing are:

(*a*) Organization of clot.
(*b*) Vascular invasion of the clot.
(*c*) Proliferation of granulation tissue.

This is followed by:

(*d*) Woven bone formation.
(*e*) More vessels penetrate the granulation tissue and/or woven bone with the formation of irregularly arranged normal bone.

Alternatively, where a fluid space has resulted, without the gel formation of a normal clot, the sequence is:

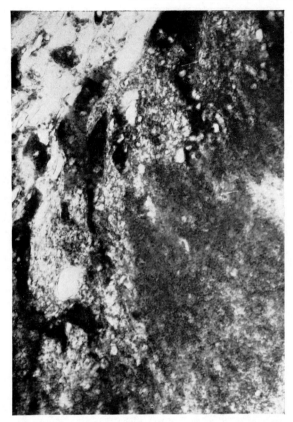

FIG. 5.35. Blood does not clot normally after the administration of an anticoagulant, but tends to separate into a fairly dense non-fibrous solid and a fluid. The solid phase is too dense for blood vessels to penetrate. In a rabbit, which had been given a high does of anticoagulant, vessels have only succeeded in penetrating the surface layers of the clot. ×200. The author thanks Mr. H. B. S. Kemp for this photograph.

(*f*) Formation of fracture cartilage, then—
(*g*) Enchondral ossification, with penetration of vessels and the formation of irregularly arranged normal bone.

In either case there is then—

(*h*) Gradual degradation of dead bone, followed by its removal by multinucleated cells (Fig. 4.31) and macrophages (Figs 5.39, 5.40). As with macrophages removing debris from soft tissue areas (Fig. 5.41) those found in the marrow can be of very variable size.
(*i*) Remodelling, which is dependent on the applied mechanical forces and also on the surrounding blood supply.

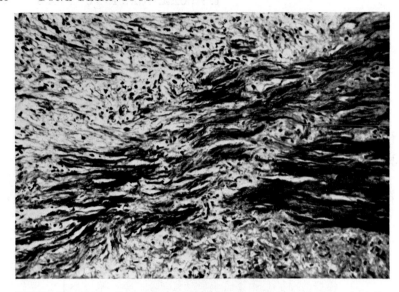

FIG. 5.36. Section of scar tissue from patient, after three weeks on anticoagulant therapy. This area presents a normal appearance. Granulation tissue is maturing to fibrous tissue, and the section has been stained to show mature collagen fibrils. × 100.

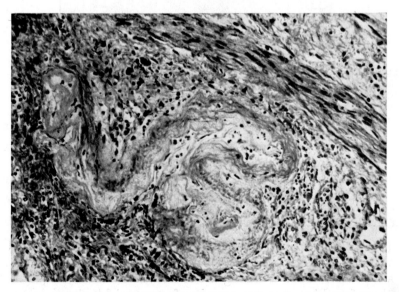

FIG. 5.37. Another area from the same section as Fig. 36. Here there is a small patch where the clot solidified abnormally. Fewer cells have been able to penetrate, and in the surrounding tissue fewer mature collagen fibrils have formed. × 100.

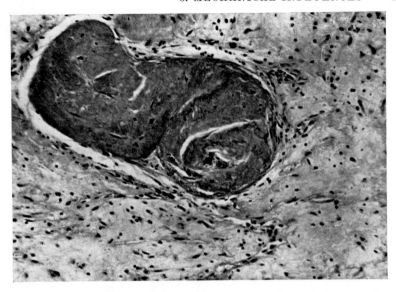

Fig. 5.38. The most abnormal part of the section. A lump of clot through which cells have been almost unable to penetrate. ×100. The author thanks Mr. J. R. P. Gibbons for the material from which these photographs were taken.

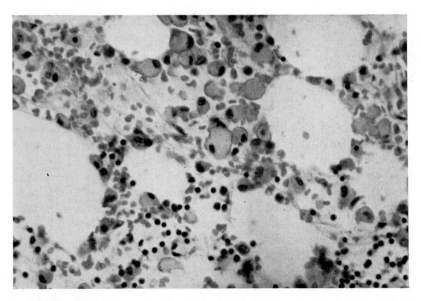

Fig. 5.39. Macrophages removing dead tissue from the vicinity of an infarct. A few fat cells (white spaces) and marrow cells can be seen. The macrophages have very variable sizes. ×200.

Q

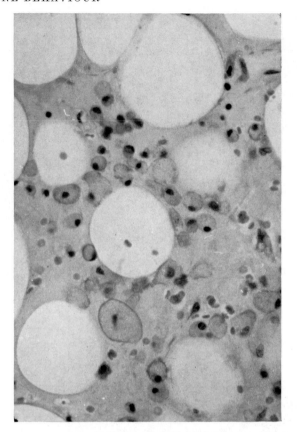

Fig. 5.40. Macrophages removing dead tissue from the vicinity of an infarct. The lesion has hindered circulation in the surrounding bone, and solids have been deposited from serum which has diffused from neighbouring vessels. ×200.

The whole of this sequence is dependent on vascular proliferation, which can be hindered by displaced muscle, or any other natural or artificial barrier, and also by movement. The result of immediate movement is to hinder clot formation and the penetration of vessels, with the gradual formation of fracture cartilage. At a somewhat later stage fracture cartilage and granulation tissue may both be converted to a stable cartilage. Later still, continued excessive shear forces could result in the formation of a pathological synovial joint.

One further point that may be mentioned is the presence of mast cells. These are commonly found in the vicinity of healing fractures, in the vicinity of minor fractures in the vertebral bodies and in the vicinity of active osteoarthritic lesions. They have also been observed in considerable numbers in some cases of fibrosarcoma. The common

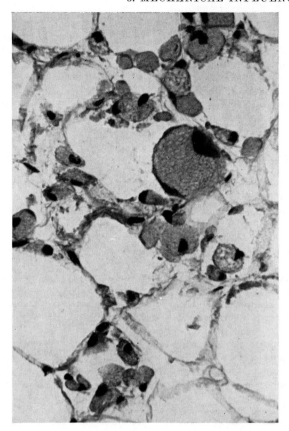

Fig. 5.41. Macrophages in fatty tissue near an operation site. They are of very variable size, apparently according to the quantity of debris they contain. ×400.

factor in all these sites is that there is an unusually prolific vascular array with a good blood flow, which is in excess of what might be expected from the combined action of systolic pressure and surrounding muscle activity. These mast cells secrete heparin, so that one might assume that their presence is associated with the need for maintaining an unhindered blood flow. The mechanism of their formation is at present quite unknown, although their distribution suggests that the stimulus for their formation is related to the stimuli that activate the formation of repair tissue.

Summary

1. The proteins of intercellular matrices are formed on the endoplasmic reticulum within cells, then extruded through sectors of the cell surfaces which

protrude and later retract. In general, fibrous matrices are extruded at the ends of elongated cells and cartilaginous matrices at the sides of more rounded cells.

2. Tensional forces acting on a tissue cause elongation of cells, and compressive and rotational forces result in rounded cells. A change in the applied forces can result in a change of shape of a cell, and therefore of the type of matrix that it produces. Metaplastic changes in tissue type and behaviour result.

3. Greater pressures affect the quality of the matrix being extruded, with the rubber-like beta-proteins being formed instead of collagen, while cell capsules are also formed. The rubbery matrix is a more efficient protection for the cells against mechanical trauma than are the gel–type matrices.

4. With a change in the forces acting on a tissue, cells are stimulated to matrix formation, cell division, or both. This is the basis of repair mechanisms in cartilage. Metaplastic changes are then an essential stage, when granulation tissue is converted first to fibrous tissue and then to cartilage.

5. When metaplastic changes are to cartilage, these changes may progress to pathological calcification and bone formation. Too great a pressure results in cell death and the formation of necrotic tissue.

6. Whereas changed forces act directly on cells in cartilage, it is the blood flow that is chiefly affected in bone. This flow is maintained partly by the pumping action from the heart, and partly by that due to muscle activity around the bone.

7. When muscle activity is decreased there is initially an increased marrow pressure. This stimulates bone removal, but without a sufficient blood flow to stimulate new bone formation, so that a condition of "disuse" osteoporosis results.

8. With a sudden increase in muscle activity after a period of inactivity, the rate of bone removal as a result of the initiation of osteonal remodelling is greater than the rate of new bone formation, so that the bone becomes temporarily more porotic. In the case of young adults who have had too little exercise during the period of growth, so that replacement of lamellar bone by osteonal bone is incomplete, "stress' fractures may result.

9. In osteoporotic bone minor stresses sometimes result in small breaks or cracks that may sometimes affect only a single trabecula. A series of such minor fractures in the vertebrae often precede the "ballooning" of the intervertebral discs.

10. The sequence of events in normal fracture healing are: organization of clot, vascular invasion, proliferation of granulation tissue, woven bone formation, remodelling to normal bone; or formation of fracture cartilage in fluid spaces without gelatinous clot, followed by enchondral ossification and then remodelling.

11. In the presence of anticoagulants, or in haemophilia, clot formation is often hindered or abnormal, with subsequent irregularities in the healing process.

6. HORMONES AND STEROIDS

In the preceding chapters hormones have rather been taken for granted. They control the quality of the intercellular matrices; they play a prominent part in all the changes in the ageing process, with growth, adolescence, maturity, the menopause and the approach to old age all under hormonal control; and temporary hormone imbalance plays an important part in the diseases that result from social stresses. The bones are closely involved in all these activities. Their main structural materials are the intercellular matrices; there are changes in the quality, quantity and distribution of all components at the main hormonal epochs; and these components are affected by many types of stress. Pathological changes may be directly on the bone, as in the production of osteoporosis; or the bones may mediate changes in other organs and tissues, because the megakaryocytes which produce the platelets that take part in thrombus formation are formed in the bone marrow.

The actions and interactions of hormones are complex. Each has a number of quite distinct actions, which are modified by interaction with other hormones, and also by interactions with their target cells. Enlightenment may sometimes be obtained by comparing the actions of natural hormones with those of synthetic compounds having related structure and behaviour. In this present chapter bone will be the centre of the discussion, but in order to preserve a balanced picture some of the effects which impinge only indirectly on the bone must be mentioned.

The hormones are in two distinct groups, those which are basically peptides, and the steroids. Only a small range of their mechanisms will be discussed. The androgenic activity and actions of the steroids on the reproductive system are outside the scope of this book. Although somewhat more relevant, water and salt balance, blood pressure and hypertension are also omitted. Steroid effects on the liver, however, cannot be ignored.

There are frequent species differences in the behaviour of the tissues towards vitamins and hormones. In particular the rat and birds have quite different hormone systems, so that although a comparison between species is a legitimate subject for the zoologist to study, it must be remembered that results obtained with the rat may well be irrelevant if the species of interest happens to be the human. In other species, differences appear to be more important for the peptide hormones than for the steroids, although care in the choice of experimental animal is also needed for investigations of the latter. The rabbit is one of the most suitable experimental animals for the investigation of steroid hormone interactions.

The peptide hormones are, so far as bone is concerned, primarily of interest in the young, and so they will be considered first. From adolescence onwards it is the steroid effects which dominate.

The Peptide Hormones

Interactions

Although to some extent and so far as bone is concerned the actions of the steroids may be considered independently of other hormone actions, except possibly for insulin, the actions of these other compounds are closely inter-related.

Insulin and vasopressin influence membrane transport processes, and as with the steroids there is evidence that the action of the peptide hormones is primarily on cell membranes (Hechter, 1955). In tissue culture experiments on mammary glands Prop (1961, 1965) found that hormones could only exert their effects on the glands in the presence of insulin. Although growth hormone needs the presence of insulin before it can act on cells, the growth hormone itself acts on those pancreatic beta cells which produce insulin, so that for any given concentrations of glucose in the body more growth hormone causes more insulin to be secreted (Campbell and Rastogi, 1966, 1967). In accord with this, high concentrations of insulin in the plasma and serum have been observed in gigantism and acromegaly. Similarly, the nitrogen-retention action of growth hormone appears to be associated with an increased requirement for insulin (Manchester and Young, 1961).

With administration of growth hormone there is a rise in serum insulin prior to a significant increase in serum glucose, but the blood sugar itself is one of the regulators for insulin production. In general it is found that the rate of insulin secretion is a continuous function of the blood sugar level (Metz, 1960). Since insulin is essential for the normal metabolism of carbohydrates, fats and proteins, low blood sugar levels lead to an inadequate human performance. Alcohol tends to induce hypoglycaemia, and it has been found that a combination of fasting and alcohol produce a very marked lowering of performance (Plechus, Chandler and Ellis, 1966).

Another group of hormone interactions involve the thyroid and parathyroid glands. Here there are three hormones to be considered, the parathyroid hormone, thyroxin and calcitonin. It has been thought that calcitonin and the parathyroid hormone provided a control for plasma calcium levels, by some action on the mineral stored in bones. This was based on experimental observations that the release of each is dependent on small changes in the calcium ion levels in the blood. It was therefore thought that a "feedback" mechanism operated. A significant action was observed in 5–10 min with the maximum effect at 20–30 min (Copp, 1964). There is now incontrovertible evidence in that the human calcitonin does not control plasma calcium (Cunliffe *et al.*, 1968), and a considerable volume of evidence that bone formation and resorption do not affect plasma calcium levels.

One piece of evidence that has been misinterpreted from time to time is that growing animals on a calcium-deficient diet become osteoporotic. Scott *et al.* (1961) and Scott (1968) have now gone a considerable way towards elucidating this mechanism. They showed that in calcium deficiency the thyroid and parathyroid glands are enlarged, but that the thyroid glands, although large, show atrophy and fibrosis and are thyroxin deficient. Without thyroid activity the full parathyroid effect on bone is prevented. They then investigated the bones and found a histological picture closely resembling that produced by corticosteroids (Kayanja *et al.*, 1965), so that there is a high probability that the osteoporosis found is primarily an adrenal effect induced by the other abnormalities. Other vitamin and hormone abnormalities have also been observed to show effects consistent with a raised plasma cortisol being a factor involved. For instance, in vitamin D poisoning, involving hypercalcaemia, the symptoms increase in pregnancy without a corresponding change in calcium levels. Pregnancy itself is known to involve an increased cortisol level.

In these fields there is still a great deal of work to be done before all the complications can be understood, but so far as bone is concerned they are of minor importance, and peptide hormone imbalance only rarely produces clinical symptoms. Other effects, such as those on the kidney, are considered to be outside the scope of this book.

Effect on cartilage

Both growth hormone and an intact thyroid are needed for the normal development of cartilage, but appear to have no specific effect on skeletal maturation. The growth hormone shows two distinct actions. It has an anabolic action in that it stimulates the production of proteins and polysaccharides, and it also stimulates the proliferation of stem cells in cartilage. The proteins and polysaccharides that are produced as a result of stimulation by growth hormone were called immature in Chapter 1, partly because they occur in the foetus and young, and partly because they are chemically less stable than the corresponding proteins and polysaccharides present in older people. This property is desirable for the active tissue turnover which takes place during the remodelling that is an essential part of growth. Davidson (1964) has found that administration of growth hormone results in a reversion of tissue composition towards that normally found in younger animals.

The action of growth hormone on the epiphyseal growth cartilage is primarily on the germinal zone cells. In rabbits, Rigal (1964) showed that, in a section through the germinal zone in cartilage, only one or two cells took up extra thymidine as they went into the predivision phase, but 50% of the cells did so when extra growth hormone was administered to the rabbits for several days before the cartilage was examined. These cells were then available to form new columns in the proliferative zone. By controlling the number of cells available for the formation of columns in the cartilage, growth hormone exerts a control over the length of those bones and the height of the individual. With too high a growth hormone level gigantism results. Congenital growth hormone deficiency causes a retardation of linear growth which is usually detectable during the first two years of life.

Observations on a girl with a calcitonin-secreting thyroid carcinoma (Cunliffe et al., 1968) have provided evidence on the part played by calcitonin in the growth process. In addition to general symptoms she showed Marfan features with elongated bones and marked Schmorl's nodes. The bone density and histological features in a bone biopsy were normal. These observations are consistent with the primary effect being on the proliferative zone of the growth cartilage.

Bone resorption

There is little or no evidence to suggest that the thyroid and parathyroid hormones have any direct effect on bone deposition, other than the general need for thyroid hormone to control glycolysis, so only bone resorption need be considered.

There are two mechanisms of bone resorption, with osteoclasts formed either by coalescence of osteogenic cells, or by fusion of macrophages. In tissue culture experiments to investigate the effect of parathyroid hormone on bone Gaillard (1955, 1959) described differences in behaviour of the two groups of osteoclasts. One group remained in the same position, while the others were free to move around. It is most probable that the fixed osteoclasts were those derived from osteogenic precursor cells.

In the type of osteoporosis caused by a lowered blood flow through the bone Jee and Nolan (1963) showed that osteoclasts formed from macrophages play a prominent role, while Burkhart and Jowsey (1967) have shown that when the production of parathyroid hormone is prevented by the removal of the thyroid and parathyroid glands that type of bone resorption does not occur. Parathyroid hormone is clearly necessary for the coalescence of macrophages to form osteoclasts. Parsons and Robinson (1969) have shown that when acting on the whole animal parathyroid hormone has an effect in 20 min, while if acting directly on the bone there is a time lag of 2 h. In tissue culture there is also the 2 h wait. The rapid mechanism must therefore be an indirect one. However, Johnson, Deics and French (1965) found that the changes in bone caused by parathyroid hormone are not secondary to changes in the level of calcium ions or the release of calcitonin, so that some form of biotransformation is the most probable mechanism.

Results from tissue culture experiments have caused some confusion. Cortisone in culture inhibits the action of the parathyroid hormone, and this was interpreted as being a direct effect on osteogenic cells. Nisbet and Nordin (1969) have clarified the situation by comparing the action of corticosteroids with that of the parathyroid hormone, separately and together, in tissue culture. Both cause bone resorption, but when corticosteroids are added to cultures containing parathyroid hormone they oppose its action. This would follow naturally from the effect of corticosteroids on macrophages, which is to inhibit their maturation and activity.

Corticosteroids

In this section some effects of cortisone and cortisol will be described. Cortisol is the most important member of the group of corticosteroids, because there is a rapidly increasing body of evidence that a raised blood cortisol is the dominant factor in the aetiology of the major degenerative diseases. Cortisone and cortisol are chemically similar and on many occasions cortisone has been used as a therapeutic agent.

Evidence is now available which shows that cortisone is almost inert physiologically and that many of the observed effects have been due to a transformation to cortisol at the cell surfaces. The cells whose surfaces mediate such biotransformations, as they have been called by Berliner and Dougherty (1961), are the cells of the reticulo-endothelial system, hepatocytes, lymphocytes and connective tissue cells. Each cell type transforms biologically active steroids into molecules that may have no activity with regard to a particular hormonal function of the original molecule; but these metabolites may have functions which

differ from those of the original molecule, and then after the transformation proceed to affect the cells responsible for the transformation.
For instance, cortisol is active in reducing the mobility of fibroblast
surfaces and inhibiting cell division. Cortisone does not have this
property, but after it has been administered to an adult approximately
a third is converted to cortisol (Jenkins and Sampson, 1966), so that the
therapeutic action of cortisone is, in practice, that of cortisol. Activity
at the surfaces of different cell types is different. At the surfaces of
fibroblasts and connective tissue cells the actions of the catabolic and
anti-catabolic steroids oppose one another, so that a determination of
which effect will dominate is partly dependent on the concentrations of
the two present. The actions on lymphocytes or megakaryocytes may
be additive, so that other steroids may enhance the effects of the corticosteroids. In the last few years Berliner and Dougherty (1960, 1961;
Berliner, 1965) have made considerable advances in disentangling the
various biotransformations which take place at cell surfaces and their
effects, and in particular those at fibroblast surfaces.

Action on intact tissues

Cortisol has a variety of actions. It disturbs the mechanisms of carbohydrate metabolism on which the maintenance of normal blood sugar
levels are dependent. The utilization of glucose is inhibited and the
metabolism of mucopolysaccharides depressed. There is an increased
release of free fatty acids from adipose tissue, with an increase in the
levels of pyruvate and lactate in the blood and a decrease in the blood
citrate. An alteration in the permeability of capillaries causes changes
in cardiovascular functions, so that electrolyte and water balance and
renal function are all affected. Another important effect is on the brain
tissue, and results in emotional symptoms which may vary from a
nervous state and depression through a chronic anxiety state to severe
psychotic episodes. Such effects have been discussed by Beck and
McGarry (1962) and others.

    To obtain detailed information about cellular and tissue changes the
effects in several animal species have been observed. In these experiments the corticosteroid most frequently used to assess the action on
bone has been cortisone, so that although the final result is qualitatively the same as if cortisol had been used, the greatest care has to be
taken over any deductions involving dose levels. In the rabbit, for
instance, it is probable that the conversion is more efficient in young
animals than in slightly older animals. Practically all steroids are involved in changes from one compound to another at cell surfaces, so that
this warning applies to the whole group of steroids, both corticosteroids

and anabolic steroids. When they are given therapeutically, there is usually an optimum dose beyond which the desired effect decreases again.

The effects of cortisone on some relevant tissues will now be considered. Unless the tissue is specifically stated to be of human origin illustrations to this chapter will be from rabbit experiments. For cartilage and bone the rabbit histology shown will be that of the lower end of the femur. In the rabbit this is the most suitable site for comparative studies.

Liver. The liver increases in size, and after 4 or 5 days of cortisone administration may be almost twice the normal weight. This is due to enlargement of individual cells. In histological sections they have a different appearance from the normal, and contain free lipid and glycogen. The liver as a whole becomes friable, and cohesion between individual cells decreases. Capillaries and ducts become inconspicuous. There are corresponding biochemical changes.

Muscle. Cortisol and cortisone reduce the protein synthetic activity in muscles. The hypotrophy induced is independent of protein intake (Goodlad and Munro, 1959), and White (1966) and Bullock, White and Worthington (1968) have further elucidated the nature of the protein metabolic dysfunction by demonstrating that ribosomes isolated from the skeletal muscle of rats and rabbits under treatment with a variety of glucocorticoids have a reduced ability to incorporate amino acids into protein *in vitro*. In intact animals muscles feel flabby, as compared with those in control animals. In the human also, both cortisone therapy or conditions associated with a raised blood cortisol produce a lowering of muscle tone, and muscle weakness is commonly observed. With cortisol there is an increase in the plasma levels of amino acids, and an interesting observation (Playfair, 1843) has been that cows produce less milk when harrassed or annoyed, but that it then contains a greater quantity of casein and is more suitable for making cheese than butter.

Growth cartilage. An immediate response to the effect of cortisone has been noted in the enlarging zone of the growth cartilage. In animals that are at the stage of rapid growth (Figs 3.2, 3.12) further enlargement towards the hypertrophic state diminishes or ceases abruptly. The cell surfaces become more prominent (Fig. 3.18; Fig. 6.1) are rounded, and the appearance of further matrix is consistent with a sluggish movement of surface prominences (Fig. 1.9). Utilization of glycine is decreased, and the further intercellular matrix which is formed is less in quantity

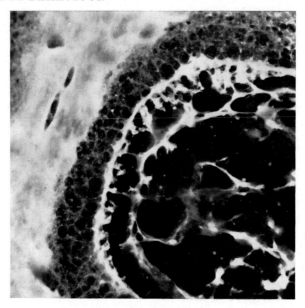

Fig. 6.1. Cell in enlarging zone of epiphyseal cartilage of rabbit which had been given cortisone. The cell surface membrane is prominent, and denser than normal. E.M. 100kV. ×5000.

but more stable. Its staining characteristics are altered (Fig. 3.18). Similar changes have been observed in human growth cartilage. Figure 3.23 showed an almost identical change in the enlarging zone in a boy, as a result of the stress involved during terminal illness.

In the adult one purpose for which prednisolone (a closely related corticosteroid, but with somewhat different side effects) is administered is to stimulate marrow activity. Its administration to children, and particularly to babies, for this purpose may not always have the desired effect. It does stimulate such marrow as is present, but it also renders the intercellular matrix of the growth cartilage more stable, so that the normal resorptive mechanisms for a young child become inadequate. Figure 6.2 shows the Harris line in a baby's vertebra, formed at the time of the acute episode for which prednisolone was first administered. Afterwards, during the period of steroid administration, cartilage resorption has been greatly reduced. Figure 6.3, at a somewhat higher magnification, shows an appearance of osteocytes and their surrounding matrix which resembles that seen in normal bone at the time of plate closure. Cartilage formed in the presence of corticosteroids often remains uncalcified or only partially calcified. Translucent zones in clinical radiographs in such cases may well indicate the presence of unchanged cartilage rather than marrow.

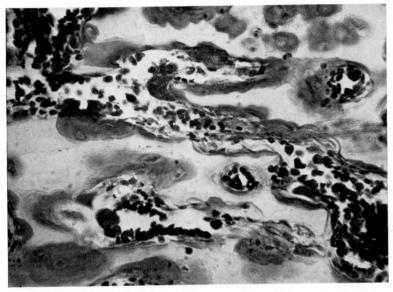

FIG. 6.3. A portion of the metaphyseal tissue formed during the time that prednisolone was being administered. The appearance of osteocytes and their surrounding matrix (more heavily stained than the cartilage matrix) resembles that more usually seen at the time of plate closure. ×200.

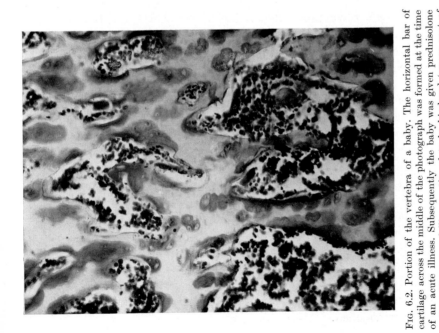

FIG. 6.2. Portion of the vertebra of a baby. The horizontal bar of cartilage across the middle of the photograph was formed at the time of an acute illness. Subsequently the baby was given prednisolone and cartilage remodelling continued to be hindered (upper part of figure). ×100.

Vessel and cell proliferation. When cortisone is given to rabbits regularly, at sufficiently high doses, the formation of new vessels and proliferation of connective tissue cells, together with the proliferation of osteogenic precursor cells from the vessel walls, ceases. Storey (1957, 1961) has observed that in the initial stages existing sinusoid vessels in bone tend to become engorged.

In the human, with the lower doses that are used therapeutically, there is a noticeable decrease in proliferation of connective tissue cells. Wound healing is hindered, and the proliferation of the fibrous plaque in rheumatoid arthritis is arrested. Cortisol produced as a result of stress has the same action, and the degree of hindrance to cell proliferation is related to the intensity of the stressful stimulus. The metaphyseal region of bone in Figs 3.23, 3.24 showed abnormalities due to the lack of vascular proliferation.

Changes in the permeability of vessel walls play a part in the anti-inflammatory action of the corticosteroids. The effect of these steroids on cells which mediate biotransformations (such as connective tissue cells, fibroblasts, lymphocytes and cells of the vessel walls) is to stabilize cell membranes, while their mobility is very greatly reduced (Dougherty *et al.*, 1961). Since channels through cells of vessel walls appear to be the normal paths for penetration from one side to another (Palade, 1961; Farquhar, Wissig and Palade, 1961) permeability of these vessels walls to the fluids which collect during the inflammatory process is decreased. Lymphocyte production is also reduced. Dougherty and Berliner have suggested that there is now sufficient evidence to show that all the anti-inflammatory actions of the corticosteroids can be explained by stabilizing of cell membranes.

Bone formation. In the presence of cortisone a small amount of new bone is laid down, but the osteoblasts are small, with scanty cytoplasm, and the amount of bone matrix per cell is less than usual. Where cells are incorporated as osteocytes their cytoplasmic processes in canaliculi are seen to be short and stumpy and there is often a visible line of demarcation between the matrix produced by one cell and the next. Such an appearance is common at the bottom of the growth cartilage during the time of plate closure. The matrix stains more heavily with haematoxylin than does ordinary bone.

In the adult the administration of cortisone or prednisolone causes less bone to be laid down by each individual osteoblast than would normally be expected. In the ageing process, as the proportion of catabolic steroids increases so the amount of matrix per cell decreases, as the bone is remodelled.

Resorptive activity. When cortisone is given to the rabbit for the purpose of following its mechanism of action in detail, it can be seen that osteogenic cells coalesce and form osteoclasts. Resorption takes place on every active bone surface (Fig. 4.21). In the metaphysis the first cells to be affected are those closest to the growth cartilage (Fig. 6.4), and the

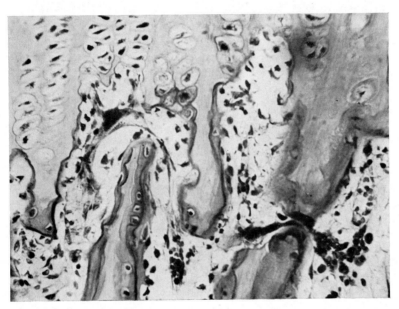

FIG. 6.4. Metaphysis of rabbit which had received cortisone for 4 days. Cartilage cells have ceased to enlarge to the hypertrophic state. Vascular endothelial cells at the base of the cartilage have coalesced to form osteoclasts which are removing the upper ends of trabeculae. ×200.

trabeculae then tend to be resorbed from both ends, so that in some areas a fragment from the middle of the trabeculae is the last to be resorbed (Fig. 6.5). These osteoclasts are very active, and after their initial coalescence a large number of cytoplasmic granules are formed (Fig. 6.6) which synthesize the enzymes responsible for bone resorption. In the final stages, when there are no more precursor cells to form fresh osteoclasts, the exposed bone surfaces remain covered by small densely staining osteoblasts. In the cortex, the bone tissue is mostly replaced by fat cells. In the inactive regions of the bone, unless osteoclast precursors are already present, there is no bone resorption.

The behaviour of fibroblasts in the presence of cortisone and cortisol has been followed in detail in cell cultures (Berliner and Dougherty, 1958). The cell surfaces became less mobile, cell processes were retracted,

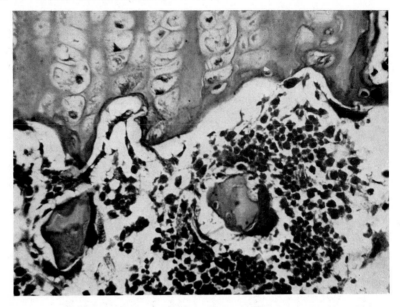

Fig. 6.5. Rabbit after 14 days cortisone. Most trabeculae in the metaphysis have been resorbed, and there is prolific red marrow. × 200.

and many cells became rounded. The cytoplasm then filled with gran-ules. Cells were later observed to become pale and many disintegrated. These fibroblasts, from both mouse and human, showed a behaviour which was the unicellular counterpart of osteoclast formation and behaviour.

In bone osteocytes also take on a resorptive function. This resorption takes place both around the cells themselves, and around cell processes passing through the canaliculi (Figs 4.29, 4.30).

In rabbit experiments with a continuous daily administration of cortisone resorptive activity reaches a maximum in 2 to 3 weeks, with active osteoclasts, and an abundance of red marrow in the active regions, but after 5 or 6 weeks there is little cell activity, and the lost bone is replaced by fatty marrow.

Osteoclast activity in the human takes place after administration of corticosteroids, or after a rise in the level of free blood cortisol, whether from a pathological cause as in the reaction to many forms of stress, or as a part of a normal physiological process, such as pregnancy. The pathological conditions will be considered in more detail in a later chapter. Here it may be noted that in pregnancy the blood cortisol rises to about 40% above the normal, with a further sharp increase associated with delivery (Appleby and Norymberski, 1957).

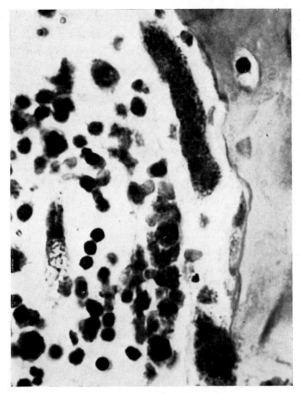

Fig. 6.6. Rabbit after 14 days cortisone. Osteoclasts derived from vascular endothelial cells in the presence of cortisol are very active. A large number of cytoplasmic granules are formed. ×400.

The marrow. Cortisol affects the bone marrow, with the introduction of a changed cell population and distribution. Where the evidence for rabbit and human overlaps it is qualitatively the same. This aspect of steroid behaviour will be considered in greater detail in a later section.

In the marrow of individuals who are in the midst of an acute osteoporotic phase—mainly women in the 50 to 70 age group—lipids are to a large extent unesterified, so that X-ray diffraction patterns of crystalline fatty acids may be obtained. Normal marrow gives only a diffuse diffraction pattern.

Anabolic and Catabolic Interactions

Except occasionally, when corticosteroids are being administered therapeutically or in Cushing's syndrome, their effects on the tissues cannot be considered in isolation. Interactions with anabolic steroids cause major modifications in the reactions of the tissues. In this chapter only those most relevant to the study of bone will be considered. These will include the effects on the liver (which would appear to influence the choice of anabolic steroids by clinicians treating osteoporosis), anabolic and catabolic interactions on bone and connective tissues, and on the bone marrow. As in the last section some very important topics, so far as patients are concerned, such as water and salt balance, blood pressure and androgenic activity will be omitted.

The corticosteroid to be discussed will again be cortisone or cortisol, partly because cortisol is the dominant factor in the aetiology of the stress diseases, and partly because insufficient is known about inter-actions involving other corticosteroids. The range of anabolic steroids chosen will be wider, although of necessity limited to the particular compounds for which factual information is available, from animal experiments and from a comparison of these experiments with human pathology. The information needed for a full understanding of the mechanisms is by no means complete, so that this is a field in which much profitable work remains to be done.

When the anabolic compounds are considered, one cannot take just one or two as representative of the group, because a number of different actions are involved, and the level of activity of each compound varies for each action. It is thus very necessary to regard each anabolic compound as a different entity.

Chemical formulae of some of the relevant steroids are:

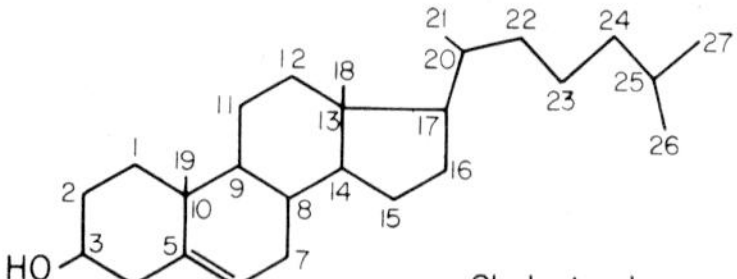

Cholesterol

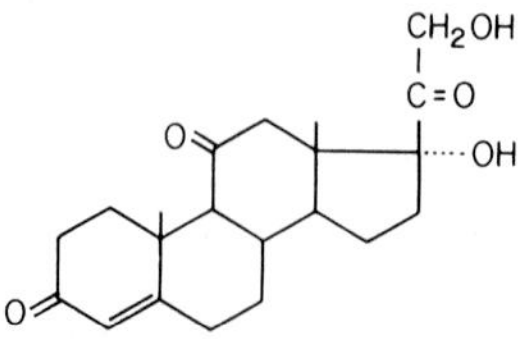

Cortisone

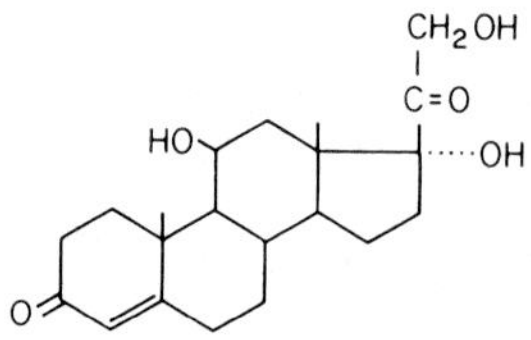

Cortisol

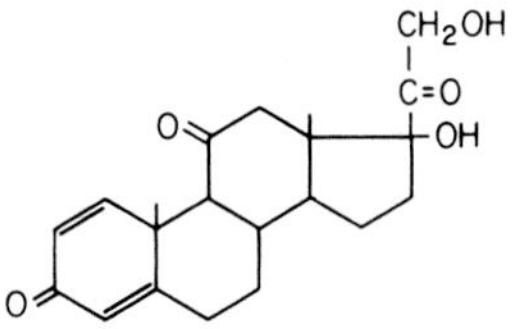

Prednisone

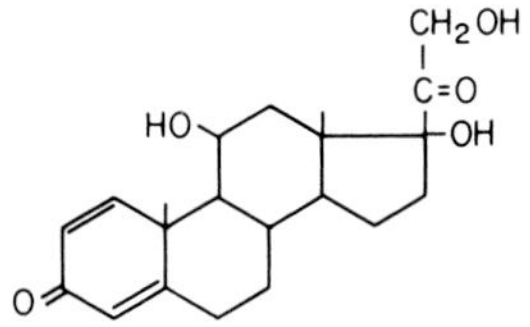

Prednisolone

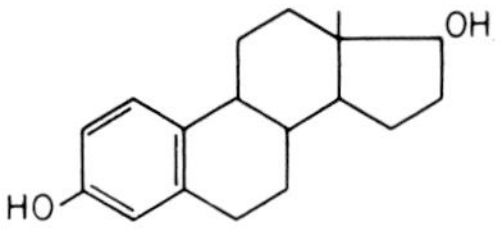

Oestradiol

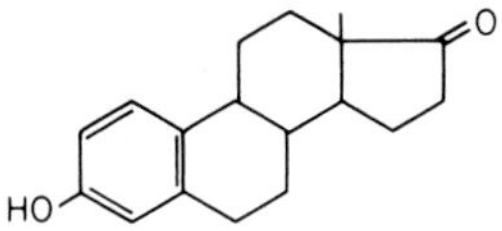

Oestrone

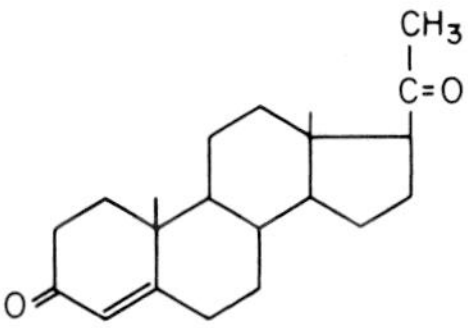

Progesterone

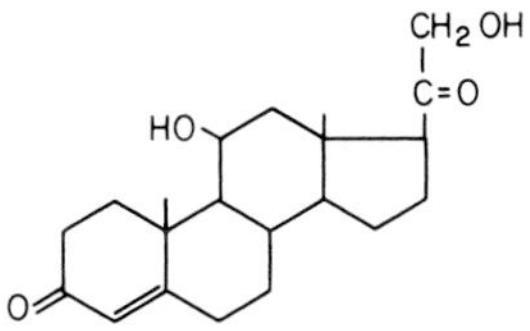

Corticosterone

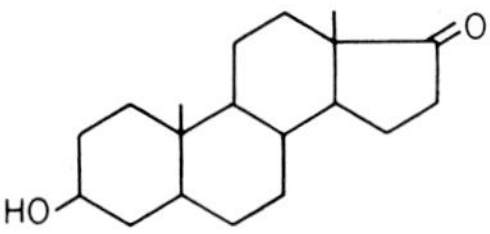

Androsterone

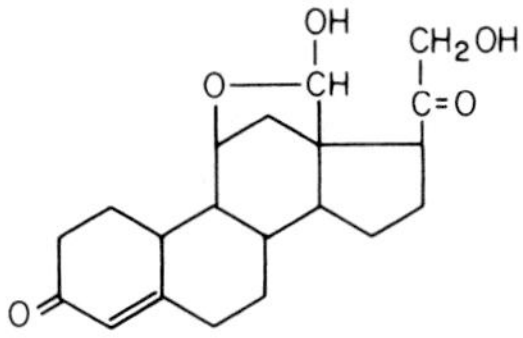

Aldosterone

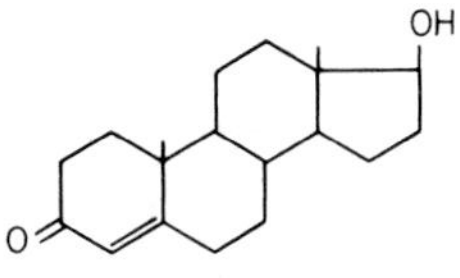

Testosterone

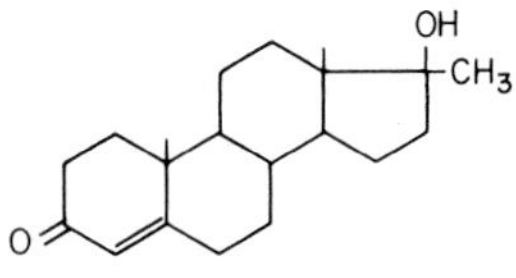

Methyl testosterone

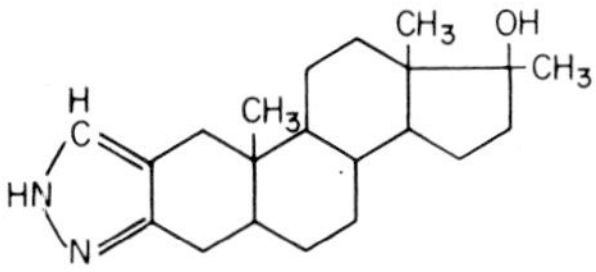

Stanozolol (Stromba)

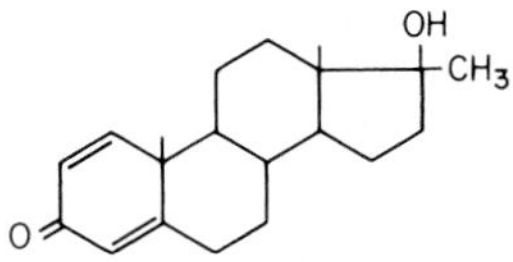

Methandienone (Dianabol)

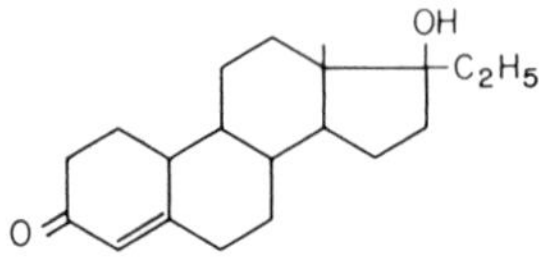

Norethandrolone (Nilevar)

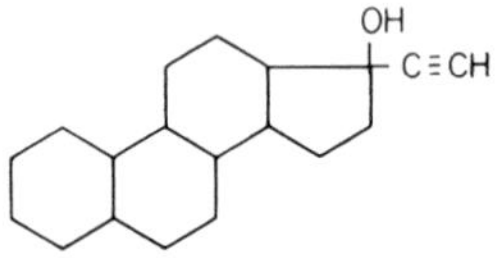

Lynoestrenol

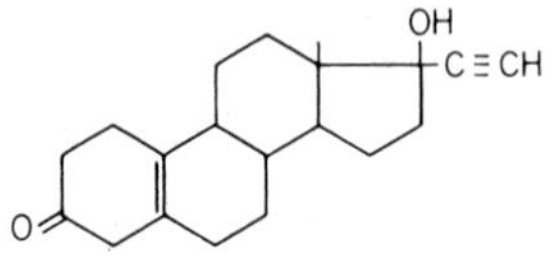

Norethynodrel

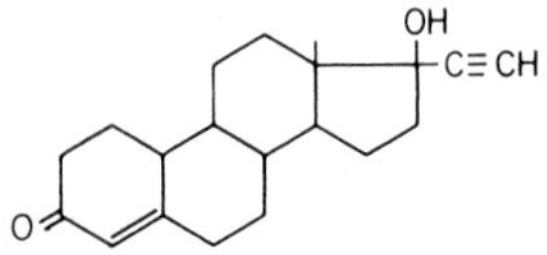

Norethisterone

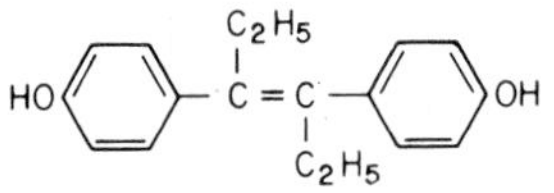

Diethyl stilboestrol

[Diethyl stilboestrol is included because, although it is not a steroid, it has as one of its actions oestrogenic properties, and has been used as a substitute for oestradiol in therapy.]

Each steroid is involved in chemical reactions and modifications at the surfaces of liver and connective tissue cells, and small differences in chemical structure may mean large differences in the properties of the products of biotransformations. These anabolic steroids have a variety of actions, some of which show considerable variation from one compound to another; some show related properties, as with the anabolic and anti-catabolic actions which are at a similar, though not identical level in each compound; and a few are linked properties. One example of this is the presence of a $17a$ methyl group, which confers oral activity, and which also causes the compounds to modify the liver function. Another probable example of a linked property is contraceptive activity and the production of abnormal sticky platelets if stimulated by cortisol. A wider range of steroids than has so far been investigated will be necessary to elucidate this point. Since they all behave as separate compounds, with separate groups of actions, anabolic steroids cannot be regarded as interchangeable in the treatment of patients.

Liver

Although on occasion biochemical changes have been reported, particularly when the $17a$ methyl group is present, such anabolic steroids as have been investigated have shown no histological changes in the liver.

When an anabolic steroid is administered after cortisone, or together with cortisone, after the liver has already been altered by cortisone (Fig. 6.7) there are considerable differences between the effects of the

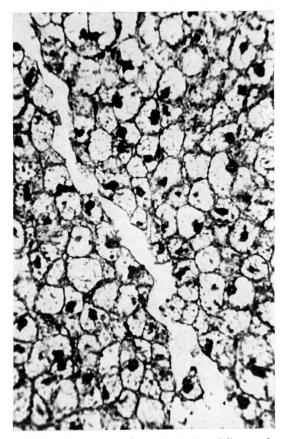

Fig. 6.7. Rabbit liver, after 2 weeks cortisone administration. Cells are enlarged, and take up little stain. Cell surfaces are altered, and their cohesion reduced, so that they readily break apart, and the liver is friable. ×400.

different compounds. Of those which have been investigated, stanozolol (Stromba), methandienone (Dianabol) and decadurabolin, even in the presence of a continued administration of cortisone, reverse the corticosteroid effect (Fig. 6.8). As the hepatic cells regain their normal appearance channels and ducts between rows of cells also become more prominent. In each case the early stages of the return to a normal appearance are around the central veins (Fig. 6.9) and the change then spreads through the remainder of the liver. This recovery is usually complete in a week, or sometimes 2 weeks. Stanozolol shows the most

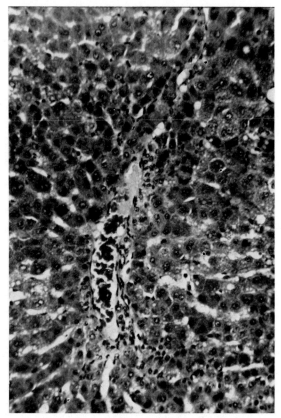

FIG. 6.8. Rabbit liver. The administration of cortisone was followed by that of methandienone (Dianabol) for 1 week. Cells have reverted to normal size and staining properties, and channels and ducts between rows of cells can again be distinguished. ×200.

rapid effect. An interesting observation has been that, whereas stanozolol does not affect the weight of the liver and cortisone causes a considerable increase, when cortisone is followed by stanozolol the weight of the liver in growing rabbits returns to the normal level, while when the stanozolol is given together with a continued administration of cortisone the recovery is only partial so far as the weight of the liver is concerned, even when the histological appearance has returned to normal. When the weight of the whole animal is considered, in their rapidly growing phase, the animals show a steady weight gain with stanozolol, but a loss in weight with cortisone. Cortisone followed by cortisone plus stanozolol shows a weight gain after the start of the administration of the anabolic steroid at about the same rate as for normal animals being given stanozolol alone, but when cortisone is followed by stanozolol, the rate of weight gain is much more rapid.

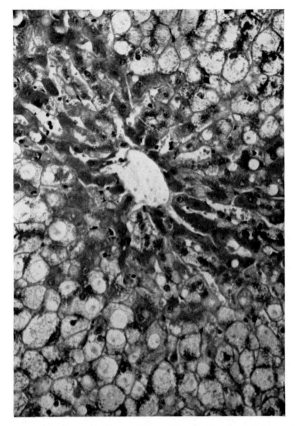

FIG. 6.9. Rabbit liver. Cortisone 14 days, followed by cortisone and stanozolol for 4 days. Cells around the central veins are in the process of regaining their normal appearance. The remaining cells contain excess glycogen, and a few fat globules can be seen. ×400.

Those compounds which reverse the effects of cortisone on the liver belong to the group most usually prescribed in treatment for osteoporosis. Wynn and Landon (1961) have shown in the case of methandienone (Dianabol) that it produced a sense of well-being and increased confidence, a change that did not occur in patients who were not symptomatically ill at the time of being given the drug. This change is not similar to the euphoria seen in some patients on cortisone. (Sometimes, cortisone may produce a psychotic state—a different phenomenon again from the mental confusion that Sholiton et al. (1961) have shown can produce a raised plasma cortisol.) Wynn (1968) has found stanozolol to show an effect sooner than methandienone.

Of this group of compounds which reverse the effect of cortisol on the liver and tend to restore a sense of well-being, methandienone has a rather low anti-catabolic activity. This combination of properties has suggested another possible use: to administer it together with a corticosteroid in order to suppress some of the undesirable side effects while allowing it to exert its anti-inflammatory action. Clinically this has met with some success in the treatment of rheumatoid arthritis, and at lower dose levels of each.

Reverting now to the effect of other anabolic steroids on the liver histology: in the time required by stanozolol or methandienone to cause a reversion to the normal appearance of hepatic cells after treatment with cortisone, some recovery of cells and vessels has been noted for testosterone, and a slight recovery for norethandrolone and lynoestrenol. None has been found for the two progestational steroids norethynodrel and norethisterone.

Anabolic action

The anabolic action, that is, the ability to increase protein synthetic activity, is the property which has given the group of anabolic steroids their name. It is related to the anti-catabolic activity, insomuch as the anabolic activity is concerned with events at the endoplasmic reticulum membranes in the cell, while the anti-catabolic activity is closely concerned with events at the cell surface and the smooth membranes. The two sets of properties tend to go in parallel more closely than most other steroid properties, but there are divergencies. Ba 36644, for example is the most anabolic of all the compounds yet prepared, although the compound with the greatest anti-catabolic activity is not Ba 36644, but stanozolol. Ba 36644 is an experimental anabolic steroid composed of 17β-hydroxy-7α,17α-dimethyl-A-nor-β-homooestrone-3,6,dione in equilibrium with its enol form. Similarly, lynoestrenol and testosterone show a reversal in properties. Lynoestrenol is slightly more anabolic than testosterone, while the testosterone is the more anti-catabolic of the two.

The anabolic action can be measured as the protein synthetic activity of the muscles, and with the more anabolic compounds its effect may also be observed histologically, since the amount of matrix produced, both protein and polysaccharide, is increased. Figure 3.17, for example, showed excess matrix in the epiphyseal growth cartilage after three weeks administration of stanozolol. This figure also demonstrated that the formation of hypertrophic cells is a result of a delicately balanced equilibrium, and that excess of either anabolic or anti-anabolic steroids may suppress their formation. Conversely, the anabolic peptide compounds favour the production of hypertrophic cells. A method of quantitatively assessing the relative anabolic activity which has been developed by Bullock *et al.* (1968), using the rabbit quadriceps muscle for analysis, has been to suppress the protein synthetic activity with cortisone, and then to give cortisone and the steroid together, thus measuring its efficiency in overcoming the anti-anabolic action of the cortisone. For one group of compounds this gave, in descending order of potency: Ba 36644, stanozolol, lynoestrenol, testosterone, methandienone, norethynodrel, norethisterone. Ba 36644 produced a considerably greater effect than any other compound even when administered at only a tenth of the dose.

Similarly, after cortisone has produced resorption cavities in cortical bone in the rabbits, these cavities are filled when the more anabolic of the steroids are administered. The proportion of matrix to cell in the newly formed bone gives a qualitative measure of the relative anabolic level. Figures 6.10, 6.11, 6.12 show the effects of Ba 36644, stanozolol

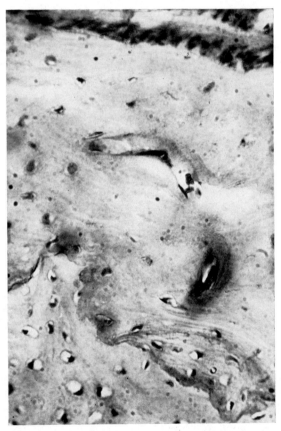

FIG. 6.10. Cortical bone from rabbit which had received cortisone acetate (15 mg/kg) for 2 weeks, followed by Ba 36644 (0·5 mg/kg) together with cortisone acetate (15 mg/kg) for 2 weeks. Bone in upper 2/3 of figure was laid down in the presence of the Ba 36644. ×200.

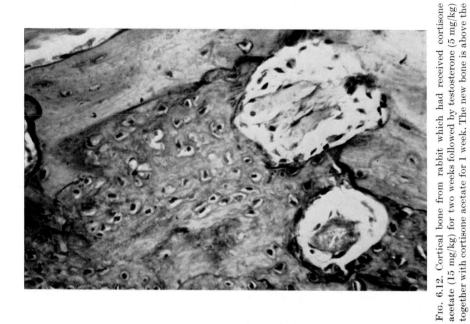

Fig. 6.12. Cortical bone from rabbit which had received cortisone acetate (15 mg/kg) for two weeks followed by testosterone (5 mg/kg) together with cortisone acetate for 1 week. The new bone is above the Haversian canal ×200.

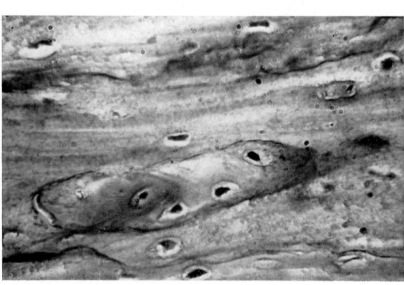

Fig. 6.11. Cortical bone from rabbit which had received cortisone acetate (15 mg/kg) for 2 weeks, followed by stanozolol (5 mg/kg) together with cortisone acetate (15 mg/kg) for 2 weeks. The strip of bone to the left of centre was laid down in the presence of stanozolol. ×400.

and testosterone. In this particular experiment (Little, 1970a) the compounds were given together with cortisone. This accounts for the bone formed in the presence of testosterone having less matrix per cell than the undisturbed bone.

Anti-catabolic action

There is no convenient quantitative method available for measuring the anti-catabolic activity, that is, the property of opposing the tendency of the catabolic steroids to suppress mobility of cell membranes and inhibit cell division in cells of the connective tissue series. Qualitatively it may be assessed by a combination of a variety of histological observations. One possible site for comparison is the rapidly growing rabbit epiphysis. Here when cortisone is given, it produces the effects shown in Fig. 3.18. This treatment can then be followed up by administering a mixture of cortisone and an anabolic compound. The most suitable bone for observing effects is the lower femoral epiphysis at the stage of rapid growth. Vessels, in the presence of an efficient anti-catabolic compound penetrate the altered growth cartilage and from the level of the bottom of the proliferative zone normal enchondral ossification is resumed, as shown in Figs 3.19, 3.20, 3.21. The more stable cartilage remains, to be resorbed later, or to form the basis of a Harris line (Fig. 6.13). With a

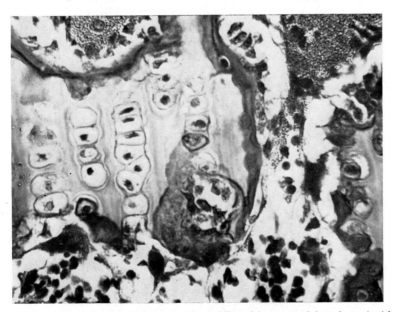

FIG. 6.13. Rabbit metaphysis. Cortisone 14 days, followed by stanozolol 14 days. An island of stable cartilage has been bypassed during remodelling and enchondral ossification. Cells have prominent outer membranes, and some chondroclastic resorption is taking place. × 250.

weaker anti-catabolic action penetration is less vigorous (Fig. 6.14). Such a survey is only roughly qualitative, since there are added complications. When testosterone is used, for example, red marrow penetrates very close to the bottom of the cartilage and the whole process is modified (Fig. 3.25). This effect was seen also in the boy's growth cartilage shown in Fig. 3.24. With Ba 36644 the anabolic action frequently takes over, with bone formation before penetration is complete (Fig. 6.15). Frequently there are areas where vessels do not succeed in penetrating, so that tongues of cartilage are formed (see Chapter 3, p. 125).

Another method of assessing the relative anti-catabolic effectiveness of the various anabolic steroids is to observe the active regions of cortical bone in a growing rabbit when cortisone and the anabolic agent are administered alternately. The result varies according to the anti-

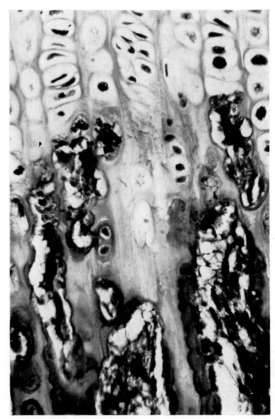

Fig. 6.14. Base of rabbit's epiphyseal growth cartilage, after cortisone and lynoestrenol had been given alternately. There has been uneven vascular penetration, but where the sinusoid vessels have penetrated this has been followed by normal enchondral ossification. ×200.

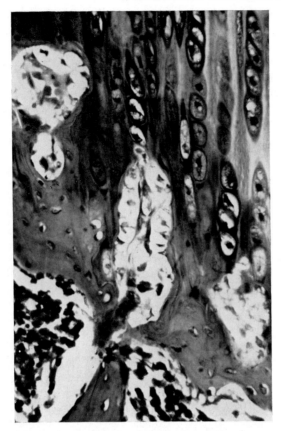

FIG. 6.15. Base of rabbit's epiphyseal growth cartilage. Cortisone acetate (15 mg/kg) for 2 weeks was followed by cortisone acetate (15 mg/kg) and Ba 36644 (0·5 mg/kg) for a further 2 weeks. The bottom of the proliferative zone shows elongated cells, while there is an abnormally high proportion of bone tissue in the new enchondral bone, which in some places (right of figure) prevents further vascular penetration. × 200.

catabolic activity of the steroid. Cortisone causes precursor cells to coalesce, form osteoclasts, and remove bone, while the anti-catabolic compounds produce more precursor cells, which may then display osteoblastic activity. When conditions are close to a balance in the level of activity, bone showing a series of arrest lines is produced, as was illustrated for lynoestrenol in Fig. 2.30. Here there were 8 cycles of treatment, and 8 arrest lines may be observed. Similar appearances in the bone in the neck of femur of patients suffering from post-menopausal osteoporosis provide evidence on the course of that condition, and suggest surges of catabolic activity with remission between episodes (Fig. 2.31).

When the steroid has a stronger anti-catabolic activity than lyn-oestrenol (e.g. stanozolol) then bone formation dominates over resorption, the strength of the bone is not decreased, and resorption cavities are not formed. But when the steroid has a weaker anti-catabolic activity precursor cells are formed that fail to go on to osteoblastic activity. These precursors become available for the next phase of catabolic activity, so that it becomes possible for more bone to be removed by this type of combination of steroids than by the action of cortisone or cortisol alone. Figure 6.16 shows a new surge of destructive

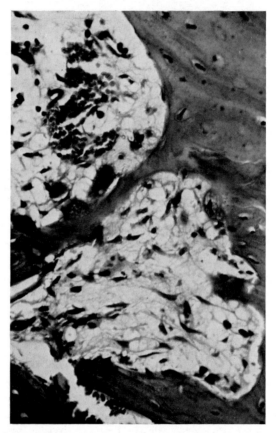

Fig. 6.16. Bone from rabbit which had received cortisone for 2 weeks followed by cortisone and methandienone for 1 week. This animal was in a group which had been additionally stressed by nearby pneumatic drills. Osteogenic cells which had started to proliferate have formed osteoclasts without laying down new bone. ×200.

activity arising in a cavity which had not been replenished by the preceding surge of anabolic activity. A large proportion of the bone can be removed by an adjustment of the timing of catabolic and anabolic actions for weaker anabolic agents. Occasionally this has happened accidentally during attempted treatment of osteoporosis, but it is an effect that could be put to use, should the occasion arise, in the removal of unwanted radioactive strontium or other bone seeking isotopes which can be excreted after mobilization. They are first deposited in active areas of bone, and it is these same active areas which would be preferentially removed in the earlier stages of a steroid-induced osteoporosis. Bone removal could then be followed by a renewal of bone deposition, if necessary accelerated by stanozolol. Loss of bone during pregnancy and in post-menopausal osteoporosis shows that bone removal can easily be accomplished in women, while in men as well the stresses associated with university examinations (Scrimshaw et al., 1966) and space flight (Mack, Vose, Vogt and LaChance, 1966) have resulted in temporary bone removal.

When cortisone has been given to young male and female rabbits, with intervals for their natural hormones to take over the anabolic action, the females have shown an apparently grossly exaggerated resorption of bone—more than might have been expected from the anabolic and anti-catabolic level of activity of their hormones. This may have been due to a further complicating steroid interaction—oestrogen doubles the time during which cortisol remains active in the serum.

In the case of the synthetic progestational compounds their relative anti-catabolic activity may be observed, in animal experiments, in liver sections. These compounds, when present together with cortisone (or cortisol) stimulate the production of an excessive number of large megakaryocytes, which release sticky platelets into the blood stream at intervals of 5 to 7 days. Within a few hours of this happening, a crop of small thrombi are deposited in the tissues. In rabbits such thrombi and their consequences are most conveniently observed in the liver. Compounds which have been compared in this way are testosterone, norethandrolone, lynoestrenol, norethynodrel and norethisterone. When vessels in the liver are plugged by thrombi, subsidiary vessels involved become engorged (Fig. 6.17). Those cells deprived of their normal blood supply die, and a necrotic patch develops (Fig. 6.18). In the case of the more strongly anabolic compounds, norethandrolone and testosterone, granulation tissue cells proliferate, and by the end of a week many multinucleated phagocytic cells are active (Fig. 6.19). By the end of the second week fibrous tissue is present (Fig. 6.20). At the other end of the scale is norethisterone. The necrotic tissue formed as a result of the combined action of this compound and cortisone is often calcified by the end of a week (Fig. 6.21), and there is not sufficient anti-catabolic potential to allow granulation tissue proliferation. Lynoestrenol

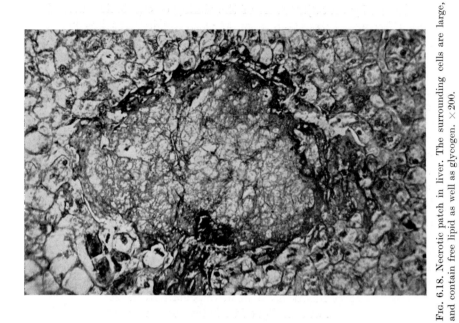

FIG. 6.18. Necrotic patch in liver. The surrounding cells are large, and contain free lipid as well as glycogen. ×200.

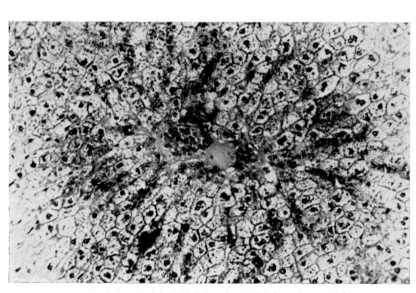

FIG. 6.17. Section of rabbit's liver showing thrombus in vessel and engorgement of surrounding capillaries. ×100.

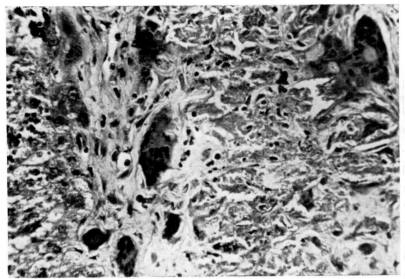

Fig. 6.19. Necrotic patch in rabbit's liver. At the end of a week many multinucleated phagocytic cells are present around each patch. ×200.

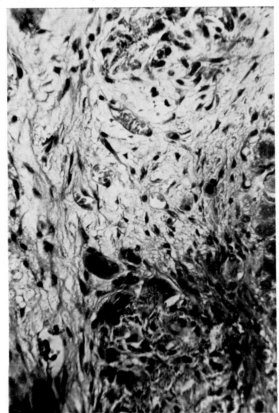

Fig. 6.20. Necrotic patch in rabbit's liver. At the end of the second week proliferating granulation tissue and fibrous tissue are behind the advancing line of multinucleated cells. This animal had been given cortisone and testosterone. ×200.

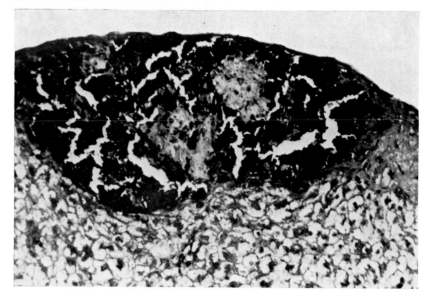

FIG. 6.21. Calcified necrotic patch near surface of liver. This rabbit had been given cortisone and norethisterone. × 200.

occupies an intermediate position, and lesions due to this compound may be partly calcified and partly replaced by granulation tissue.

The reaction of surrounding tissue to infection is also primarily an anti-catabolic property, the general rule being that the greater the catabolic level of the surroundings the greater the spread of the infection, and the greater the anti-catabolic level of the surroundings the less the spread of the infection, or the greater the degree to which it is contained. This has been observed in both low grade lung infection, and also in rabbits infected at the site of injection. With the generalized infection necrotic patches were sometimes preferentially infected. Observation on the type of person liable to succumb to an infection is in general agreement with these more precise observations. Here again, however, there are two separate effects which need to be distinguished. A high catabolic level encourages spread of infection. It also discourages the reactions of the tissues to that infection, whether they be of an inflammatory nature or a proliferation of granulation tissue. It is thus very possible for these drugs to cause an apparent improvement while they are in reality aggravating the condition.

The Marrow

Bone marrow is of two main types. Red marrow contains the active haemopoietic tissue which produces blood cells, while fatty marrow is

quiescent and as its name implies contains mainly fat cells. Haemopoietic tissue is also called myeloid tissue, and it is now generally
agreed that the main cell types found in the marrow are derived from a
single group of stem cells that can differentiate either to reticulo-
endothelial cells (and eventually to bone) or to free cells. It is possible
that the precursor cells are of reticulo-endothelial origin, although
adequate evidence on this point is lacking. Certainly, wherever in the
body sinusoid vessels are formed there seems to be the possibility of
haemopoietic activity. It is very common in the spleen and fairly
common in the liver. Similarly, in the regenerating process after all the
marrow has been removed from the shaft of a bone (Brånemark et al.,
1964), whether in the rabbit or somewhat more slowly in the human, the
cavity fills with blood, which clots. Granulation tissue and new vessels
invade from the vascular channels of the cortex; trabeculae are formed
along the lines of advance of these invading vessels; after about three
weeks the trabeculae begin to resorb and then with no cells in the vicinity
other than granulation tissue, vessels and osteogenic cells, haemopoietic tissue forms near the resorbing bone. As resorptive activity
decreases there is a gradual replacement of new tissues and red marrow
by fatty marrow.

Names given to cells have tended to vary, but the precursors of the
free cells are often called myeloblasts (e.g. Ham, 1965). These myeloblasts can differentiate to erythrocytes and their precursors, leucocytes
and their precursors or to the megakaryocytes which produce platelets.
Howell (1890) formed the opinion that the megakaryocytes arose from
small "lymphoid" cells and afterwards reproduced by direct division.
These lymphoid cells fit the description of the cells later described as
myeloblasts. Observers are now in general agreement that formation of
megakaryocytes is from small precursor cells and not by division of
mature cells. In Fig. 6.22 a number of enlarging myeloblasts can be seen
in the marrow of a rabbit which had been given cortisone. There is also a
megakaryocyte whose nucleus appears to be in the process of dividing,
although most probably it is in the process of increasing the number of
lobes of the nucleus.

In histological sections an abundance of red marrow is found in regions
of bone turnover. Most of the marrow is red in the young child, while in
the adult inactive regions of bone, within the shafts of the long bones, or
even in cavities in the cortex during quiescent phases of osteoporosis,
are occupied by fatty marrow. The lumbar vertebrae are one of the most
important sites where continuing bone turnover contributes to a
continuing presence of erythropoiesis. Since exercise is one of the
factors which determines the amount of bone turnover, it follows that
an adequate amount of exercise is also one of the contributory factors

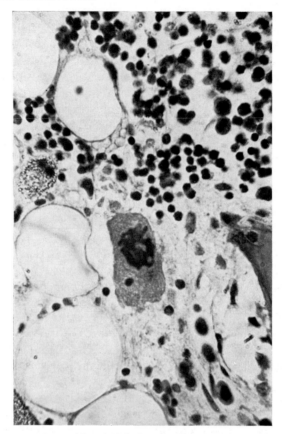

Fig. 6.22. Bone marrow from rabbit which had received cortisone acetate for 2 weeks. A number of enlarging myeloblasts can be seen. There is also a megakaryocyte whose nucleus appears to be in the process of dividing. ×400.

that combine to maintain an adequate red cell and haemoglobin level. In general it may be said that wherever there is active bone resorption, there red marrow is found. The neck of the femur shown in Fig. 2.33 is one example.

The amount of haemopoietic tissue in the marrow is also under hormonal control, and the proportions of the cell constituents vary from one steroid mixture to another. In the child, for example, the proportion of megakaryocytes to red marrow is smaller than in the adult. The interactions of steroids on the marrow are very different from their actions on the bone and connective tissue cells. With these latter the corticosteroids and anabolic or anti-catabolic steroids have an antagonistic action, while their action on marrow may be additive. The proportion of each of the main cell types, however, varies from one anabolic steroid to another. For the few steroids for which a direct comparison has so far been possible correspondence between the rabbit and human is close, so that there is a probability that results obtained with steroid and hormone trials on rabbits will be qualitatively similar to the effects to be expected when these same steroids are administered to the human.

A number of effects may be noticed when rabbits are given cortisone. There is an increase in the amount of red marrow in the vicinity of resorbing bone, and also in the vicinity of resorbing cartilage. In this red marrow, as well as an increased production of erythrocyte precursor cells, there are an increased number of megakaryocytes, many rather larger than normal. In rabbits there is evidence that it takes 4–7 days for one of these megakaryocytes to mature and release its platelets into the bloodstream. When administration of cortisone is frequent and regular (i.e. daily) cell activity gradually ceases, and after 6 to 8 weeks in a young rabbit the growth cartilage is static and all the osteoclast precursors are used up. At the same time the amount of red marrow decreases and is eventually considerably less than normal, being replaced by fat cells. These are found even in Haversian canals.

In the human such detailed histological evidence is not available, but it is known that in the active stages of osteoporosis there is an increase of red marrow in areas of active bone resorption, with a correspondingly very high proportion of fatty marrow during the later quiescent phases. Where the bone loss has been sufficient to cause some mechanical instability, sufficient to lead to a microfracture, then as the dead bone is resorbed red marrow forms around that fracture. The administration of corticosteroids is a recognized method of raising the platelet count. The proportion of cell types does not remain constant, and corticosteroids are also used to reduce the number of active leucocytes. Their action on these cells has been described by Dougherty (1952).

When other steroids are administered to rabbits together with cortisone there is an increase in cell activity, and a corresponding rise in the amount of red marrow in the active sites. Fig. 2.32 showed that with cortisone and methandienone together the cavities in the cortex could become filled with red marrow. There is also a considerable variation in the degree of stimulation of cell activity between one cell type and another. The study of this aspect of steroid activity is still in its early stages, although, it holds considerable promise for the treatment of a variety of haematological disorders.

Consequences of steroid interaction which are emerging as a topic of considerable importance are the cell changes in the marrow which result from the interaction of progestational steroids and corticosteroids. There is cell proliferation, not only near the active regions of the bone,

but often throughout the fatty part of the marrow. When these two
types of steroids are administered together there are changes in the red
and white cell precursors which vary from one progestational compound
to another and invariably the production of a large number of giant
megakaryocytes. This effect seems to be triggered off by the cortisol,
and is not produced by the progestational compound alone. The
threshold level of cortisol required to stimulate the abnormal activity
varies. It is high for some of the synthetic steroids prepared for therapeutic purposes (with a high anabolic to androgenic ratio), lower for
testosterone, and lower still for the efficient contraceptive compounds.
Figures 6.23–6.28 show typical histological appearances of the abnormal
megakaryocytes. Figures 6.23, 6.24 show the effect of lynoestrenol in the

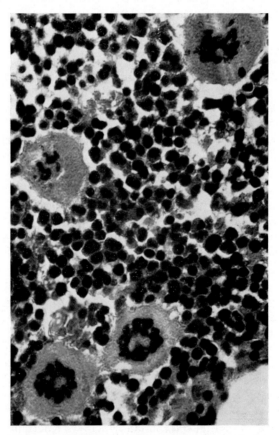

FIG. 6.23. Bone marrow from rabbit which had received cortisone for 2 weeks, followed by
cortisone and lynoestrenol for 1 week. From just below growth cartilage. There are a large
number of large and abnormal looking megakaryocytes, in an abundance of red marrow.
×400.

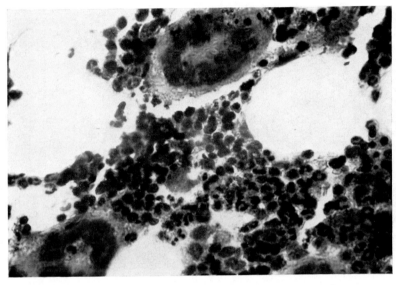

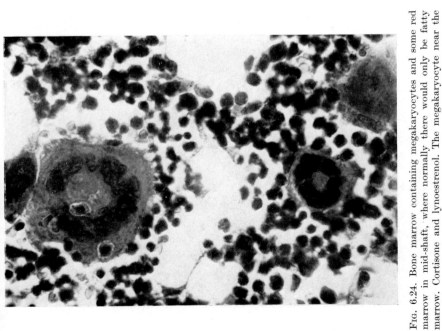

FIG. 6.24. Bone marrow containing megakaryocytes and some red marrow in mid-shaft, where normally there would only be fatty marrow. Cortisone and lynoestrenol. The megakaryocyte near the bottom of the photograph has recently shed its platelets, but the nucleus remains intact. ×400.

FIG. 6.25. Bone marrow from rabbit which had received cortisone for 2 weeks, followed by cortisone together with norethisterone for 2 weeks. Mid-shaft. The appearance of megakaryocytes and also of the surrounding red marrow is distinctive for each progestational agent. ×400.

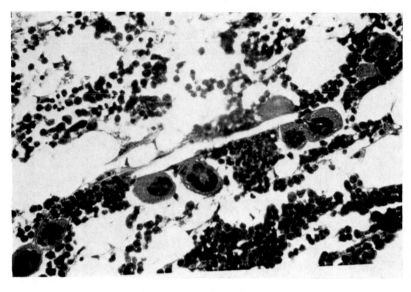

Fig. 6.27. Bone marrow from shaft of rabbit given cortisone followed by cortisone and lynoestrenol. Many megakaryocytes are attached to walls of sinusoid vessels. ×200.

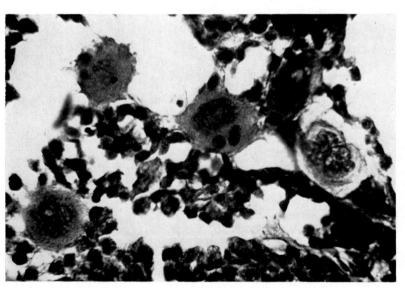

Fig. 6.26. Bone marrow from rabbit given cortisone for 2 weeks, followed by cortisone and testosterone for 2 weeks. Many megakaryocytes in this section were in the process of loosing platelets, while lesions in the liver of this animal were either at the stage shown in Fig. 6.17 or at the stage shown in Fig. 6.19. ×400.

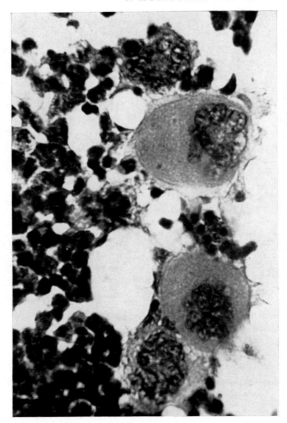

Fig. 6.28. Bone marrow from near endosteal surface, from rabbit given cortisone for 2 weeks, followed by cortisone and testosterone for 2 weeks. The nuclei of many megakaryocytes are less dense than those of normal megakaryocytes, or of megakaryocytes formed in the presence of lynoestrenol. ×400.

metaphysis and shaft respectively. With each progestational compound the effect on the marrow as a whole can be seen to be somewhat different, while the production of abnormal megakaryocytes is a constant factor. Frequently they appear in the vicinity of vessels (Fig. 6.27).

As each crop of large and abnormal megakaryocytes approach maturity, their cytoplasm takes on a bluish tinge (when stained with haematoxylin and eosin) and also has a somewhat granular appearance (Fig. 6.28). Then abnormal platelets are released (Fig. 6.29) to leave an almost bare nucleus. After a day or two a fringe of smooth pink-staining cytoplasm appears, expands and matures, until with almost completely formed platelets the cytoplasm again takes on a bluish hue when stained. In experimental rabbits a short-lived peak in the peripheral platelet count is observed soon after the release of the platelets.

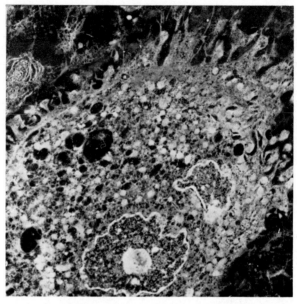

Fig. 6.29. Electron microscope photograph showing portion of megakaryocyte, in the process of shedding platelets. Low density nucleus. (Light cell on dark ground.)

The platelets released from the abnormal megakaryocytes seem to be stickier than usual and within a short time of their release numerous small platelet thrombi may be found in the tissues. The normal platelets remaining in the circulation do not coalesce, and no further thrombi are found till the next crop of abnormal megakaryocytes have released their platelets (Little, 1970b).

Sharp (1961) has demonstrated that there are two separate stages in the clumping of platelets. First reversible aggregates are formed, then later there is irreversible fusion. It would seem that with the abnormal platelets which have been described, fusion takes place very quickly to form small clumps or thrombi. These are stickier than usual, and can even stick to normal vessel walls (Fig. 2.34). They block small vessels in many parts of the body. The liver has been mentioned (Figs 6.17–6.21), and heart, kidney, diaphragm, brain (Fig. 6.30) and many other tissues may be affected. In the marrow of some experimental animals given cortisol together with progestational steroids small necrotic lesions have been observed (Fig. 6.31) suggesting that this is one cause of metaphyseal bone cysts. Together with the large numbers of small thrombi, a much smaller number of large ones are found. These have more immediately dramatic consequences, and have resulted in the deaths of a number of the experimental animals. Figure 6.32 shows a

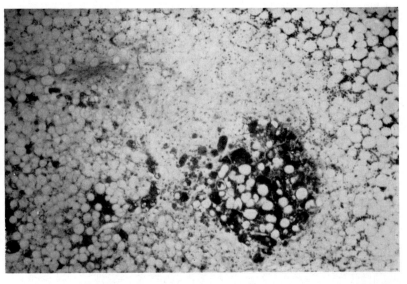

FIG. 6.31. Bone marrow in metaphysis of rabbit on cortisone and testosterone, showing darkly stained necrotic patch, proliferating granulation tissue, and unaffected marrow, with fat cells among the haemopoietic tissue. ×35.

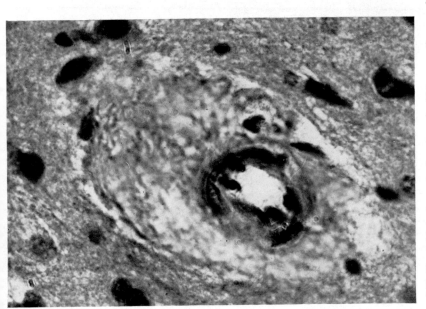

FIG. 6.30. Frontal lobe in cerebral cortex of rabbit on cortisone and norethisterone. Degenerating area around vessel. ×300.

large thrombus lodged in the liver of a rabbit that was being given cartisone and norethynodrel.

Stress causes a raised plasma cortisol, which can be above the threshold level for the steroids naturally present, and the first recorded observations of the clumping of platelets, in cases of acute infectious illness, was by Osler (1874). Examination of haemopoietic tissue in men who have died after the stress of a terminal illness has shown the same types of megakaryocyte appearance as has been found in rabbits given testosterone. Figures 6.33, 6.34 show two types of megakaryocyte in the

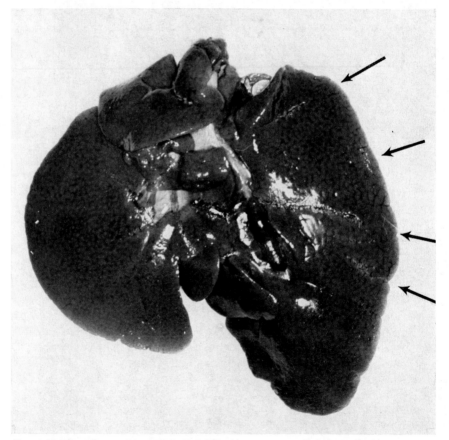

Fig. 6.32. Liver from rabbit which had been given cortisone and norethynodrel. A large thrombus lodged in the liver, and tissue surrounding the affected vessels has begun to calcify. Some of these vessels are indicated by arrows.

lumbar vertebrae of an elderly man who had been under stress during a terminal illness. The bone was osteoporotic and the number and size of megakaryocytes greater than in the normal. Fairly recently organized

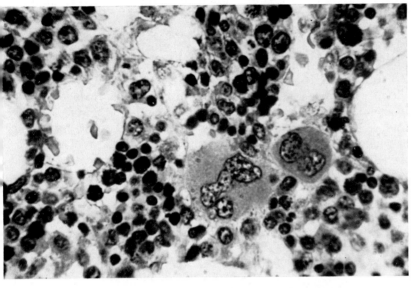

FIG. 6.34. Marrow in a lumbar vertebra of an elderly man, after a stressful terminal illness. There were many recent thrombi in the tissues. These megakaryocytes are of abnormal size and shape, and have low density nuclei (cf. Fig. 6.28). ×400.

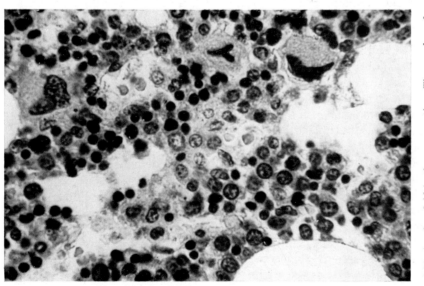

FIG. 6.33. Another field in the same section. The number of megakaryocytes in the bone was greater than normal. ×400.

thrombi were found in neighbouring tissues. The population of abnormal megakaryocytes with dense and less dense nuclei varies from one steroid compound to another.

Cell Surfaces and Membranes

Many of the effects caused by steroids on cells are as a result of the interaction with surfaces and membranes of these cells. Changes occur in the chemical form and hence the properties of both steroid and membrane.

Some examples of changes which take place at the surfaces of reticulo-endothelial cells in the liver, fibroblasts and other connective tissue cells, which have been described by Berliner and Dougherty (1961) and others are:

$$\text{cortisol} \rightleftharpoons \text{cortisone}$$
$$\text{corticosterone} \rightleftharpoons \text{11-dihydrocorticosterone}$$
$$\text{estradiol} \rightleftharpoons \text{estrone}$$
$$\text{testosterone} \rightleftharpoons \text{androstenedione}$$
$$\text{progesterone} \rightleftharpoons \begin{cases} \text{4-pregnine-20}\alpha\text{-ol-3-one} \\ \text{4-pregnine-20}\beta\text{-ol-3-one} \end{cases}$$

The half-life of the cortisol in blood is about 40 min, and twice this time in the presence of oestrogens. In an investigation of rabbit articular cartilage, Mankin and Conger (1966) have shown that injected cortisol produced a depression in glycine C^{14} incorporation within 2 h, with a recovery of function by 10 h.

There are now several lines of evidence which show that, as well as these cell membranes modifying the steroids, steroids also modify cell membranes and hence cell function. Thus the strongly anti-catabolic steroids, stanozolol and testosterone, have the effect of making cell surfaces more flexible and more labile, while with corticosteroids surface movement is sluggish to immobile, and the surfaces tend to assume their minimum areas. The anti-catabolic action is, in fact, the effect of the changes in cell behaviour resulting from the changes in surface membrane mobility. The mechanisms of cell division, matrix production and the special case of coalescence to form osteoclasts are all affected by this. So are the changes in quantity and type of intercellular matrix, although these are also partly dependent on changes in the endoplasmic reticulum.

The actions vary from one cell type to another. For instance, the anti-catabolic steroids themselves, without any interactions with corticosteroids, increase the stability of erythrocyte surfaces. This has been demonstrated by Isaacs and Hayhoe (1967) for the abnormal cells in sickle-cell disease. In this condition abnormal haemoglobin crystals distort the erythrocytes, both *in vitro* and *in vivo*, but the presence of testosterone, 17-OH progesterone or durabolin (nor-androstenolene phenyl propionate) stabilized the cell membranes sufficiently to prevent distortion. Neither prednisolone nor oestrone had this stabilizing action. The authors found that treatment with the steroids did not affect the underlying haemoglobin disorder.

The steroids probably do not exert their effect on the cell surfaces unaided. Prop (1961) has shown, in a series of tissue culture experiments, that without insulin present in the medium many, if not all, hormones are unable to act. In another tissue culture experiment, Rigal (1964) has shown that growth hormone helps to preserve marrow cells intact. This field of research is also at an early stage, and is one in which there is much that remains to be discovered.

Summary

1. The two main types of hormone are polypeptides and steroids.

2. In the body groups of compounds have closely inter-related activity. One such group is growth hormone, insulin and serum glucose; and another group includes parathyroid and thyroid hormones and calcitonin.

3. Growth hormone has an anabolic action, and stimulates the formation of proteins and polysaccharides. Those formed in the presence of growth hormone are less chemically stable than the intercellular components whose production is stimulated by anabolic steroids. Growth hormone also stimulates division of stem cells, such as the germinal zone cells of the epiphyseal growth cartilage.

4. Parathyroid hormone has a role in the maintainance of plasma calcium levels. Bone formation and removal do not affect plasma calcium levels.

5. There are two types of precursor cell which can coalesce to form osteoclasts, osteogenic precursor cells and macrophages. In the type of bone removal which is caused by a decreased flow of blood through that portion of the bone osteoclasts formed by coalescence of macrophages dominate. The presence of parathyroid hormone is necessary for macrophages to coalesce, while corticosteroids prevent the formation and maturation of the macrophages. In the formation of this type of osteoclast, therefore, corticosteroids oppose the action of the parathyroid hormone.

6. Cortisol is the corticosteroid formed by the human adrenal cortex. Stress stimulates its formation, so that it is a dominant factor in the aetiology of the major stress diseases.

7. After cortisone administration, a biotransformation at the surfaces of cells in liver, bone, connective tissue and the reticulo-endothelial system converts it to cortisol.

8. Cortisol inhibits the utilization of glucose, releases free fatty acids from adipose tissue, decreases the permeability of capillaries, affects the cerebral cortex to produce emotional symptoms. In the liver it enlarges individual cells, increases the amount of free lipid and glycogen, and causes the total weight to increase. It reduces protein synthetic activity in muscles, and increases the plasma levels of amino acids.

9. In the growth cartilage proliferative activity decreases in the presence of cortisol; intercellular matrix, although more stable, is formed in diminished quantity; and cells do not expand to the hypertrophic state. These observations are consistent with a decrease in activity of cell membranes. So are the reduction in vessel and cell proliferation, decrease in permeability of vessel walls, and other factors which contribute to the anti-inflammatory action.

10. Cortisol stimulates the coalescence of osteogenic precursor cells to form osteoclasts. It also inhibits the formation of more precursor cells, lymphocytes or macrophages. Osteoclasts have a limited life, approximately 48 h, and as the cells die they are replaced by more osteoclasts until the supply of osteogenic precursor cells is exhausted.

11. Anabolic steroids, whether natural or synthetic, interact with excess cortisol. The precise effects vary from one anabolic steroid to another. Steroids show some linked properties, as when the presence of a $17a$ methyl group confers oral activity. In general, however, anabolic steroids have to be considered as separate entities, so they cannot be regarded as interchangeable in the treatment of patients.

12. Some anabolic compounds are more effective than others in opposing the effects of cortisol on liver. Of those which have so far been compared stanozolol, methandienone and decadurabolin are the most effective. These compounds are also the most effective in restoring a feeling of well-being in patients.

13. The anabolic action of these steroids is shown by their ability to increase the protein synthetic activity of cells. In this respect cortisol has an anti-anabolic action. These opposing actions can be used to give a measure of anabolic potency. For those steroids which have so far been compared the anabolic activity, in descending order, is Ba 36644 > stanozolol > lynoestrenol > testosterone > methandienone > norethynodrel > norethisterone.

14. Steroids which oppose the tendency of catabolic steroids to inhibit cell division and suppress the mobility of membranes in cells of the connective tissue series are the anti-catabolic steroids. Evidence concerning the relative anti-catabolic action of a group of steroids may be obtained in a number of ways. Among these are the administration of catabolic and anti-catabolic steroids alternately or simultaneously to growing animals, with observation of the resulting histological pattern in the bone, and the local reaction to infection. In the case of those progestational steroids which stimulate thrombus formation, the organization of necrotic patches caused by deposition of these thrombi varies from fibrous scar tissue to calcification, according to the anti-catabolic level. The relative anti-catabolic activity of those compounds which have so far been compared is: stanozolol > Ba 36644 > testosterone > lynoestrenol and methandienone > norethynodrel > norethisterone.

15. Changes in the histological appearance of bone which are seen in patients under stress have been simulated by administering cortisone and anti-catabolic steroids alternately to animals. The precise effect on the growth cartilage and metaphysis varies from one anti-catabolic steroid to another, the histological appearance of growth cartilage after testosterone administration being closely similar to the changes seen in bones of boys who have died after stressful episodes. Similarly, the alternation of cortisone with a weak anti-catabolic steroid results in the loss of a large proportion of bone tissue, comparable with the effects seen in acute post-menopausal osteoporosis or incorrect timing of doses during steroid therapy.

16. Bone marrow contains haemopoietic tissue and fat cells. Haemopoietic

tissue may also be formed in other parts of the body where sinusoid vessels are present (e.g. the liver and spleen). It is observed in regions of bone turnover, while fatty marrow is found in quiescent parts of the bone. Haemopoietic activity is partly under hormonal control. Effects vary from one steroid or steroid combination to another. Cortisone administration initially increases erythrocyte and platelet production and decreases lymphocyte numbers and activity.

17. The interaction of excess corticosteroid with progestational compounds (including testosterone) produces abnormal megakaryocytes which in turn form abnormal platelets. Normally there are two separate stages in the clumping of platelets. Reversible aggregates are formed first, while later there may be irreversible fusion. The abnormal platelets are sticky, and fuse immediately. The resultant thrombi are mostly small, but some larger ones are formed. All are deposited very soon after formation.

18. The threshold level of cortisol required for the formation of abnormal megakaryocytes, sticky platelets, and thrombi varies from one progestational steroid to another. It is high for some of the synthetic steroids used for therapeutic purposes, lower for testosterone, and lower still for efficient contraceptive compounds.

19. The main sites of action of steroids are cell surfaces and membranes. Steroids modify these membranes, and the membranes initiate steroid biotransformations, thus modifying the steroids and their subsequent properties. Corticosteroids cause the surface movements of connective tissue cells to become sluggish, while anabolic and anti-catabolic steroids render the membranes more flexible and labile. Modes of action vary from one cell type to another. Insulin plays a part in steroid and cell membrane interactions.

T

7. SOME EFFECTS OF STRESS

The stress-induced and degenerative changes which affect the connective and hard tissues include those pathological conditions that are such a frequent accompaniment of ageing that they have been mistaken for that process. They can occur at any age, but because of hormonal changes at the menopause and in the elderly these people are more sensitive to the effects of stress, although some old people remain active and healthy for up to 30 years after these changes have taken place.

The hormonal balance in the body is complex, and stress—primarily emotional—affects it in a number of ways. When some of the metabolic inter-relationships are considered, it can be seen that a change in one parameter could have a multiplicity of effects. Minor variations are responsible for many of the differences between individuals in their mental and emotional make-up, as well as their reaction to stress, and their racial differences. The main pathway by which stress affects a person is through the hypothalmus and the pituitary gland, and the most important change has been found to be a rise in the level of cortisol in the blood. Many of the effects which follow from this are reversible, including those psychotic symptoms that might be mistaken for mental disease, but the consequences of thrombus formation and deposition tend to be irreversible.

Bone is involved in several ways. Most hormones have some effect on its formation and removal. Additionally, not only do deposited thrombi affect the bone tissue itself, but an essential stage in the mechanism of formation of platelet thrombi is the action of certain steroids on the marrow, to form the abnormal megakaryocytes which produce sticky platelets.

Metabolic Inter-relations

In considering hormone balance, many separate but related facts have to be taken into account. The list given in the Appendix contains a number of facts which are reasonably well established.

The list is by no means complete, and only those facts which might be relevant in the present context are included. Others may be found in books such as "Animal Hormones" by Lee and Knowles (1965), and specialized endocrinology textbooks.

With such a wide range of inter-related mechanisms it is essential when pursuing investigations in this field to rely on actual observations as far as possible, and to check all speculations and hypotheses. It is necessary that every observed fact should be accounted for. Otherwise it is very easy to treat inaccurate or incorrect hypotheses as if they were fact, and so reach quite erroneous conclusions. Any hypothesis intended to account for conditions which involve some of these mechanisms, such as vascular disease, osteoporosis or chronic bronchitis, should be checked to ensure that it does not contradict established facts. In general it is better to seek an understanding of biological mechanisms, rather than to rely on facile correlations. Such methods can only give a correct answer when *all* the relevant information is fed into the process, and with such a large number of variables there is a high probability that some which are essential, if the correct deductions are to be made, will be overlooked. Some common errors in reasoning are best seen in actual examples.

(*a*) It is widely "known" that sugar causes dental caries. If one surveys the literature on the subject hundreds of papers state this as a result of investigations where the sugar was taken in conjunction with starch. A much smaller number of papers have been written which provide evidence that sugar alone does not influence the incidence of caries, but that some starches do.

(*b*) There has been concern over the increase of thrombotic episodes in women of child-bearing age. Accordingly, the deaths from thrombosis in that age group for a period of a year were examined. It was found that there were no deaths from thrombosis in women who were not taking contraceptive steroids and had not had a child during the year. There were an approximately equal number of deaths among women taking contraceptive steroids and those having children. The conclusion that was widely reported was that these contraceptive agents were no more dangerous than having a child. But those were not the only relevant facts. Given the additional information that all the women who during that period died of thrombi after child-birth were taking stilboestrol to prevent lactation (this compound affects pituitary secretion), and that there is evidence that the administration of stilboestrol for this purpose increases the incidence of non-fatal thrombi (Oliver and Boyd, 1961; Daniel, Campbell and Turnbull, 1962), a more realistic conclusion would have been that women of child-bearing age, whether or not they have children, are not likely to die from thrombi unless they are taking drugs which affect the hormone balance.

(*c*) It is sometimes said that because people who are coronary risks tend to smoke more heavily than people of equivalent age who are not at risk, smoking is one of the contributory causes of the condition. But other facts are known. One is that stress is the cause of rises in serum cholesterol and cortisol, and the clotting rate, which bring a person into the category of coronary risk. Another is that one reason for smoking is that the individual concerned feels that it helps to reduce mental stress or tension. Further, although non-smokers who "experiment" with a cigarette show the transitory rise in plasma cortisol associated with novelty, smoking does not effect cortisol levels of habitual smokers (Hökfelt, 1961). It is thus not surprising that the German Institute for Industrial and Social Medicine have found that those members investigated who were in the "at risk" category and who were also heavy smokers suffered less from headaches and heart trouble than non-smokers who were "at risk".

These three examples are chosen as ones where the members of the medical and dental professions working on the problems tend to have a personal emotional involvement. In such cases it sometimes helps to apply the same argument to a non-controversial topic. Thus, an analogous statement with the type of reasoning used in reaching the conclusion that smoking is a contributory cause of coronary heart disease would be "because people with acute infections take antibiotics more frequently than other categories of person, therefore antibiotics are one of the causes of acute infection".

It will be appreciated that there is no place for a theory based solely on the use of one technique. It must be remembered that statistical methods are merely one of the ways of obtaining suggestions which might possibly provide a short cut to a knowledge of the type of evidence that would lead to an elucidation of the mechanisms of the subject under discussion. Before attempting this short cut it would be as well to study the reasoning involved, in a work such as Dodgson's "Symbolic Logic" (1896).

Stress

Stress, in the sense in which it is commonly used, activates

(a) the adrenal medulla to liberate adrenalin (A132, A133*),

(b) the anterior pituitary gland, initiating a more complex series of events (A4, A7, A32, A80, A104) that include activation of the adrenal cortex.

Situations which provoke stress reactions include many of emotional origin, trauma, pain (Shenkin, 1964), acute infection (Bassoe et al., 1965) or illness (Sholiton et al., 1961), and terminal illness, in particular cancer

*Numbers preceded by "A" refer to points listed in the Appendix, pp. 289–296.

(Werk *et al.*, 1964). The unpleasant emotions are stressful: anger, fear and jealousy, with apprehension and anxiety being particularly potent. Stimuli such as dental appointments (Shannon, Isbell, Prigmore and Hester, 1962) or merely entering hospital as normal controls in an experiment (Mason *et al.*, 1965) cause an increased corticosteroid level, while the greater stress of university examinations (Scrimshaw *et al.*, 1966) or space flight (NASA, 1967) produce higher levels and a temporary negative nitrogen balance. Bureaucratic control is another cause of stress. Thus, coronary thrombosis as a cause of death of farmers in the Scottish borders was almost unknown until the post-war form-filling era. Within a few years it had become the most frequent cause of death among these farmers (G. Rutherford, 1955, pers. comm).

The pleasant emotions, joy, love and a tranquil state are not stressful. Neither is a "hectic life" if it does not involve the stressful emotions or excess physical stress (Chapman *et al.*, 1966). In an extensive survey these same authors have also shown that high cholesterol levels are not accounted for by blood pressure, physical activity, smoking habits or body weight. Novelty tends to be a factor, so that individuals can become psychologically adapted to a situation (Mason, 1959; Davis *et al.*, 1962). Conversely, when an activity such as smoking has been used to relieve stress, withdrawal tends to produce a more severe reaction.

There is abundant evidence that individuals react to potentially stressful situations differently (Davis *et al.*, 1962; Tesse *et al.*, 1965; Bursten and Russ, 1965; Scrimshaw *et al.*, 1966). The degree of reaction reflects personality differences, while variations in hormonal make-up result in different effects dominating. There are variations between men and women, as for example the fact that women have a lower susceptibility to severe cardiovascular disease and chronic bronchitis; there is often a familial tendency to, say, longevity or coronaries; elderly people, after their level of adrenal and gonadal anabolic hormones begins to fall (at the age of 60–70, and 40–50 for female gonadal steroids) react to smaller stressful stimuli; and many racial differences have also been observed.

These racial differences are undoubtedly the result of differences in hormonal make-up, (e.g. A101, A102, A103). Thus, when the incidence of cerebral vascular disease and coronary heart disease were compared in South Africa (Walker and Seftel, 1962) it was observed that there was little difference between the sexes for cerebral vascular disease, but that it was more common in the Indian than in the white population. By contrast, the incidence of coronary heart disease was about the same for the Indian and the white, but it was far more common in men than in women.

Nordin has compared the incidence of osteoporosis and pathological fractures in the elderly in several countries, and differences are again significant. The most striking differences are between the main ethnic groups. In Africans and Negroes post-menopausal and senile osteoporosis are very rare. These people retain a fairly high level of growth hormone throughout their adult life (A103). In countries such as the United Kingdom and Finland there is a fair amount of osteoporosis together with pathological fractures, predominantly in women. The Indians and Japanese have a far higher proportion of post-menopausal and senile osteoporosis, and the incidence in Japan is possibly the highest in the world. In Japan, too, a high proportion of men are affected, as compared with India. G. C. Robin (1968, pers. comm.) has compared Orientals with Western races among the inhabitants of Jerusalem, and observed that the pathological fractures of the hip which are a complication of osteoporosis are more common in women, but that they occur to a lesser extent in white men and to an intermediate extent in Oriental men. The ratio of female to male is approximately 2:1 for the white and 1·3:1 for the Oriental.

In the same way that there are differences between the Indians and the Japanese, there are indications that there are racial differences within Europe. When the incidence of femoral neck and wrist fractures were compared for cities in England (Buhr and Cooke, 1959), Switzerland (Schlettwein-Gsell, 1966) and Sweden (Alffram, 1964) the incidence in England and Switzerland is fairly high, but in Sweden it is approximately double that in the other two countries. Alffram (1964) came to the conclusion that this represents a real biological difference, and this would seem to be borne out by the differing incidence of other conditions such as Paget's disease (Price, 1962) and chronic bronchitis.

One must always remember that there are other factors to take into account beside the dominant genetic and hormonal differences, and Schlettwein-Gsell's observations (1966) provide a timely reminder. In Switzerland, although osteoporosis and its consequent fractures are fairly common in the city (Basel) they occur far less frequently in the inhabitants of mountainous regions, and are very rare among the men in those regions. The amount of exercise taken by these people undoubtedly plays a part, and so may the less harassed live in those surroundings. Both Nordin (1966) and Schlettwein-Gsell (1966) have aimed at explaining their findings in terms of dietary differences. An additional finding in Nordin's survey was a widespread prevalence of rickets and osteomalacia in India. This is undoubtedly partly nutritional in origin, but there is the fact that other racial types, also with nutritional deficiencies, do not show such a marked response to a low intake of vitamin D. In Great Britain, for example, Indian and Pakistani immigrants have a higher level of late rickets and osteomalacia than can be accounted for by a simple nutritional deficiency. Symptoms tend to develop at puberty and during pregnancy, and the length of time spent in Great Britain has been found to be irrelevant. This osteomalacia is often calciferol-resistant, and Swan and Cook (1971) have come to the conclusion that in these people there is a defect at some point in the conversion of vitamin D_2 to its physiologically active metabolite.

Within any one racial group, however, there are wide differences in the manner in which the effects of stress show themselves. This is due to the interplay of a range of factors which include hormonal differences between individuals, their general state of fitness, the amount of exercise they take, the amount of sugar in their diet, and the frequency, duration and intensity of stressful episodes. Since several different metabolic pathways are involved there is the probability that two or more manifestations of stress will occur simultaneously. With this array of variables there is no satisfactory alternative to a systematic survey of the mechanisms involved. The main outline is known, but many details await elucidation.

Stimulation of the adrenal medulla

Adrenalin is released, and acts rapidly. It decreases the blood supply to the gastro-intestinal tract, and increases the blood supply to the muscular system (A134). There is an increase in the amount of available oxygen, while acid waste products that would hinder muscle activity are removed more rapidly. At the same time the liver provides extra glucose (A136). The two together provide increased energy for immediate flight, fighting, or other excessive physical exertion. This primitive reaction occurs even when the modern situation allows of no energetic response. When adrenalin is released repeatedly, and without subsequent physical activity, interference with the normal functioning of the digestive tract can lead to the formation of *gastric and duodenal ulcers* or *ulcerative colitis*.

Adrenalin also causes free fatty acids, lipoproteins, cholesterol, triglycerides and phospholipids to be released into the blood stream (A138–A140). Simultaneously the clotting time decreases (Friedman *et al.*, 1958). Macht (1952) showed that in healthy people, both male and female, acute apprehension or fear and intense worry markedly accelerated blood coagulation. Such effects are useful to initiate healing after trauma, but can aggravate problems caused by the deposition of thrombi. Lecithin facilitates the aggregation of platelets (A144), while factors which contribute to the deposition of fibrin are also enhanced.

Adrenalin converts glycogens to glucose (A136), thus providing a rapid rise in available energy. It stimulates the secretion of ACTH, which releases cortisol (A137). This cortisol has more than one effect. It helps to restock glycogen supplies, and also enables the adrenalin to mobilize lipids in quantity (A138, A141). The concentration of cholesterol in the serum can vary widely during the course of a few hours (A139, A140) (Peterson *et al.*, 1962; Wolf *et al.*, 1962). Cortisol shows similar fluctuations with changing emotional states (A143) (Bliss *et al.*, 1956; Bunney *et al.*, 1965).

Deposition of lipids

Circulating lipids are held in suspension by proteins present in the blood, but under certain conditions they may be deposited as free fat or cholesterol crystals on vessel walls. Observation of the nature and distribution of these deposits suggests that several contributory factors are involved. The most obvious is that the quantity of lipids held in the blood should rise above normal. Another appears to be that some haemolysis of red cells should have taken place. In the arteries and around prosthetic replacements lipid deposits are commonly observed at sites where there is, or has been, turbulence or stagnation. They are not found in vessels where the flow of blood is smooth. Before the age of about 50 coronary artery disease is often not associated with a more generalized atherosclerosis. It is probable that a chemical released from erythrocytes damaged in regions of turbulent flow, is involved in the mechanism of fat deposition.

Once lipids have been deposited they are surrounded by fibrous tissue, or in pneumatized bone by osseous tissue (Fig. 7.1) (Simonetta, 1949; Altes, 1966; Beaumont, 1967b). Lipids deposited on artery walls, together with their sequellae, have been shown to be benign (Mitchell *et al.*, 1964). The coronary artery disease from this cause is symptomless; whereas coronary heart disease, with no greater amounts of cholesterol deposition and an equivalent decrease in diameter of the lumen of the arteries, has serious consequences (Mason, 1963). One additional factor is thrombus deposition. Mitchell *et al.*, (1964) have found that the deposits which lead to undesirable symptoms are not the fatty streaks but plaques with quite different appearances. They have also ascertained that thrombi cause the plaques, associated with clinical symptoms, but plaques do not cause thrombi. An important difference between the male and the female is that in the latter there is less proliferation of fibrous tissue in response to any given stimulus, so that for a given amount of cholesterol deposition the narrowing of the lumen of the coronary arteries is less. It takes a larger thrombus, therefore, to block the coronary artery

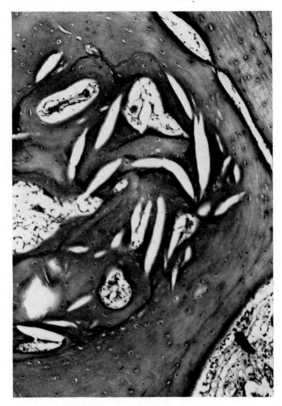

Fig. 7.1. Cholesterol deposited in a pneumatized hen bone after operative interference with the air supply. Granulation tissue formed around the cyrstals (which occupied the areas now seem as empty elongated spaces) and ossified. Later the whole cholesterol nodule was surrounded by a layer of lamellar bone. × 100.

in the woman, so that there is a smaller probability that she will show the symptoms of *coronary heart disease*.

Pituitary stimulation

Stress activates the anterior pituitary gland, and since this gland has a number of functions the further effects produced by stress may be diverse, with very different symptoms from one individual to the next.

The alternating rhythm of oestrogen and progesterone production (A4) may be temporarily affected. Bliss *et al.* (1956) have also shown that interspersed with the bursts of high adrenal activity resulting from emotional stress there may be bursts of high oestrogen output. In the body it has been found (Ullberg and Bengtsson, 1963) that oestrogens accumulate selectively in the ovarian follicles, endometrium and adrenal cortex, and that there is also a fairly high concentration in the brain. Since peptide hormones and steroids affect the mobility of cell membranes there is a possibility that the concentration of oestrogen in the brain directly affects the mental state.

Over activity of the thyroid gland is another possibility. An increased thyroid production can sensitize the tissues to adrenalin (A114). Mental stress and anxiety are commonly cited as the cause of *thyrotoxicosis,* in which restlessness and over activity are combined with tiredness and an actual physical weakness. Again there are emotional symptoms. Witte (1966) has reported cases of *acute hyperthyroidism* which were in response to known stressful stimuli. Women are more commonly affected.

When stress activates the pituitary gland, the most frequently observed effects are those which are consequent upon the release of ACTH. This in turn activates the adrenal cortex, and the result is a rise in the level of cortisol in the blood (A32). In mice, an increase in the weight of the adrenal in stressed animals (those of lower social status in a group) has even been observed (Christian and Davis, 1957). The increase in corticosteroids during stress is predominantly of unbound steroid (Knigge and Hoar, 1963), and it seems most probable that it is the unbound cortisol which is responsible for the various effects which have been observed. The increase is maintained for a longer period when excess oestrogens are present (A38), or during fasting (A39).

It has been said that for some people "food acts as a sedative" (Wright *et al.,* 1968), and it is worth considering the effect of sugar on cortisol mechanisms. Those cited in the last section point to two possible routes whereby sugar can counter, at least to some extent, the effects of stress. The effect of excess cortisol on the brain is either euphoria, or emotional symptoms varying, according to the degree of stress, from a *nervous state and depression* through a *chronic anxiety state* to *severe psychotic episodes* (A69). The brain is also dependent on an adequate level of blood sugar, and both rational thought and emotional stability are impaired when the level of sugar drops (A99). One action of sugar, therefore, is to help restore emotional stability and the ability to assess a situation objectively, thereby directly reducing a major cause of stress. At the same time, the balance with insulin is such that an increase in sugar increases the insulin output, and this in turn reduces the effect of cortisol on cell surfaces.

Exercise also helps to reduce the harmful effects of stress. Morris *et al.* (1953) and others have shown that men in physically active jobs have a lower incidence of coronary heart disease, and in milder form, than men of similar age in equivalent sedentary jobs. An explanation of these observations, and others like them, was provided when Cornil *et al.* (1965) demonstrated that muscular exercise by untrained normal men is accompanied by a significant fall in plasma cortisol levels.

Cortisol has a wide variety of actions, many of them due to its effect on cell membranes. The effects on cells in the brain are mentioned in the Appendix (A69), and these may be modified by the presence of abnormal quantities of hormones, steroids and related compounds. Thus, euphoria tends to be more common in the male than in the female. In the presence of progestational compounds the severity of episodes of depression is increased (Grant and Pryse-Davies, 1968), so that women who take effective contraceptive agents when under stress tend to be suicide risks. The more severe effects, which require hospital treatment, need to be distinguished from genuine mental disease. Patients revert to normal behaviour and normal reactions when the cell membranes are restored to normal. In many instances, particularly in the elderly, administration of anabolic steroids has had the desired effect (Wynn and Landon, 1961; Wynn, 1968).

Cortisol affects the proliferation of connective tissue cells (A56), and the production of intercellular matrices (A47, A76). As a result of this Plotz *et al.* (1950) have reported that skin incisions in cortisone-treated patients fail to repair normally. The lack of adequate repair mechanisms in the skin has also led to the production of *purpura* in patients treated with corticosteroids (McConkey *et al.*, 1965) similar to that seen in elderly people who exhibit other symptoms that could be caused by stress. *Muscle weakness* is also observed, together with osteoporotic symptoms. One type of *osteoporosis* is the result of the direct action of corticosteroids on bone, as was described in Chapter 6, while the whole subject of osteoporosis will be considered in greater detail in Chapter 8. Yet another effect of cortisol is to decrease inflammation, both by reducing the permeability of capillaries and by the destruction of lymphocytes (Dougherty, Berliner and Berliner, 1962). Normally the cause of inflammation is not affected, and the lack of its effects may actively help, for example, the spread of an infection. Zweifach, Shorr and Black (1953) have also suggested that disturbances in cardiovascular function may be due to the alteration in the permeability of capillaries, while this may also be a contributory cause of *chronic bronchitis*.

In the case of conditions such as *asthma* and *allergy* in children, Harper (1962) has shown that they are prominent in a definite genetic type with characteristic appearances. He has further been able to demonstrate beyond reasonable doubt that those manifestations in children are stress-induced. He has followed a substantial number of cases where symptoms have disappeared when children moved into almost stress-free surroundings, but recurred when the stressful stimuli were temporarily renewed.

Many of the changes which result from an excess of cortisol are reversible, but there is one important mechanism which often produces irreversible results (A79). The effects of the production of platelet thrombi will be considered further in the next section.

Thrombi

The mechanism of thrombus formation was described in Chapter 6. The interaction of a raised plasma cortisol with other steroids can result in a changed manner of formation and maturation of megakaryocytes, followed by the production of abnormally sticky platelets. These platelets adhere to one another to form thrombi which then adhere to the walls of arteries and veins. For each episode of stress many small thrombi may form, and occasionally there is a more massive one that produces dramatic results.

In their survey Mitchell *et al.* (1964) showed that, for white people living in Great Britain, the fatty streaks are not closely related to age, but that the plaques that result from thrombi were not common before the age of about 35 in men and 50 in women. They were often found in areas of turbulence, the carotid, femoral and pulmonary arteries each being an important site. Fibrin from the blood is often deposited on platelet thrombi, with the possibility of emboli breaking loose and blocking vital arteries. Those from the carotid artery are particularly dangerous, since they may deprive portions of the brain of their blood supply, and sometimes cause blindness when they lodge in vessels behind the eye.

Small thrombi lodge in arteries and veins in many parts of the body. Most organs or tissues have, or can develop, an alternative blood supply, but parts of the heart and brain lack a collateral circulation, and damage done as a result of thrombus or embolus deposition is irreversible. *Cerebral vascular disease* and *coronary heart disease* are thus the most serious consequences of stress. Minor vascular damage in the brain frequently shows as a *headache* although, apart from women taking progestational steroids and related compounds, headaches are more usually the result of muscular tension.

The effects of *venous thrombosis* vary according to the site in the body. The bones, as well as being the organs upon which stress acts in order to produce thrombi, are themselves vulnerable to an impaired blood supply. When the flow of blood through a bone is hindered by deposits in vessels, often enlarged during their subsequent organization, the result is commonly known as *senile osteoporosis*.

Occasionally massive thrombi are deposited in bone, so cutting off a sector and causing *avascular necrosis*. A common site for this is the head of the femur. When the blood supply to a portion of the bone is cut off osteocytes and other cells die and that portion of the bone becomes necrotic. The articular cartilage remains alive and chondrocytes tend to proliferate so that it becomes thicker than normal. Around the periphery of the lesion an active repair process commences with vascular activity, osteoclastic activity and new bone formation. The frequency of occurrence of avascular necrosis has risen considerably since the mid-1950s, and d'Aubigne (1964) has found that in a high proportion of the cases there has been a prior administration of corticosteroids, for a variety of conditions. Burrows (1965) has pointed out that when the administration of the corticosteroid is accompanied by that of another steroid (e.g. methyl testosterone or contraceptive steroids) avascular necrosis may occur in several sites almost simultaneously. Avascular necrosis of the hip under such circumstances is frequently bilateral. Such thrombus formation is not the only possible causative mechanism for avascular necrosis. In some instances Jones (1971) has demonstrated the presence of fat globules in bone capillaries. In these cases he also found that large fat droplets were present in the liver.

In the animal experiments described in Chapter 6 it was found that for each steroid there is a threshold level of cortisol above which the changes that lead to thrombus formation are found. This threshold is considerably lower for synthetic progestational compounds than it is for naturally occurring hormones. Post-mortem investigations by Irey, Manion and Taylor (1970) point to a similar conclusion. In women who had died from thrombi produced as a result of taking progestational steroids they found multiple thrombi, but no evidence of the atherosclerosis that is a frequent accompaniment of the thrombi produced by stress in the presence of natural hormones alone. Normally one would only expect to find such thrombi in women in this age group after a serious illness. This abnormally high level of thrombus formation was well recognized by 1962, and there were frequent reports in such publications as the British Medical Journal and the Lancet. Salmon, Winkelman and Gay (1968) have pointed out, for instance, that there is no record of vertebrobasilar occlusion in otherwise healthy young women except for those who have taken contraceptive steroids.

These steroids have more than one action. Grant (1968) has found that headaches and mood changes are the main initial complaints, but that after a while vascular reactions turn out to be the most frequent and troublesome complaint. The incidence varies with the progestational steroid used, but in the first year is in the range of 30% to 60% of the individuals concerned. It is well recognized that the progestational component in contraceptive agents is primarily responsible for depression and psychological effects (Brit. Med. J. 1969), although oestrogens also have an effect on cells in the brain. The situation over vascular lesions is more complex, since three separate mechanisms are involved. So far as deposits from the blood are concerned the first step is thrombus formation as a result of the production of abnormal platelets. This is mediated by the progestational steroids. Once these thrombi have adhered to vessel walls fibrin and more platelets can adhere to them. The changes which produce this secondary deposition are sensitized by oestrogens (Bolton, Hampton and Mitchell, 1968). The third change, which seems to be present in all women taking these steroids is a hyperplasia of the vessel walls (Irey *et al.*, 1970). This last effect could mean that in due course the incidence of coronary heart disease and chronic bronchitis in these women will be nearer that in men, as compared with normal women. More important, this internal proliferation will occlude vessels and so produce violent circulatory disturbances.

There are a number of other late effects of vascular occlusion as a result of taking these steroids, but here it is the effect on bone that is of immediate interest. There is an almost total lack of published data, so that this discussion is mostly concerned with points that need to be watched. The increase of infarcts has already been mentioned, and this is the only immediate effect that is likely to be noticed. The others are long-term.

Another possible effect is due to the direct action of the steroids on bone. In the adult an unsuitable alternation of anabolic and catabolic steroids results in a reduction of the amount of bone tissue present in a bone. This is the mechanism in post-menopausal osteoporosis. It can occur in younger people who are receiving corticosteroids as treatment for rheumatoid arthritis and other conditions, and it is also possible for contraceptive steroids to have the same effect. In the adolescent the situation is more complicated, since the natural mechanism of plate closure in bones involves an alternation of anabolic and catabolic levels. During this period there are minor menstrual irregularities that normally disappear spontaneously—it takes about three years to achieve a stable pattern. When these apparently necessary irregularities are artificially stabilized by the administration of steroids, or when children take progestational steroids as an adjunct to fornication, the alternation is disrupted. Bone remodelling is therefore liable to be affected. As a result of longer periods with raised catabolic steroid levels, the bones may become unduly porotic, and in the long-term abnormalities in remodelling and the maturation of bone can lead to arthritic changes. The hip joint is particularly susceptible.

The formation of minor thrombi in young women would also lead to the development of porotic bones, by exactly the same mechanism as operates in senile osteoporosis. Descriptions of radiological appearances and bone histology of individuals taking these steroids are almost completely absent from the literature, so that this would be a useful field of investigation. A point of academic interest would be to ascertain the ease with which the histological appearance of abnormal megakaryocytes from tissue obtained at post-mortem can be correlated with the specific steroids or other compounds taken by the victim. Further problems may well arise if compounds are used which are designed to affect the pituitary gland directly, since in that case all the metabolic pathways could be disorganized.

Summary

1. In considering hormone balance many separate but related facts have to be taken into account. Some of the facts necessary for an understanding of stress and its effects on bone are listed. These properties include:

(a)   those related to the activity of the anterior pituitary gland;
(b)   those related to the activity of the adrenal cortex;
(c)   those concerned with the production and properties of cortisol,
(d)   and the anabolic hormones,
(e)   growth hormone,
(f)   insulin,
(g)   thyroid hormone,
(h)   and parathyroid hormone;
(i)   those related to the activity of the adrenal medulla and adrenalin; and
(j)   those related to the activity of the neurohypophysis.

2. The need for ascertaining mechanisms of such complex interactions is discussed, together with rules for the development of viable theories.

3. Causes of physiological stress reactions are most frequently the stressful emotions, particularly apprehension and worry. Physical stress can be a contributory cause.

4. There are individual, familial and racial differences in the reactions to stressful stimuli, as a result of underlying hormonal differences. There are also differences between male and female, and in elderly people. Thus, the Negro who has a larger proportion of bone tissue is almost immune to osteoporosis, while the different fat metabolism of the Indians and Pakistanis leads to a greater susceptibility to osteomalacia. There are differences between racial groups within the main ethnic types. Elderly people, with a more precarious anabolic/catabolic balance, are more susceptible to the effects of stress than younger people.

5. An immediate reaction to stress is the release of adrenalin from the adrenal medulla. It decreases the blood supply to the gastro-intestinal tract, and increases the blood supply to the muscular system. When adrenalin is released repeatedly and without subsequent physical activity, ulcerative lesions of the gastro-intestinal tract may develop.

6. Adrenalin also causes lipids to be released into the blood stream, and subsequent release of cortisol from the adrenal cortex allows them to be mobilized in quantity. Fatty deposits on blood vessel walls which may result from the presence of these lipids are benign. Once deposited they are surrounded by fibrous tissue, and the higher anabolic level in the male causes a greater decrease in the lumen of vessels in men than in women.

7. Both cholesterol and cortisol are released into the blood as a result of stress. Their levels show parallel fluctuations with changing emotional states.

8. Stress also activates the anterior pituitary gland, with several possible effects:

(a) The alternating rhythm of oestrogen and progesterone production may be temporarily affected. Excess steroid may affect cells of the brain directly, leading to depression or psychotic symptoms.

(b) Excess thyroid hormone may be produced, giving rise to thyrotoxicosis or acute hyperthyroidism, depending upon the level of stimulus.

(c) ACTH may activate the adrenal cortex to produce excess cortisol.

9. The excess cortisol may be partly controlled by muscular exercise or by an increased sugar intake.

10. Cortisol has a number of different effects:

(a) It may induce euphoria; or depression, anxiety and psychotic symptoms.

(b) Its catabolic action may lead to skin lesions, muscle weakness and post-menopausal osteoporosis.

(c) It decreases the effects, but not the causes, of inflammation, by reducing the permeability of capillaries and destruction of lymphocytes.

11. Many of the changes which result from an excess of cortisol are reversible, but thrombus formation can have irreversible consequences. Thrombi formed as a result of stress are usually small, but occasionally more massive ones are produced.

12. In arterial disease the fatty lesions are benign, but plaques that result from thrombi cause clinical symptoms. Cerebral vascular disease and coronary heart disease are the most serious of the consequences of these stress-induced thrombi. The effects of venous thrombi vary according to the site in the body.

13. In addition to massive damage to the brain, lesser consequences of vascular lesions are headaches and migraines.

14. In bone, multiple small thrombi produce an almost irreversible senile osteoporosis. Occasional larger thrombi or emboli which block vessels leading to a sector of bone cause avascular necrosis. This is more common when steroids are being taken.

15. Contraceptive steroids have an exceptionally low cortisol threshold level for thrombus formation, and a high proportion of women are affected (one survey showed 30% to 60% in the first year). Headaches and mood changes are early symptoms.

16. The progestational steroids produce abnormal platelets which readily coalesce to form thrombi, and the oestrogens sensitize other blood clotting factors. These steroids also induce hyperplasia of vessel walls.

17. Contraceptive steroids can induce abnormal effects in bone. It is possible that when adolescents take contraceptive agents these will interfere with the normal processes of remodelling and plate closure, and so lead to other lesions later in life.

Appendix

In considering problems associated with hormone balance, many separate but related facts have to be taken into account. This list gives 150 such facts that are reasonably well established. Only those relevant to problems dealt with in this book are included, but even for this it is by no means a complete list.

A1. Under nervous control: anterior pituitary gland and adrenal medulla; and indirectly, adrenal cortex and thyroid.

A2. Primarily under chemical control: neurohypophesis, pancreas and parathyroid.

A3. The central nervous system controls the anterior pituitary gland by way of the hypothalmus. The immediate control by the hypothalmus is chemical, by way of connecting vessels passing through the pituitary stalk.

A4. The anterior pituitary gland produces gonadotrophic hormones, which in the adult female stimulate the alternate production of *oestradiol* and *progesterone*.

A5. In the adult male the gonadotrophic hormones stimulate the production of *testosterone* by the testis.

A6. The hormones whose production is stimulated by the gonadotrophic hormones then proceed to suppress the formation of the latter.

A7. Among the hormones *oestradiol, progesterone, testosterone* and *cortisol* are steroids, while *growth hormone* and *calcitonin* are polypeptides.

A8. All hormones have more than one action.

A9. Related steroids, whether natural or synthetic, exhibit their different properties in different proportions. Thus, *testosterone* is both anabolic and androgenic, while for *stanozolol* at any given anabolic level the androgenic properties are lower than those of *testosterone* by a factor of about 8.

A10. Testicular hormones are more strongly anabolic than ovarian hormones.

A11. There tend to be variations from one species to another in the precise steroids produced by a gland. Thus:
(a) *Testosterone* is formed in the testis in man, and the prostate secretes *acid phosphatase*; while in the rat the testis produces *androstenedione*, and the prostate secretes *alkaline phosphatase*. When acting on bone these hormone systems induce a different pattern of cell behaviour, one manifestation of which are the open epiphyses in adult rats.
(b) *Cortisol* is produced by the human adrenal cortex and *corticosterone* in the rabbit. So far as bone is concerned these two corticosteroids have very similar properties. The difference observed in cell behaviour between the bones of rabbit and man is that although the same actions occur they are seen more quickly in the rabbit.

A12. Androgenic properties are those which lead to male development and oestrogenic properties are those which lead to female development.

A13. The level of *progesterone* and *oestrogen* is at its lowest just prior to menstruation.

A14. One method of reducing post-menopausal symptoms has been to give *oestradiol*.

A15. The action of *prolactin*, one of the gonadotrophic hormones, together with *insulin* and *cortisol,* is among the requirements for lactation.

A16. Progestational compounds suppress the formation of *prolactin*.

A17. *Oestrogens* lower *cholesterol* and elevate *phospholipid levels* in serum. *Androgens* reverse these effects.

A18. *Diethyl stilboestrol* has some of the actions of the oestrogens, but it is not itself a steroid.

A19. *Diethyl stilboestrol* decreases serum *cholesterol* levels, but increases thrombus incidence (Oliver and Boyd, 1961; Daniel *et al.*, 1962).

A20. *Stilboestrol* is a *pituitary* suppressant. In the *stilboestrol* series of compounds it is impossible to dissociate oestrogenic activity from pituitary suppressant activity (Dodds, 1961).

A21. Suppression of the pituitary by *stilboestrol* is only temporary. In prostatic cancer return of symptoms is detectable 3 days after stopping the maintenance dose.

A22. *Diethyl stilboestrol* administration causes an increase in Factor IX level (Daniel *et al.*, 1968).

A23. Both *oestradiol* and *testosterone* first stimulate bone growth, and then later cause closure of the epiphyseal cartilage plate. In this they are showing anabolic properties.

A24. Castration leads to excessive growth of the long bones.

A25. The anterior pituitary gland produces an adrenocorticotrophic hormone (*ACTH*) which stimulates the adrenal cortex. Acute stress increases the production of *ACTH*.

A26. The production of *ACTH* is suppressed by *cortisol*.

A27. The adrenal cortex produces *aldosterone, cortisol,* and small quantities of *oestrogens, androgens* and *progestogens.*

A28. The precise methods of control of *aldosterone* secretion are not yet known. It is partly controlled by *ACTH*, and partly by the level of *potassium* ions in the blood.

A29. *Aldosterone* regulates the concentration of *sodium* ions in the blood by promoting re-absorption in the kidney.

A30. With a deficiency of *aldosterone* excess *sodium* is excreted and there is a rise in the level of plasma *potassium*. This leads to muscle and cardiac weakness.

A31. With an excess of *aldosterone* there is salt and water retention, with an expansion of plasma volume and a fall of plasma *potassium*. This also leads to muscle weakness.

A32. The level of *cortisol* in the blood is primarily controlled by the level of *ACTH* (Dougherty and White, 1944).

A33. There is a diurnal variation in the secretion of *cortisol*.

A34. The half-life for disappearance of *cortisol* from the plasma is 78–120 min.

A35. Muscular exercise causes a fall in the plasma *cortisol* levels (Cornil *et al.*, 1965).

A36. The plasma cortisol level is very low during a hypnotic trance (Sacher *et al.*, 1966).

A37. Pregnancy involves an increased *cortisol* level. There is simultaneously an increase in the plasma binding capacity (Appleby and Norymberski, 1957).

A38. *Oestrogen* treatment increases the half-life of plasma cortisol by a factor of about 2. It is accompanied by a 4-fold rise in the concentration of protein binding sites (Mills, Schedl, Chen and Bartler, 1960).

A39. Fasting increases the half-life of plasma *cortisol*. After 4 days it is up by a factor of about 2. This facilitates extra mobility of carbohydrate to produce energy. There is little increase in the number of protein binding sites.

A40. There are biotransformations at cell surfaces. Thus, in the human when *cortisone* (inactive) is administered a third of it is converted to *cortisol* (active).

A41. The peak value of plasma *cortisol* is 2 h after the administration of *cortisone*, and 1 h after the administration of *cortisol*.

A42. Liver is the most important site for the conversion of *cortisone* to *cortisol* and *prednisone* to *prednisolone*. The efficiency of *cortisone* to *cortisol* is approximately a third, and of *prednisone* to *prednisolone* about 90% (Jenkins and Sampson, 1966).

A43. Proteins and polysaccharides present in the surrounding fluids modify biotransformations. Thus, chondroitin B taken up by fibroblasts inhibits the transformation of *cortisone* to *cortisol* but not *cortisol* to *cortisone*.

A44. *Cortisol* causes *glycogen* to be formed in the liver, and as the *cortisol* level in the blood rises, so does the amount of *glycogen* in the liver. This *glycogen* is the main source of blood *glucose*.

A45. An increased *cortisol* is accompanied by an increase in adipose tissue.

A46. *Cortisol* does not affect the peripheral utilization of *glucose*, or the peripheral action of *insulin* on the uptake of *glucose*.

A47. *Cortisol* hinders protein production. With the administration of a single dose an effect is found within 2 h and recovery in 10 h.

A48. With *cortisol* there is an increase in the plasma level of amino acids.

A49. *Cortisol* increases the level of *pyruvate* and *lactate* in the blood. It decreases the blood citrate level.

A50. Some de-esterification takes place in the marrow fat of post-menopausal women during each osteoporotic episode.

A51. *Cortisol* causes a rise in *free fatty acids, cholesterol, phospholipids* and *triglycerides* in serum. Changes in *serum lipids* are secondary to increased mobilization of free fatty acids from adipose tissue.

A52. The effect of *cortisol* in releasing *free fatty acids* from adipose tissue is overcome by the simultaneous infusion of *insulin* (Jenkins *et al.*, 1964).

A53. The main effect of *salicylate* is to depress *free fatty acid* release from adipose tissue (Carlson and Ostman, 1961).

A54. *Insulin* has no effect on increased plasma *cortisol* during pregnancy and delivery.

A55. *Cortisol* reduces the number of circulating eosinophils in the blood.

A56. *Cortisol* reduces the mobility of connective tissue cell membranes, and hence the proliferation of connective tissue cells and vascular proliferation.

A57. *Cortisol* inhibits the abnormal proliferation of granulation tissue cells in rheumatoid arthritis.

A58. Most patients with rheumatoid arthritis receive adequate suppression of inflammation on a smaller dose of *corticosteroid* when *methandrostenolone* (Dianabol) is given in addition (Clark and Mills, 1962).

A59. *Cortisol* suppresses *calcium* absorption from the gut.

A60. *Cortisol* suppresses *vitamin D* absorption from the gut.

A61. *Cortisol* reduces the permeability of capillaries, and so affects the cardiovascular functions, electrolyte and water balance, and renal function.

A62. *Cortisol* reduces inflammation.

A63. In the early stages of continuous *cortisol* administration, the number of red cells and platelets is increased, and the number of active lymphocytes reduced. Later all haemopoietic activity tends to be suppressed and red marrow is replaced by fatty marrow.

A64. *Cortisol* induces lysis of lymphocytes. There is reduced mitosis and loss of cytoplasm.

A65. *Cortisol* prevents macrophages from maturing and inhibits their activity.

A66. *Cortisol* hinders cell division of fibroblasts, and induces morphological changes which tend towards the disintegration of the cells (Ruhmann and Berliner, 1965).

A67. *Cortisol* encourages osteogenic cells to turn into osteoclasts.

A68. *Cortisol* stimulates the formation of enzyme-secreting organelles in fibroblasts and osteoclasts.

A69. The effect of *cortisol* on the brain is either euphoria or emotional symptoms varying from a nervous state and depression through a chronic anxiety state to severe psychotic episodes. The precise effects produced depend upon the level of activity of other hormones, such as *growth hormones, androgens* and *oestrogens,* and other related chemicals which may be taken, such as *synthetic progestational compounds,* which also affect cell membranes in the brain.

A70. Some *anabolic* compounds counter the effect of *cortisol* on the liver.

A71. Other *anabolic* compounds in the presence of *cortisol* cause the proportion of free lipids to increase in hepatic cells.

A72. Some *anti-catabolic steroids* increase the stability of erythrocyte surface membranes. Neither *prednisolone* nor *oestrone* have this stabilizing action.

A73. *Anti-catabolic* (anabolic) *steroids* counter the catabolic effect of *cortisol* and encourage the proliferation of connective tissue cells and vessels.

A74. *Anabolic* compounds (steroid or polypeptide) counter the effect of *cortisol* on intercellular matrix production.

A75. After cessation of *cortisone* administration there is a surge of *anabolic* activity (Storey, 1957).

A76. All *steroids,* whether anabolic or catabolic, encourage the production of stable intercellular matrices, in the sense that they are less easy to resorb, whereas *peptide* hormones, such as *growth hormone,* cause a more labile matrix to be formed.

A77. The presence of a 17*a* methyl group in steroids confers oral activity. It also causes the compounds to modify liver function. This is an example of a linked property.

A78. *Cortisol* together with an anabolic steroid tends to increase the amount of haemopoietic tissue. The proportion of cell types varies from one anabolic steroid to another.

A79. *Cortisol* and *progestational steroids*, acting together, and above a threshold level of free *cortisol* which varies from one *progestational steroid* to another, stimulate the production of abnormal megakaryocytes and platelets. The latter coalesce almost immediately to form thrombi.

A80. The anterior pituitary gland produces *growth hormone*.

A81. *Growth hormone* has an anabolic function, but in its presence a comparatively labile matrix is produced.

A82. This matrix formation is associated with an increased requirement for *insulin* (Manchester and Young, 1961).

A83. *Growth hormone* stimulates the rate of division of stem cells.

A84. *Growth hormone* controls both the rate of growth and the metabolism necessary for growth.

A85. The *pancreas* produces *insulin*.

A86. The rate of *insulin* secretion is a continuous function of the blood *glucose* level (Metz, 1960).

A87. *Insulin* lowers the concentration of *glucose* in the blood.

A88. *Insulin* facilitates the entry of *glucose* into cells. The transfer mechanism is non-enzymatic (Hechter, 1955).

A89. In the absence of *insulin* the blood *glucose* rises, and extra water is excreted. This condition is diabetes mellitus.

A90. With the administration of *growth hormone* there is a rise in serum *insulin* prior to a significant increase in serum *glucose*.

A91. For any given concentration of *glucose* in the body more *growth* hormone causes more *insulin* to be secreted (Campbell and Rastogi, 1967).

A92. *Growth hormone* needs the presence of *insulin* before it can act on cells.

A93. *Insulin* promotes fat anabolism.

A94. *Insulin* is essential for the normal metabolism of carbohydrates, fats and proteins.

A95. Many hormones are unable to act except in the presence of *insulin* (Prop, 1961).

A96. Disorders other than those involving the blood sugar level can be present in diabetes.

A97. *Alcohol* tends to induce *hypoglycaemia* (Plechus *et al.*, 1966). For a given level of alcohol the effect tends to be greater in the Negro than in the white.

A98. *Alcohol* combined with fasting produces a very marked lowering of performance (Gibbons, Plechus, Chandler and Ellis, 1966).

A99. The brain is the organ most dependent on an adequate level of blood *sugar*—both rational thought and emotional stability are impaired when the level of sugar drops.

A100. There are differences between individuals in their hormonal balance which affects their physique and mental outlook.

A101. There are also inter-racial differences. Thus, with a similar blood glucose:
(*a*) The Bantu has lower serum *insulin* than the white.
(*b*) The Bantu has lower renal *insulin* clearance than the white.

(c) The Bantu has higher *growth hormone* than the white.

(d) The Bantu has lower *cholesterol* and *triglycerides* than the white.

(e) The Bantu has lower *free fatty acids* than the white.

(f) Indians* have *insulin* and *growth hormone* similar to the white.

(g) Indians* have *cholesterol* and *triglycerides* similar to the white.

(h) Indians* have lower *free fatty acids* than the Bantu.

(Rubenstein *et al.* 1967).

A102. In the Bantu a comparatively high level of *growth hormone* is maintained throughout life, whereas in the white it decreases at the time of adolescence.

A103. Distribution of hair also shows racial differences, as do many other characteristics.

A104. The anterior *pituitary* gland produces *thyrotrophic hormone,* which stimulates the thyroid gland to produce *thyroid hormone.*

A105. The production of *thyrotrophic hormone* is suppressed by *thyroid hormone.*

A106. *Thyroid hormone* production is stimulated by cold and depressed by heat.

A107. *Thyroid* activity increases during puberty and adolescence.

A108. In deer *thyroid hormone* enhances the growth of the antler.

A109. *Thyroid hormone* controls the basal metabolic rate (the rate of oxygen consumption in the production of energy gives a measure of this).

A110. *Thyroid* excess raises the blood *glucose* (compensatory mechanisms tend to obscure this effect).

A111. The consequences of a low *thyroid hormone* level include:

(a) fall of pulse rate,

(b) fall of respiration rate,

(c) prolonged reaction time,

(d) low red cell count.

A112. A high *thyroid* level is more common in females. Its consequences include:

(a) increased pulse rate,

(b) little change in respiratory rate,

(c) reaction time not shortened,

(d) enhanced excitability, irritability and emotional lability,

(e) increased sweating,

(f) muscular weakness.

A113. The *thyroid* is thought to secrete two active compounds, *thyroxine (tetra-iodothyronine)* and *tri-iodothyronine.* There are probably biotransformations affecting these, with the latter being the more active compound.

A114. An increased *thyroid* level sensitizes the tissues to *adrenalin.*

A115. *Thyroid hormone* is one of the requirements for growth. A lack of it leads to cretinism.

A116. In controlling body growth *thyroid* hormone acts in conjunction with, or sensitizes the tissues to, *growth hormone.*

A117. In *calcium* deficiency the thyroid gland shows *thyroid hormone* deficiency (Scott *et al., 1961).

A118. A high *calcium diet* causes goitre if the iodine intake is low.

A119. A high calcium intake is also associated with a high incidence of hyperthyroidism in adolescence, if the iodine intake is low.

* Indians from India.

A120. *Thyroid hormone* is necessary for the formation of adequate quantities of *chrondoitin sulphate*.

A121. With a decrease in *thyroid hormone* production there is a rise in blood *cholesterol*. Conversely, excess of thyroid hormone lowers the level of cholesterol in the blood.

A122. In *calcium* deficiency the adrenal releases excess *cortisol*.

A123. Without *thyroid* activity the *parathyroid* effect on bone is prevented.

A124. The *thyroid* also secretes *calcitonin*.

A125. *Parathyroid hormone* controls the level of blood *calcium*.

A126. Removal of the *parathyroids* causes a drop in the serum *calcium* level which leads to tetany.

A127. The rate of secretion of the *parathyroid hormone* is governed by the plasma *calcium level*.

A128. *Parathyroid hormone* prevents re-absorption by the kidney tubules of *phosphate*, so that more is excreted and the blood level falls.

A129. The *phosphate* level in blood controls the *calcium* level. A fall in phosphate causes an increase in calcium.

A130. *Parathyroid hormone* is necessary for macrophages to coalesce and to form multinucleated cells.

A131. When acting on the whole body the *parathyroid hormone* takes 20 min. When acting directly on bone in tissue culture it takes 2 h. The action would therefore seem to be through some intermediary (not either serum calcium or calcitonin).

A132. The *adrenal medulla* is activated by sympathetic nerves which are under the control of the *hypothalamus*.

A133. Physiological quantitities of *adrenalin* are produced only at times of stress.

A134. The actions of adrenalin include:
(*a*) Dilatation of the bronchi.
(*b*) Relaxation of the intestinal tract and contraction of the sphincters.
(*c*) Contraction of small blood vessels of skin and bowel, dilatation of those supplying striated muscle.
(*d*) An increase in the rate of the heart.
(*e*) The power of each cardiac contraction is increased, so that a greater volume of blood is ejected at each beat.
These factors add up to a rise in the blood pressure.

A135. An excess of *adrenalin* causes sweating and a sensation of fear.

A136. *Adrenalin* converts liver and muscle glycogens to glucose and lactate.

A137. *Adrenalin* stimulates the secretion of *ACTH*, releasing *cortisol* (which helps restock liver glycogen).

A138. *Adrenalin* is necessary to mobilize lipids (Wool, Goldstein, Ramey and Levine, 1954).

A139. *Adrenalin* causes an immediate rise in the plasma level of *free fatty acids,* and a delayed rise in serum *cholesterol* and *phospholipids*.

A140. Alterations in serum *cholesterol* and *triglycerides* occur within 60 min of stress (Wolf *et al.,* 1962).

A141. *Cortisol* is necessary for *adrenalin* to mobilize lipids in quantity (Shapir and Steinberg, 1960).

A142. Lipid concentrations in the blood are not markedly affected by diet.

A143. Concentrations of cortisol can vary widely during the course of a few hours.

A144. A lipoprotein (lecithin) which is released at the same time accelerates the coagulation time of blood (Bolton *et al.*, 1967).

A145. The neurohypophysis secretes *vasopressin*.

A146. *Vasopressin* has the effect of controlling the osmotic pressure of extracellular fluids.

A147. The secretion of *vasopressin* is controlled by the concentration of sodium chloride in the blood.

A148. An insufficient secretion of *vasopressin* is the cause of diabetes insipidus.

A149. Nicotine stimulates the release of *vasopressin*.

A150. Like *insulin, vasopressin* influences membrane transport processes.

8. DEGENERATIVE CONDITIONS

So far the properties of bone and closely associated connective tissues have been considered—the types of cells, their reactions to their surroundings, and the intercellular matrices they produce. Factors that have been shown to affect these properties are blood flow, with a consequent variation in the proportion of oxygen, carbon dioxide and other chemicals, vitamins and trace elements, physical forces, hormones and steroids, and stress, which affects the proportions and action of the hormones. It has also been suggested that many of the degenerative conditions met with as an apparent part of the ageing process are caused by variations in these factors.

Now that the use of antibiotics has reduced the incidence of infections, it is these degenerative and stress-induced diseases that have become the major causes of disability and death. Non-orthopaedic conditions commonly met with are arterial and coronary heart disease, chronic bronchitis and emphysema, and cancer. Some aspects of the cancer problem impinge on orthopaedics, and these will be considered in the next chapter. Arterial and coronary disease and chronic bronchitis have been mentioned in previous chapters dealing with fundamental mechanisms. In this chapter some of the common orthopaedic conditions will be discussed, in terms of their mechanisms.

In practice, those which most frequently lead to in-patient treatment are fractures and trauma; osteoarthritis, particularly of the hips and feet (hallux valgus); and prolapsed intervertebral discs. Conditions often met with in outpatients are osteoporosis, which is a common cause of low back pain, and rheumatoid arthritis. Another degenerative condition, usually asymptomatic, is the presence of pathological calcifications. In this chapter the mechanisms of osteoporosis, osteoarthritis, disc and vertebral lesions which might lead to back pain, and pathological calcifications will be discussed. Three other degenerative conditions will be included. Dental caries is not strictly connected with bone, but it is closely related and very widespread; while decompression sickness and Paget's disease are of limited incidence. The aetiology of the latter is still obscure, and suggestions will be made as to how further information could be sought.

Dental Caries

The treatment of dental caries is very different from that of other degenerative conditions so there is a tendency to forget that they are related. The unique properties of teeth are due to the fact that their hard tissues protrude though the mucous membrane, so that once they have erupted it is not possible for those parts of the tooth without access to a direct blood supply to be repaired by natural means. Because of this dentists use very different techniques from those employed by doctors.

Dental structure

Dental pulp. In the central part of a tooth is the pulp, containing fibrous tissue, blood vessels and nerves. The blood vessels penetrate as far as the odontoblasts on the inner dentine surface, and from there outwards nutrients and chemicals that are necessary to maintain the organic components of the dentine and enamel travel by diffusion processes. Problems can be caused by any hindrance to this diffusion process.

Dentine. The main body of a tooth is dentine, which is covered by enamel. Dentine is formed by a layer of odontoblasts, that normally remain quiescent on the inner surface of the dentine once its formation is complete. Processes from these cells pass through tubules in the dentine to the base of the enamel, and facilitate the transport of fluids and chemicals. Odontoblasts belong to the same family of cells as fibroblasts and osteoblasts, and are activated by the same stimuli. Thus, trauma to a tooth stimulates further dentine formation, and an irregularly arranged dentine, the equivalent of fracture callus, is laid down behind the damaged area. Osteogenic cells and fibroblasts can be stimulated to produce proteolytic enzymes, and so can odontoblasts.

The texture of dentine is very similar to that of bone tissue. It is a fibrous structure containing collagen and other proteins and polysaccharides. The organic component is the continuous phase, and may occupy up to 50% of the total volume. It is the fact that this organic component is the continuous phase, and that it has the properties of a gel, which gives dentine its resilience. In the connective tissues the gel structure is only maintained by continued cell activity. If the supply of nutrients ceases, or waste products cannot be removed from the cells these cells die, and the tissues maintained by them lose their gel characteristics. With death of odontoblasts and other cells in the pulp dentine loses much of its resilience and becomes brittle.

Enamel. The outer layer of a tooth is the enamel, which is laid down by ameloblasts before the tooth erupts. When the tooth emerges through the gum the ameloblasts die, and after this no further deposition of enamel is possible and worn, damaged or decayed enamel cannot be replaced. The proportion of mineral in enamel is much higher than in dentine or in bone, but although it occupies only about 5% of the volume the organic component is again the continuous phase, with mineral crystallites laid down in an organic sponge. The organic component of enamel is different from that of dentine or bone. There are no well-organized fibres and it contains beta-proteins in place of collagen. Figure 1.37 shows a cross-section of enamel matrix as first laid down and Fig. 1.38 the appearance immediately before calcification takes place. This change was in the calcifiable matrix laid down on top of the more stable structural components The horseshoe arrangement of "prisms" is typical. At the surface the prisms bend over so that the calcified denser protein forms a continuous surface layer in a well-developed tooth.

The major component of each part of the enamel matrix is a beta-protein, with X-ray diffraction patterns corresponding to the mature and dense beta-proteins. It would appear, therefore, that whereas dentine owes its resilience to the fact that its organic matrix, present in the continuous phase, is a gel; the enamel owes its resilience to the fact that both major protein components, also present in the continuous phase, are rubbers. To maintain gel properties a fairly closely defined fluid medium must be maintained, with correct chemical components supplied by the cells. To maintain the rubbers in enamel, and prevent them becoming brittle, all that is required is that they should remain wet.

Carious lesions

There is more than one type of carious lesion. In enamel caries the enamel itself is invaded and destroyed by bacteria; while at other times cementum (the outer covering of the root of the tooth) and dentine may become necrotic and have this necrotic material invaded by bacteria. The latter process resembles the infection of necrotic areas elsewhere in the body, and differs only in the fact that teeth tend to be more vulnerable. Enamel caries is clinically more important and has an interesting mechanism.

Well-formed teeth, with an adequate supply of vitamin D present during their formation, are less susceptible than poorly formed teeth (Mellanby, 1930, 1934). An adequate supply of fluoride is also required during the time of tooth formation, and Aslander (1963) has shown that even in a population with a very high caries incidence most lesions can be prevented by a correct diet during the time of tooth formation. Darling (1956, 1958) has shown that lesions spread from defects in the surface, and the better formed the tooth the fewer the defects. It is also apparent that too hard a toothbrush and too vigorous brushing could create defects.

The destructive agents that can penetrate through these weak points are acids and bacteria—there is an abundance of evidence for this, but less work has been done on the actual mechanism of their attack. It can be shown that the organic component is attacked first (Little, 1959), that the crystallites are as likely to be washed away as to be dissolved away, and that it is the less dense protein that is vulnerable. This helps to explain why it was reasonable to amend the statement "sugar causes caries" to "some starches cause caries" (see p. 275). The latter may contain proteolytic compounds which would help to initiate the lesion. One would expect such a lesion to advance slowly.

There remain the characteristic and fairly rapidly developing lesions. It can be shown that susceptible teeth have the protein in a less chemically stable form than normal (Little, 1962), which would facilitate the spread of these lesions. In such a tooth the less dense protein of the prism cores is even more susceptible to acid attack than is the similar protein in healthy teeth from skeletons nearly 2000 years old. There is plenty of circumstantial evidence that the incidence of dental caries is affected by the degree of stress to which the individual is subjected, and sometimes this can be put on a quantitative basis. Thus, in the early 1960s a Melbourne dentist correlated stressful incidents with the start of rapidly developing lesions, and found that they could be detected clinically three weeks after the initiating event (Sutton, 1965). He had a practice in the business district, and during the time he was making these observations currency restrictions were imposed. During the period before the financial change $\frac{1}{8}$ of his patients developed new lesions, and during an equivalent period after the change $\frac{1}{4}$ developed new lesions, of the rapidly progressing type that could be correlated with stressful situations. In the last chapter it was shown that the most important effect of stress is a rise in the level of excess cortisol in the blood. This cortisol stimulates connective tissue cells to produce proteolytic enzymes. There is also a physiological rise during pregnancy, while the changing patterns of hormone secretion mean that there is often a series of temporary rises in cortisol level during adolescence. It is these three groups of individuals, adolescents, pregnant women and people under stress who most frequently develop carious lesions. One may assume that enzymes diffusing from odontoblasts in a phagocytic phase have partly degraded protein in the neighbouring enamel.

Osteoporosis

The term osteoporosis is non-specific, all it means is that there is too little osseous tissue present in the bones. It could be due to too little or too slow bone deposition or to too fast or too great bone removal, and there is the possibility that several mechanisms may be operating simultaneously. There are indications that the clinical conditions loosely referred to as "osteoporosis" involve at least three separate mechanisms, and the terms disuse, post-menopausal and senile osteoporosis have been used. For an understanding of the various causes of osteoporosis all the mechanisms which contribute to bone formation and removal need to be taken into account. Some possibilities are rare, and in practice a few combinations are found to dominate.

As well as the degree of bone loss that may be regarded as pathological, there is a loss of bone with increasing age that may be regarded as a normal physiological process. Everyone begins to lose bone from the age of about thirty-five, with a gradual increase of the size of the marrow spaces. In middle age there are endocrine changes, and a period of involution starts. As well as loss of bone mass there is also a loss of muscle mass and changes in brain, liver, kidney and other organs. When the loss of bone outstrips the changes in muscles and other tissues it can be regarded as a pathological entity.

In older people the apparently normal or physiological loss of bone that parallels changes in muscle and other tissues involves bone within the cortex as well as enlargement of the marrow space and loss of trabecular bone. This produces a change of gait, but it is only when the loss of bone has outstripped other changes that it is regarded as a clinical senile osteoporosis. The symptoms that are observed are backache, fractures, and a change in walking and running habits. In this chapter we are concerned with those osteoporotic changes that may be regarded as pathological.

Recognizable descriptions of pathological osteoporosis date back at least as far as the sixth century. In one part of his treatise on medicine Aegineta (sixth to seventh century A.D.) deals with the treatment of those fractures near the head of the thighbone which fail to unite, and in another part he writes of the type of "arthritis which affects the vertebrae and many other sites" and describes the disease as being occasioned by a "preter-natural humour" and a "weakness of the parts" meeting together. His description mostly fits senile osteoporosis, although one or two passages could equally well refer to post-menopausal osteoporosis. That the difficult fractures of the hip tend to be associated with "old and cholleric" people has long been recognized (Lovve,

1634), but post-menopausal osteoporosis does not seem to have been described as a separate entity until Albright's work was published in the 1940s (Albright, Bloomberg and Smith, 1940; Albright, *et al.*, 1941). Albright recognized that there is a decreased anabolism in osteoporotic subjects, that the balance of anabolic and catabolic hormones is disturbed in both post-menopausal and senile osteoporosis, and that disuse is often a superimposed complication (Albright, 1947).

Each of these three main types of pathological osteoporosis that are recognized clinically—disuse, post-menopausal and senile—has a distinctive mechanism. They rarely occur completely independent of one another, except for those cases of disuse osteoporosis due to immobilization of a limb, poliomyelitis or some other cause, but frequently one mechanism is dominant.

Disuse osteoporosis

Disuse is used to describe that type of osteoporosis which is caused by a diminished flow of blood through the bone, as a result of a lowering or cessation of normal muscle activity around that bone. Immobilization in plaster or paralysis are frequent causes, but a lowered muscle tone as a result of the action of corticosteroids, or the hindrance of blood flow through the muscle by thrombi (Fig. 2.36) would also have the same effect.

With a sudden diminution or cessation of the rate of flow of blood through a bone there is initially an increased pressure within that bone. With a continued lack of muscle activity it takes approximately 2–3 weeks before a pressure balance is restored (Geizer and Trueta, 1958; Trueta, 1964). Until the pressure balance, and thus the amount of carbon dioxide within the bone, is restored to normal the production of phagocytic osteoclasts is stimulated. The effects of the extreme pressure may also include damage to some of the membranes covering the osseous tissue in the cortex, thus initiating extra osteonal activity. Figures 5.25, 5.26 showed cutting cones of osteoclasts enlarging Haversian canals in the cortical bone of an experimental animal. At the same time as this additional bone resorption is taking place the lower amount of available oxygen reduces osteoblast activity, and even when the pressure balance is restored to normal and excess resorption ceases the level of osteoblast activity remains below normal. One characteristic of this type of osteoporosis is that osteones remain only partially formed. When there is a total loss of muscle activity and a state of equilibrium has been reached, the proportion of osseous tissue in bone is reduced to about half its normal quantity. Should muscle activity be resumed, as when the plaster is removed from an immobilized limb, the increased flow and thus the increase in available oxygen stimulates osteoblast activity and the quantity of bone tissue is restored to normal. The rate of bone formation, however, is only about a tenth of the rate of bone removal (Johnson, 1964), so that the time for recovery is correspondingly longer.

When disuse is superimposed on senile osteoporosis the effect tends to be magnified, and Albright et al. (1941) observed that old women are more susceptible than men of comparable age to the harmful effects of immobilization. Jowsey (Jowsey et al., 1965; Jowsey, 1966) has established that the degree of immobilization afforded by bed-rest causes a considerably increased resorption and decreased bone formation in osteoporotic subjects, but only a slight change in normal people. Conversely, the effect of increased muscular exercise may be magnified when osteoporotic subjects are considered. These differences are the result of the interplay of a number of different mechanisms.

In Chapter 4 it was shown that the cells which remove bone when the blood flow is reduced are osteoclasts derived from macrophages. Unlike osteoclasts derived from osteogenic cells these phagocytic osteoclasts will also remove dead bone when it has reached a stage of partial degradation. (At that stage no osteogenic cells are available for osteoclast formation.) Figure 4.24 showed such osteoclasts removing dead bone from a fracture site. In senile osteoporosis there is frequently a higher proportion of dead bone present than normal. This is less readily removed than normal because excess corticosteroids present prevent the macrophages from maturing. A somewhat similar situation was simulated in experimental animals (Little and de Valderrama, 1968) by immobilizing the oscalcis by removing a portion of the Achilles tendon. Those animals which were additionally given cortisone showed less removal of bone than those in which the macrophages were able to act freely. But when a patient is relaxing in bed the cortisol level often drops, so that macrophages can mature and coalesce to form osteoclasts which remove the dead bone that is present. Under such conditions one may find the core of a trabecula being removed (Fig. 8.1), so presenting a histological appearance which for a time superficially resembles hyperparathyroidism. In hyperparathyroidism phagocytic osteoclasts are unduly stimulated, so that tissue containing dead and moribund cells is selectively removed.

Post-menopausal osteoporosis

The mechanism of post-menopausal osteoporosis involves the direct removal of bone tissue by the interaction of anabolic and catabolic steroids. It frequently occurs in women 5 to 10 years after the meno-

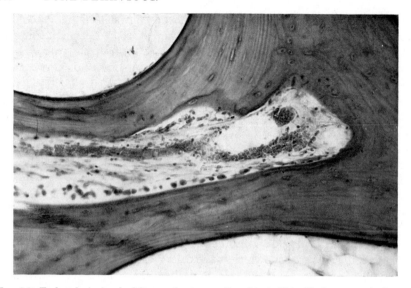

Fig. 8.1. Trabecula in head of femur of osteoporotic subject. This elderly woman had spent several weeks in bed prior to the removal of the femoral head, and a number of trabeculae showed selective removal of dead bone from the core. ×200.

pause (Albright *et al.*, 1940), but it can occur in individuals of any age who have taken steroids for therapeutic or other purposes.

In a general way, Aegineta (sixth to seventh century A.D.) had recognized that there was a metabolic cause for the osteoporosis that occurs in middle-aged women and in the elderly, and that the stimuli were sometimes physical, while sometimes "sorrow, care, watchfulness, and the other passions of the mind (can) excite an attack of the disorder". But it was not until details of endocrine activity had been discovered that Albright (1947) was in a position to say that the condition was one of decreased anabolism and that in ageing there is a decrease in anabolic activity; while a few years later more precise investigations (Reifenstein, 1957) showed that men have a higher anabolic level than women, that women produce a smaller quantity of anabolic hormones after the menopause, and that a further decline in the production of both anabolic and catabolic steroids begins at the age of 70 to 80, the proportion then tending to get more out of balance. The mechanisms of post-menopausal and senile osteoporosis, although both are stress-induced effects, are different, and so will be discussed separately.

In the condition which is usually called post-menopausal osteoporosis, there is an imbalance between anabolic and catabolic steroids in the body which has a direct effect on the bone. Cushing's syndrome and continuous corticosteroid therapy produce such an imbalance, and may be considered first. A continuous high level of corticosteroid tends to inhibit phagocytic bone removal, to inhibit osteoblast activity and to encourage osteogenic precursor cells to coalesce to form osteoclasts. These factors taken together lead to a smaller quantity of bone that is not easily resorbed and a lower level of osteogenic cell activity. In the case of Cushing's disease Albright (1941) found that treatment with testosterone in order to restore the anabolic level led to a clinical improvement. Synthetic steroids, which are now available with a higher anti-catabolic level and lower androgenic level than testosterone, are more satisfactory.

In women after the menopause the situation is different. At the time of the menopause there is a reduction in the level of anabolic steroids, while the level of catabolic steroids remains much the same (Reifenstein, 1957). Superimposed on this are periods of stress which tend to be recurrent. Reactions to stress show considerable individual variations, so that the levels to which blood cortisol rises vary. The situation, then, is that during periods of stress there is a rise in blood cortisol. The effect of this is to inhibit osteoblast activity and the differentiation of osteogenic precursor cells to osteoblasts, and at the same time to cause those osteogenic precursor cells to coalesce to osteoclasts. All the available evidence is consistent with this coalescence being an irreversible process. When the cortisol level drops to normal more osteogenic precursor cells are formed, which in the now anabolic climate differentiate to osteoblasts and form new bone. The vigour of this action depends upon the anabolic level of the steroids present, although Storey (1957) has provided evidence which suggests that in the period immediately after the cortisol level returns to normal there is a brief surge of anabolic activity.

The overall effect of these processes depends upon the combination of cortisol level, anabolic level, and the timing of the alternation between these. In the presence of a strongly anabolic and anti-catabolic agent such as testosterone, the bone removed during periods of stress is quickly restored in the intervening periods. Data provided by Mack et al. (1966) suggests that bone resorption which occurred during the Gemini flights was replaced in about 4 days and that for the succeeding 10 days there was a continuing surge of anabolic activity.

When the anabolic level is comparatively low, as is the case in women after the menopause, a situation can arise, with unfortunate timing, when the surge of cortisol with stress inhibits osteoblastic activity and stimulates osteoclastic activity, then in the intervening period osteogenic precursor cells proliferate in a rather sluggish manner, so that before new bone formation takes place a new phase of resorption commences, with the new osteogenic precursor cells available for osteoclast formation (cf. Fig. 6.16). In this way it could be possible for a great deal

x

of bone, and particularly trabecular bone to be removed. Animal experiments have been performed in which this type of behaviour has been simulated (Storey, 1958; Little, 1970a), and in some instances a large proportion of the bone tissue was resorbed in the course of a few weeks. Although it is possible to lose far more bone by the alternation of anabolic and catabolic steroids than in disuse, it is only rarely that natural hormones alone produce a catastrophic loss of bone. The problem might arise more frequently if certain synthetic steroids were administered during a period of prolonged stress, and with intermittent timing.

Figure 2.33 showed a typical appearance of the upper part of the shaft

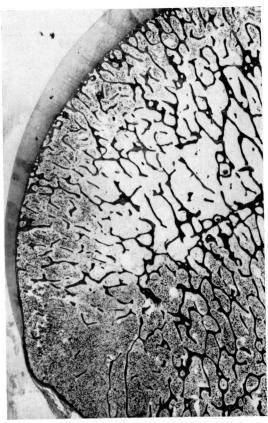

Fɪɢ. 8.2. Head of femur from a woman with post-menopausal osteoporosis. This was taken during an active phase, and there is an abundance of haemopoietic tissue. In the area where there has been little or no weight-bearing, nearly all the trabeculae have been resorbed. This weakens the structure and could lead to an intracapsular fracture. Because of the effect of raised cortisol concentrations arthritic changes that would normally be caused by inadequate use of the hip are minimal. ×35.

and neck of femur of an osteoporotic subject during an active phase, and Fig. 8.2 is a section of the head of femur from another subject. The trabecular appearance in the neck of femur was shown in Fig. 2.31. During active phases of the disease there is an abundance of red marrow, because resorbing bone tissue provides nutrients in the surrounding area for cell proliferation. During quiescent phases the marrow spaces are filled with fat cells.

Reports on the efficiency of natural and synthetic anabolic steroids for treatment of post-menopausal and senile osteoporosis have varied widely. In those instances where there has been an increase in bone tissue sufficient to show on clinical X-rays one may assume that the anabolic steroid was being administered in such a manner as to consistently increase that overall anabolic level. Nordin (1964) has reported that dominant symptoms are backache in patients in the sixth and seventh decades, and fractured hips in the eighth and ninth decades. The latter are typical of senile osteoporosis. He and others have further reported that anabolic agents relieve the backache. The alternation of anabolic and catabolic conditions affects trabecular bone more than cortical bone, and it is the trabecular bone in weight-bearing situations that is most likely to suffer microfractures or even major fractures (cf. the crush fracture in a vertebra shown in Fig. 5.30).

High catabolic levels produce effects other than this direct action on the bone. Treatment with anticatabolic steroids is therefore likely to produce a clinical improvement in these cases, whether or not there is an increase in the amount of bone tissue. When the alternation of catabolic and anabolic conditions is not the major cause of the osteoporosis, or in the subsequent quiescent stages when a decreased muscle efficiency prevents renewal of the total quantity, replacement of osseous tissue would not necessarily be expected. Apparently contradictory results are often reported. Tillis (1961), for example, reported improvement with methandrostenolone (Dianabol) treatment in most but not all cases. By improvement he meant not so much an improvement in quantity of bone but in such ways as relief of pain, increased sense of well-being and mental alertness, and disappearance of symptoms of fatigue and listlessness. In the quiescent stages, when symptoms due to a raised cortisol level are not present, anabolic steroids are without noticeable effect (Wynn and Landon, 1961; Wynn, 1968). Even when an increased quantity of bone is not reported there is usually no further diminution in quantity (Henneman and Wallack, 1957).

Since hormone imbalance is a generalized condition, other symptoms may be expected. One sign which has been reported is the increased transparency of the skin (McConkey, Fraser and Bligh, 1965), so that in more severe cases the appearance of the back of the hand may give an indication of the state of the bones. There is also an effect on intestinal absorption, particularly of fats and fat-soluble components of food. Nordin (1961) has estimated that 15% of patients with osteoporosis also suffer from steatorrhea. Calcium absorption is affected (Caniggia *et al.*, 1963), and also vitamin D absorption, so that a by no means unusual complication of osteoporosis is osteomalacia. This can normally be corrected by increasing the quantity of vitamin D in the diet, and choosing a diet with a low phytic acid content.

Senile osteoporosis

Senile osteoporosis is also due to stress. Unlike post-menopausal osteoporosis it affects both men and women, and it is usually found in an older age group. The age of incidence is lower in the Oriental than in the white. In senile osteoporosis the cause is thrombus deposition in minor blood vessels. Stress, of a sufficient degree of severity, or a sufficiently high level of corticosteroid administration—Rosenberg (1958) has commented on the fact that there seems to be a threshold dose level for cortisol administration in rheumatoid arthritis above which pathological fractures become a serious complication—causes changes in megakaryocytes in the bone marrow (Figs 6.33, 6.34) which result in the production of sticky platelets that coalesce to form thrombi. Sometimes these thrombi partially block vessels, where they are soon invaded by fibrous tissue. Figure 2.35 showed a vessel in a lumbar vertebra, and Fig. 2.36

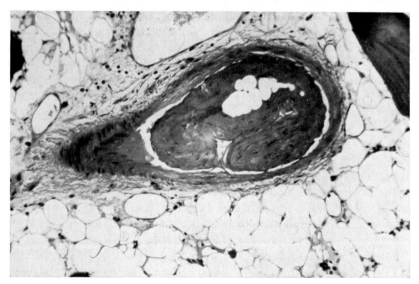

FIG. 8.3. Bone removed at operation from a patient with rheumatoid arthritis. A recently formed thrombus blocks a vessel in cancellous bone. ×200.

one in an adjacent muscle. Smaller vessels may be completely blocked. Figure 8.3 shows a newly formed thrombus in cancellous bone. This was in bone removed at operation from a rheumatoid patient. No necrotic tissue is formed, because there are alternative pathways for the flow of blood. The vascular network within a bone provides alternative routes to nearly all sectors of vessels, so that it is only when a main supply artery is blocked that an area of avascular necrosis develops. When only the smaller vessels in cancellous bone are involved, the result is to diminish the total flow of blood, and so induce the type of bone removal that is also found in disuse osteoporosis.

When a vessel in compact bone is blocked the results are somewhat different. Figure 8.4 shows a recently formed thrombus in such a bone, and Fig. 8.5 a later stage. Deposited material has calcified—more densely than the surrounding bone—and osteocytes in this bone which have been deprived of their source of nutrients die.

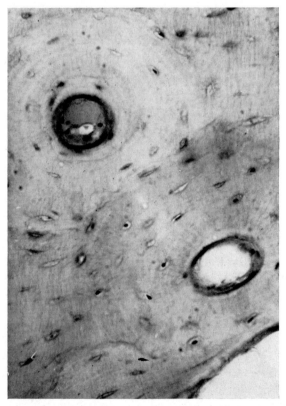

Fig. 8.4. A recently formed thrombus in compact bone of an elderly person. The Haversian canal is blocked. Some osteocytes in the surrounding bone are still viable, but others have died. ×200.

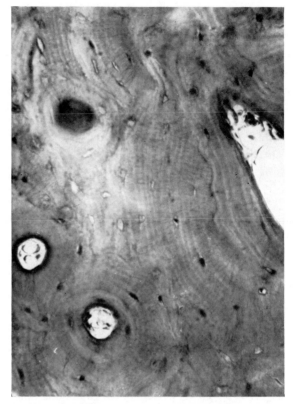

Fig. 8.5. Blocked Haversian canal in another area of compact bone. All osteocytes dependent upon that canal are dead. The deposited material is heavily calcified. × 200.

Other characteristics of bone in senile osteoporosis are the result of the raised blood cortisol levels. As bone turnover proceeds the lowered blood flow means that there is inadequate replacement of resorbed bone. Where resorption has taken place the breakdown products of the matrix provide the necessary nutrients for cell proliferation, and areas of haemopoietic tissue are found. Diffusion through vessel walls, however, is hindered, and osteocytes in both cortical and trabecular bone may die. While the cortisol levels remain above normal macrophages do not mature, so that the normal mechanism for removing dead and moribund bone remains inactive. One frequently finds, therefore, not only dead but also intact trabeculae (Fig. 8.6 is typical), and new bone laid down over dead bone (Fig. 8.7). When the individual relaxes, or if for any reason the parathyroid level is increased, then a considerable amount of the dead bone may be removed in a short time. In quiescent phases the bone is surrounded by fatty marrow.

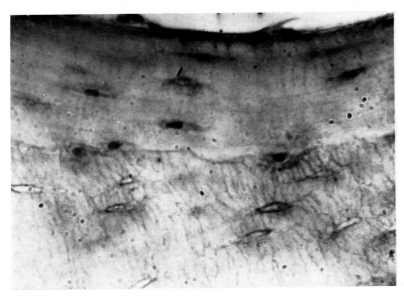

Fig. 8.7. Trabecula in the neck of femur of another osteoporotic subject. Osteocytes in the core of the trabecula are dead, and their lacunae and canaliculi have enlarged. The trabecula is covered by a layer of viable bone. ×400.

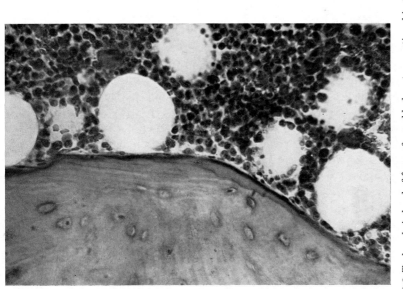

Fig. 8.6. Trabecula in head of femur from elderly osteoporotic subject. Many osteocytes are dead, and a thin layer of new bone has been laid down over the moribund tissue. The marrow spaces are filled with haemopoietic tissue. ×200.

Vitamin C deficiency

A few years ago a high incidence of severe osteoporosis among young Bantu men in the Johannesburg district was reported (Seftel *et al.*, 1966). Young men are in the age group least susceptible to osteoporosis, particularly when, as in the present instance, they are physically active. They have a good blood flow through their bones, and so the conditions for a disuse osteoporosis are absent. They also have a high testosterone level, augmented in Negroes by a high growth hormone level, and so the mechanisms of post-menopausal osteoporosis cannot operate. They had none of the accompanying symptoms of hyperparathyroidism or senile osteoporosis. Further, their osteoporosis tended to be present as an acute condition associated with the consumption of illicit liquor. Careful investigation showed that an excessive iron intake derived from the containers used for brewing the liquor interfered with ascorbic acid metabolism, so that the amount of vitamin C in leucocytes was decreased. The quantity available to the tissues was thus reduced to a level where osteoporosis and in a few cases other scorbutic symptoms developed (Lynch *et al.*, 1967).

More commonly a lack of vitamin C has to be remembered as a possible contributory cause to osteoporosis in the elderly, particularly when the individuals concerned live alone, and do not have sufficient vitamin C in their diet.

Pathological fractures

Post-menopausal and senile osteoporosis are most readily recognized by a typical ballooning of the intervertebral disc (Fig. 5.27), the mechanism of which will be discussed in the section on intervertebral discs. Symptomatically they commonly present as pain, particularly low back pain, and as pathological fractures. The main sites at which these fractures occur are the vertebrae, where there is a constant bone turnover throughout life; the head and neck of femur which is subjected to the stress of weight-bearing; and the wrist, which frequently sustains minor trauma.

The severity of such pathological fractures varies. In some instances, in weight-bearing bones, it may be limited to a single trabecula. Figure 5.29 showed a re-fracture of one such trabecula. Fluids from damaged vessels have killed marrow cells in the vicinity. In Fig. 8.8 is another such trabecula, showing the early stages of callus formation, with a more advanced stage shown in the trabecula in Fig. 8.9. Sometimes scattered trabeculae may be damaged, and in the low magnification picture shown in Fig. 8.10 their location is indicated by the small patches of

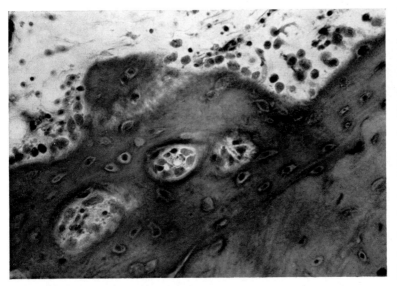

FIG. 8.9. Another fractured trabecula. The fracture callus is in the process of consolidating. ×200.

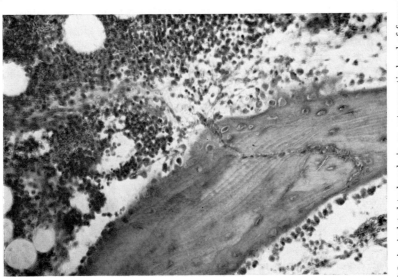

FIG. 8.8. An isolated trabecula in an osteoporotic head of femur has fractured. Early stages of callus formation may be seen on the right. ×100.

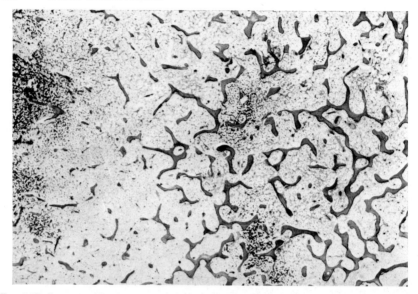

Fig. 8.10. Low magnification photograph of osteoporotic head of femur. Transverse section. Areas of haemopoietic tissue in centre of figure indicate the positions of three fractured trabeculae. ×35.

haemopoietic tissue. At a later quiescent stage they are seen as scattered abnormally shaped trabeculae (Fig. 8.11).

Figure 5.30 showed a crush fracture of a vertebra, with extra bone in the area of healing. Sometimes only a part of a vertebra is affected. Figure 4.18 showed woven bone formation in one such area, while Fig. 8.12 shows macrophages removing dead tissue from a similar site. In the spine such fractures result in temporary episodes of pain and a shortening of the stature.

In a survey in Oxford, Buhr and Cooke (1959) found that in the elderly there was a sharp rise in the number of pathological fractures of the hip in both men and women, the age of onset of the "epidemic" in men being approximately 10 years later than for women (i.e. 70+). Fractured wrists, on the other hand, were a female speciality. Alffram and Bauer (1962) in their study of forearm fractures have pointed out that this fragility involves trabecular bone more than cortical bone. Some broken arms are due to genuine trauma, and as a measure of this they compared the ratio of metaphyseal to shaft fractures. For the male this ratio changes only slightly through life, but for the female it changes from 3:1 in children to 72:1 in the aged.

More than one pattern of hip fracture is discernible. The two dominant types of pathological fracture are intra-capsular and extra-capsular. The former is due to a gross loss of trabecular bone, which is almost

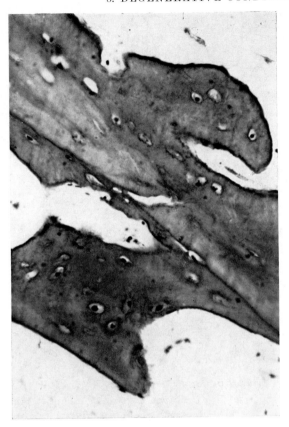

Fig. 8.11. Trabecula in lumbar vertebra. Its abnormal shape is due to the fracture callus around it. This is the final quiescent state. ×200.

entirely absent in the non-weight-bearing regions (Fig. 8.2). Trabeculae that are left show the multiple arrest lines that indicate an alternation of anabolic and catabolic conditions (Fig. 2.31), and the appearances are typical of post-menopausal osteoporosis. Robin, Bar-Maor and Winberg (1963) have shown that the peak incidence for this type of fracture corresponds with the ages at which post-menopausal osteo- porosis is most common, and that it is most frequent in women. In extra-capsular fractures there is not usually such a gross loss of osseous tissue. Instead one tends to find a great deal of dead bone that has become brittle, and a very frequent finding is evidence that this osteocyte death, when in the cortex, has been caused by the plugging of intra-cortical vessels by small thrombi. Robin et al. (1963) have also shown that whereas the peak age for intra-capsular fractures is 50 to 70, the number of extra-capsular fractures rises sharply beyond the age of 60.

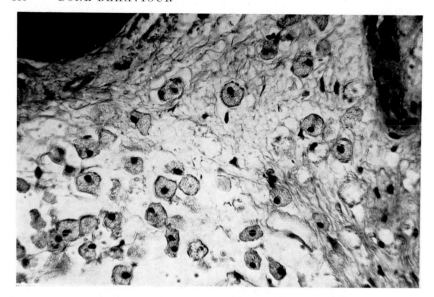

Fig. 8.12. Vertebra, near site of recent crush fracture. Debris is being removed by macrophages. ×200.

Decompression Sickness

This condition, also known as Caisson disease, is due to the release of small bubbles of gas in the blood stream. The most common sign is the pain known as the bends, which Fryer (1969) has shown is limited to those sites in bone where the venous outflow through cortical bone is susceptible to obstruction. Most frequently there are no lasting ill-effects, but sometimes the bubbles of gas cause a region of bone to be deprived of its blood supply for a sufficient length of time for cell death to occur.

Areas of avascular necrosis may occur in the head and neck of the femur, the head of the humerus, and sometimes the lower end of the femur and the upper end of the tibia. Infarcts may also arise in the medulla of the femur, humerus and tibia. These are all sites where the collateral circulation may be inadequate. The sequence of events is death of the area of bone concerned, possibly with some crushing in weight-bearing situations, followed by proliferation of repair tissue in the surroundings. This is usually partly woven bone and partly fibrous tissue. If a band of fibrous tissue is formed subsequent repair processes are hindered or prevented. Some debris is removed by macrophages (cf. Figs 5.39, 5.40).

Another factor which needs to be remembered when examining

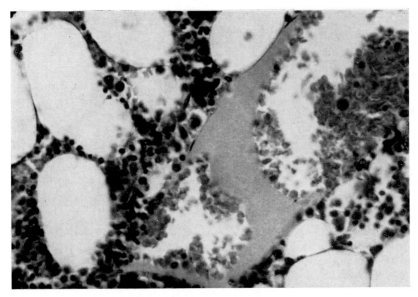

Fig. 8.13. A blocked vessel in the epiphyseal zone of a long bone. Death occurred several days after a decompression incident. Regions of avascular necrosis were present in other areas of bone in this patient, as a result of previous incidents. ×200. The author thanks the late Dr. D. I. Fryer for the material from which this figure was taken.

histological sections of bone from decompression sickness is that the individuals concerned have very frequently been under stress. The pain from the bends may have lasted several hours or days, and apprehension may have created more stress. Thrombus formation is therefore a possible complicating factor in some very severe cases. Figure 8.13 shows a blocked vessel in the epiphyseal region a few days after a decompression incident. More frequently the raised cortisol levels sustained over a period of time, while the blood flow is low, may interrupt diffusion of nutrients to the osteocytes, with resultant osteocyte death. Particularly in men it is then probable that some of the dead trabeculae will be covered with new bone before the macrophages become active again. The type of situation illustrated in Fig. 8.14 may then arise, where a dead trabecula is partly covered by a layer of living bone, macrophages are transporting debris through the marrow, and phagocytic removal of the dead bone tends to be limited to sites unprotected by new bone.

Paget's Disease

This bone condition was first described accurately by Paget (1877), and an expanded description of its mechanism was given by Johnson in 1964. The main abnormality is in the bones, and there have been few

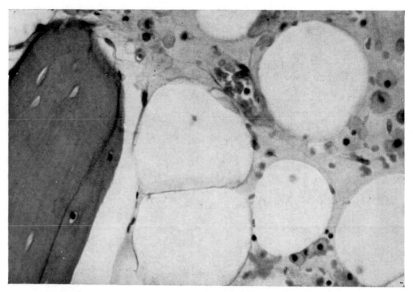

FIG. 8.14. Head of femur from a case of Caisson's disease. A dead trabecula is partly covered by a layer of new bone. Macrophages are transporting debris from a nearby infarct through the marrow. Phagocytic removal of dead bone in this section was limited to sites unprotected by new bone. ×200. The author thanks the late Dr. D. I. Fryer for the material from which this figure was taken.

definite indications of associated disease or disability, other than local pain during excessive bone remodelling, and in some severe cases a deleterious effect upon the heart when arterio-venous shunts have increased the blood flow.

The initial lesion in long bones is usually in the diaphysis, with a larger effect on the endosteal surface. The rate of advance may vary from 1 mm to 10 mm per month, and it "may go so fast that dissecting osteitis is seen, like that of hyperparathyroidism, and the repair is a non-calcifiable malacic bone" (Johnson, 1964). Following immediately behind the chisel edge of cutting cones is a proliferation of "loose connective tissue" in which focal islands of immature bone develop 5–10 days later.

A detailed examination of the cell mechanisms involved shows that the most outstanding feature of Paget's bone, in which it differs from both normal and osteoporotic bone is the great proliferation of vessels in the affected areas. In order to visualize these vessels clearly L. H. Pimm (1967, pers. comm.) has used a perfusion mixture of barium sulphate (Micropaque) and Berlin blue. This fills the arterial vessels and many of the bone sinusoids, and those that are not filled with perfusion medium contain packed red cells. Figure 8.15 shows a typical

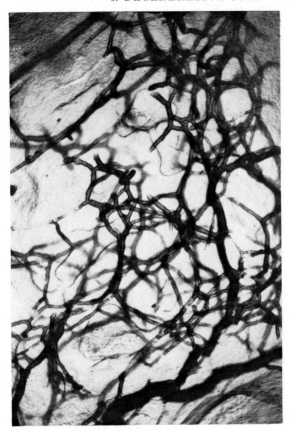

FIG. 8.15. Three hundred micron section through perfused bone from Paget's disease. Vessels which are filled with perfusion medium, are present as a branched disordered entanglement. ×35.

disordered entanglement of vessels with many side branches. Many of the terminal vessels have a diameter only slightly larger than a single erythrocyte, and they frequently lie behind active osteoclasts (Fig. 8.16). Such vessels are only rarely seen in normal bone.

Within the lesions there are only a limited number of types of cell behaviour. In the active stages the dominant characteristics are of the proliferation of vessels and of the proliferation of cells from the vessel walls (Fig. 8.17). It is to these cells that the terms "loose connective tissue", "fibrous proliferation" and so on have been applied. These cells, in the vicinity of bone, behave as osteogenic precursor cells, differentiating to osteoclasts or osteoblasts according to their local conditions (blood flow, and partial pressures of oxygen and carbon dioxide). The irregular profusion of vessels leads to irregular bone resorption, frequently giving

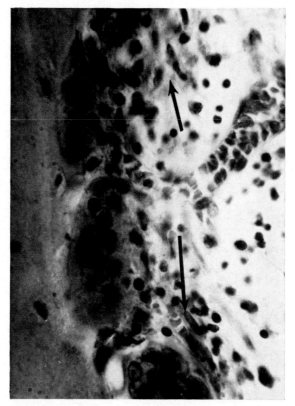

FIG. 8.16. A row of active osteoclasts in cortical bone in Paget's disease. Behind the osteoclasts are blood vessels with diameters of the order of one erythrocyte. Two are arrowed. A rather larger supply vessel is seen on the right. ×400.

rise to characteristic resorption cavities. Figures 8.18, 8.19 show cavities in bone containing vessels and both osteoblasts and osteoclasts, surrounded by equally characteristic irregularly laid down bone (as indicated by the more heavily stained arrest lines). Nearly all the cells in the section through the cavity shown in Fig. 8.20 are vascular endothelial cells. This appearance is possible because the osteoclasts which produce the cavities have only a limited life.

All cell activity is very exuberant. An indication of this is given in Fig. 8.21 where, not only have a large number of cells coalesced to form the osteoclasts, but cells between it and the bone surface, together with several osteocytes, are apparently displaying a resorptive activity. The result of this type of cell activity is that the shape of bones may be greatly distorted but the overall form remains intact. In this Paget's disease shows a difference from the uncontrolled cell proliferation of a

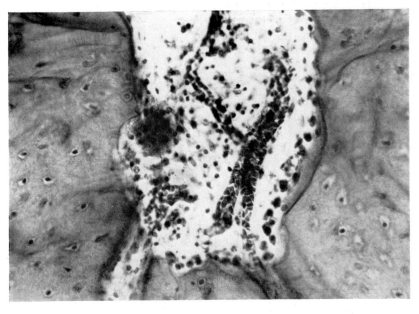

FIG. 8.18. Typical irregular bone cavity in Paget's disease, containing vessels, osteoblasts (bottom) and osteoclast (top of cavity). It is surrounded by irregularly laid down bone. ×200.

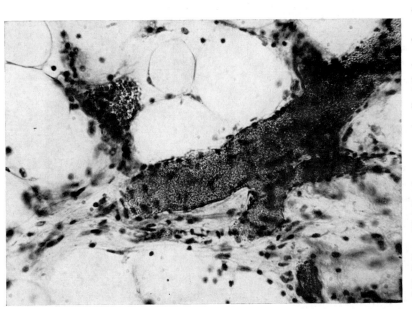

FIG. 8.17. Cells proliferating from a vessel wall, at the boundary of a Paget's lesion in bone. The vessel is filled with perfusion medium. ×200.

Y

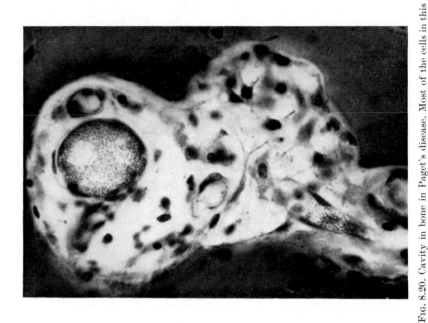

FIG. 8.20. Cavity in bone in Paget's disease. Most of the cells in this section are vascular endothelium, and all are derived from this source. One cell shows a mitotic figure (towards bottom of figure). ×400.

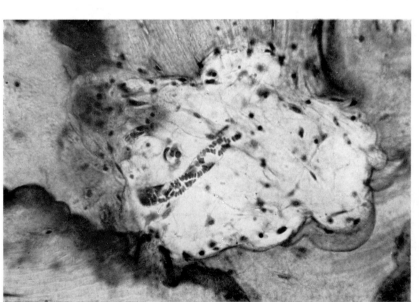

FIG. 8.19. Irregular cavity in bone in Paget's disease, containing vessels and cells derived from the vessel walls. In the irregular bone surrounding the cavity there are heavily staining arrest lines. ×200.

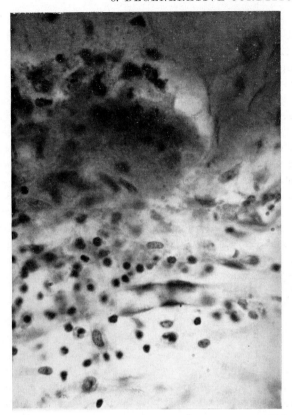

FIG. 8.21. A large osteoclast in Paget's disease. At top of figure cells between it and the bone surface, and also the neighbouring osteocytes, are displaying resorptive activity. ×400.

sarcoma. The effects of immobilization may be dramatic. In Paget's disease increased osteoblastic and osteoclastic activity usually go on simultaneously, but if a bone is immobilized the decreased blood flow, through a maze of vessels that are frequently of small diameter (though anastomoses between large vessels may lead to the shunting of a high proportion of the available blood), may cause a complete cessation of osteoblastic activity, while cell proliferation and osteoclastic activity go on unchecked.

To establish that all the observed effects in Paget's bone can be accounted for by the increased rate of proliferation of vessels and cells in the affected areas does not explain the condition, but it does enable questions to be asked for which satisfactory answers could give the explanation. There are a number of facets of the problem which still await careful investigation.

One immediate problem is that lesions are localized. The condition involves the proliferation of vessels and cells from vessel walls. This is something that is usually controlled by hormones, so that one might expect all the bone to be affected, as is the case in osteoporosis. Instead there are separate lesions, sometimes only one, with the distribution showing a maximum occurrence in those regions of bone subjected to mechanical stress. Price and Goldie (1969) have shown that the excessive proliferation that leads to sarcoma formation involves the right femur more often than the left. In addition to hormonal stimulation of the cells, a requirement for proliferation is the presence of nutrients which are supplied by resorbing bone, and also oxygen. It might seem that for the excessive proliferation of Paget's disease there is a threshold amount of these chemicals from the bone that must be present before the condition is triggered off. (This could be analogous to the situation where a threshold level of cortisol and other steroids are required before abnormal megakaryocytes are produced.) Once the extra activity is started, enzymes from the plentiful supply of osteoclasts will keep up the quantity. In support of this suggestion is the fact that autografts of normal bone are converted to Paget's bone. Also, a careful search by Johnson (1964) has shown that in the initial lesion, ahead of the leading osteoclasts is a region he describes as pre-Paget's bone, in which the characteristic fluorescence of one of the bone matrix components is absent. This component has presumably been leached out by the enzymes from osteoclasts, and might be the local limiting factor.

When one considers the systemic aspects, there are a number of observations which suggest that the possibility of Paget's disease being a stress-induced condition is one worth pursuing. There is a tendency for the occurrence of familial cases, and also a well-marked racial specificity, including England and Western Europe (Price, 1962; Price and Goldie, 1969). It is rare in Scandinavia and among other racial types. This racial specificity is found with osteoporosis, chronic bronchitis and other stress-induced conditions and would seem to reflect a genetic difference. Again the majority of cases start after the age of 40, and a third start after 60. This is the age when most conditions involving excess cell proliferation decrease, but it is the age at which stress-induced illnesses become prominent. Metastatic calcifications of blood vessels are also associated with Paget's disease (Price, 1962). They are frequent accompaniments of osteoporosis and other stress conditions.

If the hypothesis that Paget's disease is a stress-induced condition is correct, then one would expect periods of remission. These are observed. Figure 8.22 shows a histological illustration of this, with normal lamellar bone, in contact with quiescent fatty marrow, laid

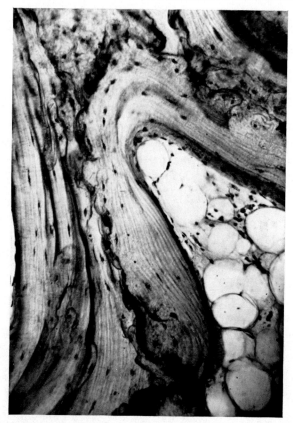

FIG. 8.22. A quiescent phase in Paget's disease. Normal lamellar bone, in contact with fatty marrow, has been laid down over irregular Paget's bone. ×100.

down on irregular Paget's bone. Paget (1877) himself was the first to provide evidence of a possible metabolic pathway, when he observed "he had taken various medicines, but none had done any good, and iodine, in whatever form, had always done harm". More recently, an apparent association of Paget's disease with Hashimoto's thyroiditis has been reported on a number of occasions (Luxton, 1957; Price, 1962; Cooke, 1966). This suggests that the action of thyroid and peptide hormones should be investigated further.

Osteoarthritis

In the present context osteoarthritis is being considered as a condition with a purely mechanical origin, although its subsequent course may be partially modified by the prevailing anabolic or catabolic level of the individual. The cause is a faulty distribution of forces across a joint. Faulty mechanics may be either congenital or acquired. Congenital dislocation of the hip and Perthes disease often lead to arthritic hips later in life. Figure 4.13 showed a radiograph of a femur with the head set at an abnormal angle. The result has been that weight-bearing is concentrated over too small an area of the joint. Mechanical imbalance can happen in almost any joint as a result of trauma, or as a result of excessive pull of muscles around that joint. When a person keeps muscles in the hands tensed for too long a period arthritic lesions may develop in the finger joints. There are various other possible causes of the initiating lesion (e.g. Sokoloff, 1969). The sites which give rise to most clinical problems are the hip, because it is an important weight-bearing joint, and the fore-feet, because of the very high proportion of the population affected.

The greatest number of acquired deformities are those produced by unsuitably shaped and ill-fitting shoes, and in recent years hallux valgus has become the commonest orthopaedic condition requiring hospital treatment. Figure 8.23 shows the positions of the toes in a pair

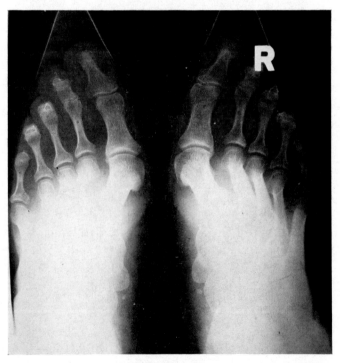

FIG. 8.23. Radiograph showing the position of a woman's toes in a pair of fashionable shoes

of fashionable shoes. Such an abnormal angle causes a portion of the articular cartilage to be uncovered so that it ceases to be subject to the intermittent pumping action which helps to convey fluids and solutions through the cartilage gel. Tendon pull still remains, and the final result is a large arthritic osteophyte known as a bunion. Shine (1965) has investigated the feet of the population of St. Helena, where many inhabitants prefer to go barefoot, and others take to wearing shoes at different ages. Abnormal angles of deviation of the big toe were almost entirely absent in those who did not wear shoes, and the proportion of the others who showed a large increase in the angle of deviation increased linearly with the time they had been wearing shoes. The observed deviations were approximately twice as great in females as in males when the fit of the shoe was comparable. A contributory factor for this might be the lower muscle strength in the female as compared with the male.

Fashion is the main problem, particularly with children's shoes. The attitude of some manufacturers has been expressed thus

(Hicks, 1965) "(evidence) suggests that if a woman can reach the age of 20 years with a big toe angle of less than 10° she is unlikely to develop bunions in old age . . . To produce a marketable shoe for teenage children it was thought that a big toe angle of 10° was a reasonable compromise between fit and fashion".

Cartilage changes

The initial lesion in osteoarthritis is a breakdown of the gel structure of the articular cartilage. This breakdown is usually from a mechanical cause, but occasionally it is chemically initiated. Such chemical initiation can occur after the effusion of blood into a joint. Figures 8.24, 8.25 are taken from an experiment where this has been simulated (Guicciardi and Little, 1967). Near the base of the articular cartilage the matrix which has lost its gel structure may become calcified, and in this illustration (Fig. 8.23) the calcification front is more heavily stained than the rest (haematoxylin is attached to free phosphate radicles). Minor trauma results in cell death, and at a later stage there is vascular invasion of areas where recovery of the gel structure does not take place, followed by ossification.

In many arthritic processes the earliest changes take place in the non-weight-bearing areas of a joint, such as the hip (Harrison, Schajowicz and Trumeta, 1953), or in the non-articulating parts of a non-weight-bearing joint (cf. Fig. 8.23). These are the areas where the intermittent pumping action which assists the flow of fluids through cartilage is missing. Hence the gel structure becomes inadequate and any minor

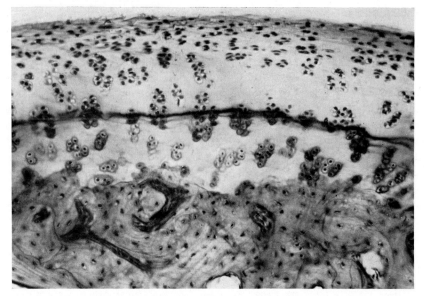

FIG. 8.24. Cartilage in rabbit's knee, 2 weeks after blood had been injected into the joint. The lower part of the cartilage is lightly calcified, the heavily stained line showing the calcification front. In one patch of the articular cartilage cells have died, and no longer take up stain. × 100.

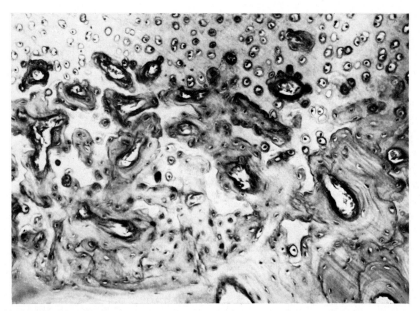

FIG. 8.25. Base of cartilage in rabbit's knee. At a later stage vessels invade the region of altered cartilage, and enchondral ossification takes place. × 100.

trauma may result in a complete breakdown of the affected area and consequently cell death. It is also possible for the components of the intercellular matrix to break down into saccharides that provide a suitable stimulant for cell division. Under these conditions rows of cells or cell nests may be formed. This can happen at any level in the cartilage. Figure 5.21 shows the edge of a changed arthritic area half way through the cartilage, and Fig. 5.22 cell nests near the surface. This mechanism allows repair to take place wherever in the cartilage it is needed. New cells, and surviving cells if the conditions become less acidic, extrude new matrix components to restore the gel structure. Figure 5.21 showed, in a non-weight-bearing area, collagen fibrils lined up normal to the surface. This is a very common observation (Little, Pimm and Trueta, 1958).

The next stage in these non-weight-bearing areas, if a suitable mechanical balance is not restored, is some calcification of the matrix near the junction with underlying bone, followed by ossification (Figs 4.2, 8.25). In regions of cartilage that were originally weight-bearing, the lower part of the cartilage is often more resilient than the upper and middle layers. Here a frequent observation is that vessels penetrate through weak points to the degraded middle sector of the cartilage, and then spread laterally, to form a new layer of bone in the middle of the cartilage.

When the pressure, whether due to weight-bearing or muscle pull, on cartilage is increased cells react to protect themselves. This is demonstrated very clearly in the illustrations to Chapter 5. Sometimes the effect of a combination of pressure and a rotary movement is to stimulate the formation of a rubber-like beta-protein, and newly extruded material is shown in Figs 5.17, 5.19. When first extruded it is more heavily stained by haematoxylin. Should the cartilage subsequently become calcified patches containing the beta-protein remain uncalcified (Fig. 8.26). A greater pressure kills cells, and Fig. 5.20 shows the state of affairs where cells in the lower half of the articular cartilage have succeeded in protecting themselves, while cells in the upper half have been killed. Once all the cells are dead the remains of the cartilage are abraded away, and the surface layer is bone. Osteocytes soon die, and as the bone is damaged granulation tissue cells proliferate (Fig. 8.27).

When repair tissue is formed in the vicinity of cartilage it spreads over the neighbouring surface (Fig. 5.5) and into defects. Where the surrounding physical forces are suitable there is a metaplastic change to cartilage (Figs 5.6, 5.7). The direction of the cell activity is thus towards repair, and making good the damage, so that if the mechanical balance is restored the articular cartilage, and hence the joint, can revert to normal function. In these attempts at repair, however, the shape of the bone

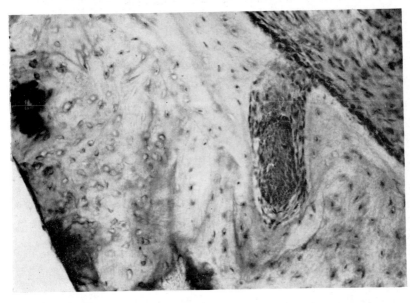

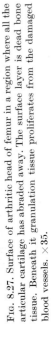

Fig. 8.27. Surface of arthritic head of femur in a region where all the articular cartilage has abraded away. The surface layer is dead bone tissue. Beneath it granulation tissue proliferates from the damaged blood vessels. ×35.

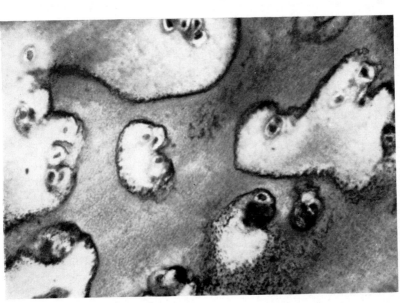

Fig. 8.26. Calcified articular cartilage in elderly human. When conditions in an arthritic joint are such that the articular cartilage calcifies, those areas occupied by the rubber-like beta-protein remain uncalcified. The portions of this calcification with a granular appearance are calcium carbonate. ×200.

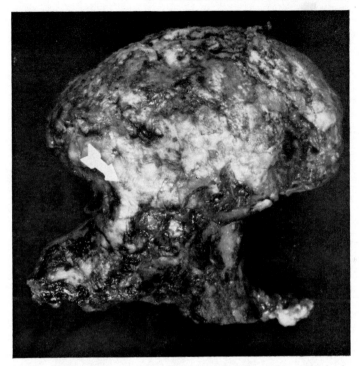

Fig. 8.28. Arthritic head of femur. Parts of the upper surface are completely denuded of cartilage and fibrous tissue. There is an equatorial overgrowth of tissue, and new fibrocartilage shows as light patches (arrowed).

may change and sub-chrondal bone may give rise to problems. Figure 8.28 shows an arthritic head of femur. Part of the upper surface is completely denuded of cartilage and fibrous tissue, there is an equatorial overgrowth of tissue, and the lighter areas (one is arrowed) are now fibrocartilage. This changed shape in itself would hinder or prevent a complete restoration of normal articulation and function.

Osteophyte formation

The success of attempts to form new cartilage depends upon the congruity of the joint, and where there is inadequate contact the cartilage is eroded from below, with vascular invasion followed by replacement by bone. Where there is uneven contact repeated attempts may be made to form a new cartilaginous cap. Figure 8.29 shows three such layers of secondary cartilage. The outer layer is still fibrous, and is the latest formed by proliferating repair tissue, the middle layer has been converted into recognizable cartilage, while the inner layer has responded to increased forces by producing extra matrix, still heavily staining

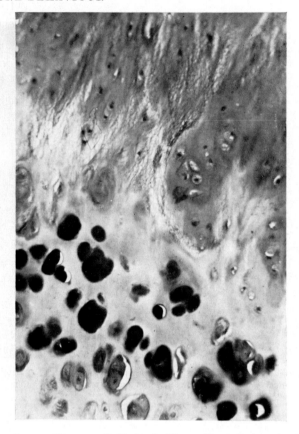

Fig. 8.29. Secondary cartilage on arthritic head of femur. The outer layer is still fibrous, the middle layer has been converted to cartilage, while the inner layer has responded to altered forces by producing extra matrix, heavily staining and therefore of comparatively recent origin. ×200.

and therefore of comparatively recent origin. The result of erosion on one side and cartilage formation on the other is to remodel the bone in the direction of a more congruous joint. It is on this type of remodelling that the success of an osteotomy depends. Figure 8.30 shows subsequent changes on the side of new cartilage deposition. The line of bone down the centre of the photograph is the original osseous base of the articular cartilage. To the left of this is a small patch of fibrous tissue, where the osteogenic factor did not reach granulation tissue formed at an earlier stage of the process in time for it to differentiate into bone. The original cartilage is now replaced by bone, and over it is a layer of cartilage formed from proliferating granulation tissue. The distribution of haemopoietic tissue shows where active remodelling is in progress.

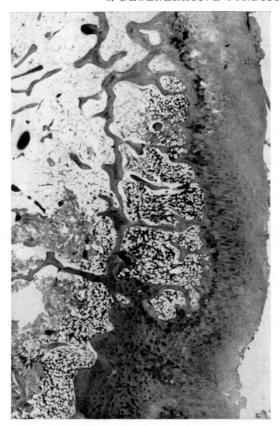

FIG. 8.30. Arthritic head of femur. Early stage in osteophyte formation. The line of bone down the centre of the figure is the original osseous base of the articular cartilage. To the left of this is some sparse fibrous tissue. The distribution of haemopoietic tissue shows where active remodelling is in progress. ×35.

Around the perimeter of bones near joints ligaments are often attached, and the tensional forces exerted by their pull can sometimes rupture vessels as effectively as the pressures operating in weight-bearing areas. Remodelling then results in the bone becoming elongated along the direction of the force applied by the ligament. During the process of formation of an osteophyte, while remodelling is taking place, the new bone is often filled with haemopoietic tissue. When re-modelling has reached a stage when the pull exerted by the ligament has eased, the haemopoietic tissue is gradually replaced by inert fatty marrow, and the surface is usually covered by fibrous tissue. A fully formed osteophyte may be quite large and irregular, but its shape reflects the direction of applied forces during its formation. Such bony excrescences are stable (as indicated by the presence of fatty marrow), and although produced by identical cellular mechanisms to the remodelling aimed at improving joint congruity are liable to prevent a successful outcome of any subsequent remodelling processes.

The progress of arthritic changes depends not only on the presence or absence of weight-bearing and the tension provided by tendons and ligaments, but also upon the hormonal state of the individual. With a high catabolic level, such as produces post-menopausal and senile osteoporosis, the proliferation of granulation tissue is hindered, while any intercellular matrix components formed in the presence of a raised blood cortisol are chemically more stable than normal. Because of this, a frequent observation in cases of intracapsular fractures is the remarkably normal appearance of the cartilage in spite of the action of unfavourable forces across the joint. Even previous microfractures and minor fractures in the head of the femur show little effect on the cartilage. In Fig. 5.18 only a single row of cells in the cartilage had been affected by changed forces across the joint. These cells were a little way below the surface, and this seems to be the most vulnerable level in articular cartilage. On occasions when damage to articular cartilage is temporary, and of a minor nature, some damage may be seen in this area, with little or no cell reaction elsewhere (Fig. 8.31). The surface layers may break away, and the congruity of the surface be restored later without further destruction.

Although corticosteroid levels in osteoporosis prevent gross arthritic changes mechanical imbalance may well be present, so that there are stresses and tensions at the insertions of ligaments and tendons. The formation of osteophytes is prevented, but cell activity is present and the matrix breakdown products stimulate the formation of haemopoietic tissue. A patch or ring of this red marrow, containing few or no bony trabeculae, often forms in the head of the femur at this level (Fig. 8.2), and may extend from the surface to the weight-bearing trabeculae. This ring of non-osseous tissue in the bone seems to be the osteoporotic equivalent of an osteophyte, and is one of the predisposing factors for an intracapsular fracture.

Bone changes

The cartilage changes and osteophyte formation which are typical of osteoarthritis occur in joints in both weight-bearing and non-weight-bearing sites, but the accompanying bone changes are more severe in weight-bearing than in non-weight-bearing joints. These bone changes are stimulated by the presence of chemical breakdown products of the cartilage, broken blood-vessels and microfractures. The pressure

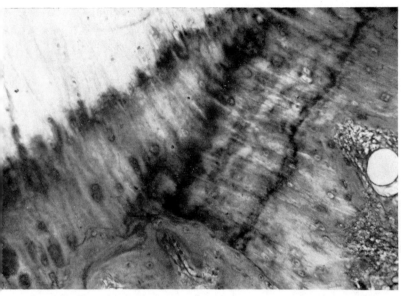

Fig. 8.32. Local pressure on toe joint has caused a crack, with some displacement, in the layer of bone at the base of the cartilage. The lower part of the cartilage has calcified, and the appearance of more heavily stained lines in this calcified cartilage suggests that there have been at least three separate traumatic episodes. ×200.

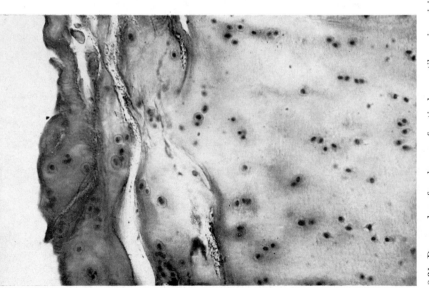

Fig. 8.31. Damaged surface layers of articular cartilage, in a joint with few signs of other cartilage changes. ×100.

of a shoe on a toe joint, for example, may apparently result in the layer
of bone and calcified cartilage at the base of the articular cartilage
being crushed (Fig. 8.32). The spread of damage is, however, limited
(Fig. 8.33). In weight-bearing situations the weakening caused by initial

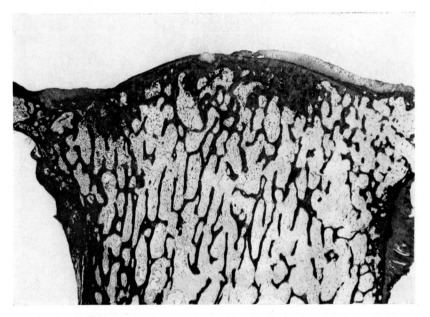

Fig. 8.33. Big toe. Patches of dense bone tissue below damaged cartilage indicate the extent
of bone damage. ×35.

damage results in further fractures and microfractures until a considerable portion of the bone is affected. The area shown in Fig. 8.34 is in the
middle of the head of femur, and shows the lower border of a damaged
region. Non-weight-bearing portions of the head of femur or the acetabulum show changes similar to those in the big toe.

   Most of the cell reactions observed in arthritic bone are of the types
which have already been described. Rupture of vessels and trabeculae
results in the proliferation of granulation tissue, and degradation of
tissue provides an ample supply of carbohydrates and other chemicals
to sustain cell proliferation. Figure 4.10 showed very exuberant cell
proliferation on the surface of a trabecula in an active region. Remodelling leads to changing areas of weakness and further crush fractures in
the weight-bearing zones. Changes are marked by frequent arrest lines
such as those seen in the bone tissue in Fig. 8.34. Figure 4.19 showed
ordinary and woven bone on either side of a trabecula in the region of

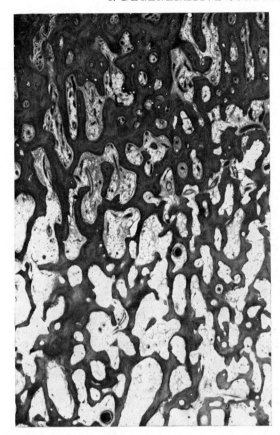

FIG. 8.34. Arthritic head of femur. This area is in the middle of the head, showing that in a weight-bearing joint the bone damage spreads at least this far. Severe involvement is seen in the upper part of figure ×35.

active remodelling. In some parts the bone becomes almost compact, and irregular osteonal remodelling is then observed (Fig. 2.9).

In the regions where remodelling is taking place there is usually a profuse array of vessels which remain open (Fig. 8.35) and with a good blood flow. This is typical of wound healing and fracture healing, and regions of bone where this type of blood vessel proliferates invariably contain mast cells. It has been assumed that these secrete chemicals which stimulate the vessels and blood flow. As the granulation tissue around these vessels is replaced by marrow and sinusoid vessels, and where they are in areas containing a high proportion of osseous tissue, the contents of a confined marrow space may well include an artery with its accompanying nerve and several sinusoid vessels. Any hindrance to the venous return can cause a build-up of pressure in the sinusoid

z

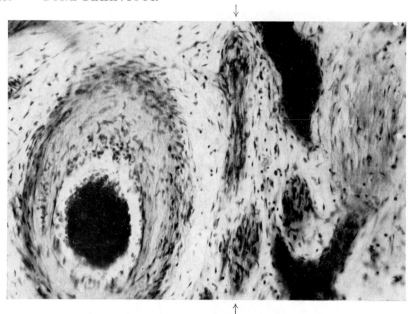

FIG. 8.35. Nerves (arrowed), accompanying an artery, are between that artery (left) and sinusoid vessels (right). The vessels contain a dark perfusion mixture. ×200.

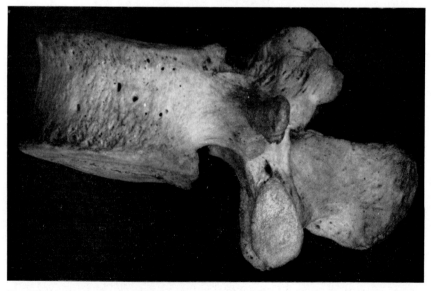

FIG. 8.36. An isolated human vertebra. There is a cavity to the right of the vertebral body through which the spinal cord passes.

vessels (Fig. 8.35) and hence exert pressure on the nerve. Trueta (1968) has provided an abundance of evidence that pain in osteoarthritis is due to a build-up of pressure within the bone in the vicinity of active vessels. Similarly Fryer (1969) has shown that the pain in bends is also due to pressure, while Anderson, Curwen and Howard (1958) and Anderson and Naylor (1961) have shown that toothache is also a pressure-induced pain—this time from osmotic pressure. In the case of osteo-arthritis of the hip immediate relief from pain has been obtained by drilling the head of femur and thus releasing pressure between the trabeculae, and also by the release of pressure during an osteotomy.

Where there is too large an area of cell death in the marrow cysts de-velop. These may be filled with granulation tissue or fluid. In those which fill with fluid fracture cartilage often proliferates, while the granulation tissue in other cysts differentiates to fibrous tissue in places where the osteogenic factor is unable to penetrate. Around the peri-phery woven bone is formed, so that eventually the fibrous cysts are surrounded by a shell of bone.

The cumulative effect of all these changes which have been described is to modify the cartilage and bone on either side of a joint towards a new congruity and to fit in with the new set of mechanical conditions and forces acting across that joint. Figure 4.15 showed the trabecular changes after an osteotomy designed to assist this process. In the cases shown in Figs 5.8, 5.9 the one after an infarct and the other after an electrical burn, complete recovery of function has been achieved. In the case of arthritic joints such results can also be obtained, providing that the mechanical balance is restored before the growth and establish-ment of osteophytes that mechanically hinder recovery.

Intervertebral Disc Lesions

The main weight-bearing part of the spine is the column consisting of the vertebral bodies and intervertebral discs. Figure 8.36 shows an isolated vertebra. Trabeculae within the bone tend to be either vertical or horizontal, and normally there is a layer of denser bone adjoining the disc. This is shown in the histological section in Fig. 8.37. This trabecular arrangement in a weight-bearing bone means that there is almost constant remodelling, and so the marrow within the vertebrae consists mostly of haemopoietic tissue. In the adult it may be the main source of blood cells. The cartilaginous tissue, the disc, which separates the vertebrae provides flexibility and acts as a shock absorber. It has three main components. Immediately adjacent to the bone is the cartilage end plate, which in appearance resembles articular cartilage (Fig. 8.38). Between the cartilage end plates are the nucleus pulposus in the

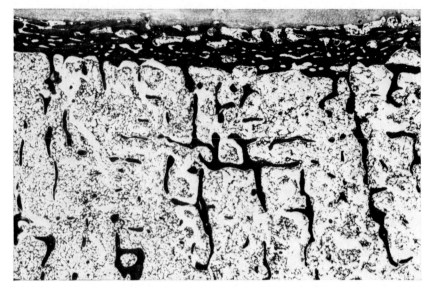

FIG. 8.37. Section through a normal vertebral body. Trabeculae tend to be either vertical or horizontal. There is a layer of denser bone adjoining the disc (upper part of fig.). Haemopoietic tissue is present in the marrow spaces. ×35.

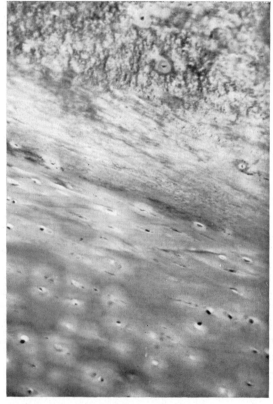

FIG. 8.38. Cartilage end plate from elderly subject. Its appearance resembles articular cartilage. Top of fig. is the adjoining nucleus pulposus, stained to show the dense beta-protein. ×100.

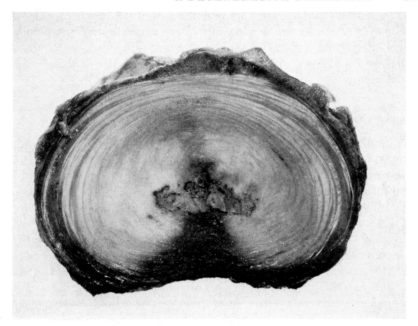

FIG. 8.39. Transverse section through intervertebral disc, with the nucleus pulposus surrounded by an orientated annulus. There are some minor degenerative changes in the central part of the nucleus pulposus.

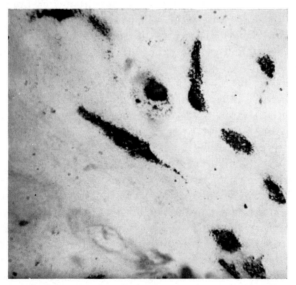

FIG. 8.40. Section of prolapsed lumbar disc tissue, taken at operation and placed in a culture medium containing tritiated uridine. The isotope has been taken up in cells which were active at the time the tissue was taken. Cells at bottom left were mature and inactive, and are therefore unlabelled. ×400.

central regions, and the annulus fibrosus around the perimeter. Figure 8.39 shows a transverse section of a disc, with the nucleus pulposus surrounded by an orientated annulus. Typical cells in a healthy nucleus pulposus were shown in Fig. 2.25, and the appearance of these cells in the electron microscope in Figs 2.27, 2.28, 2.29.

Lumbar disc lesions

The commonest defects in the vertebral column are found in the lumbar regions. The mechanisms involved in defects in the cervical region follow a similar pattern. Sometimes the lesions produce acute clinical symptoms, but more often a less severe lesion produces a "low back pain". The precise causes of the low back pain, which is very prevalent, are not known, but it does seem probable that they are multiple. Disc lesions are frequently painful. Sometimes it can be shown that pressure on a nerve root is responsible, and Nachemson (1969) has provided evidence that a connective tissue reaction around a nerve root is painful, and that sufficient acid is present in a degenerating disc for a chemical pain stimulus to operate. Microfractures or a hindered blood flow through the vertebral body could also lead to pain.

The disc is an avascular tissue and, as for articular cartilage, diffusion alone is unable to provide an adequate cell nutrition. A pumping action provided by the action of neighbouring muscles is also required. In order to protect the cells from the minor trauma that may be regarded as a normal part of life further exercise is required to induce the production of the rubber-like proteins. Once an adequate distribution of the rubbery beta-proteins is complete any minor cell destruction tends to remain localized. Figure 5.15 shows the edge of such an area, with adjacent cells remaining viable. In a series of lumbar disc lesions investigated by Taylor (1964), the unaffected tissue of the nucleus pulposus adjacent to changed tissue was observed to contain a smaller proportion of the beta-proteins than did normal disc tissue obtained at post-mortem from subjects of equivalent age.

Scandinavian workers have shown that at times the lumbar intervertebral discs can be subjected to very high pressures (Nachemson, 1971), and it seems most probable that an inadequate development of the beta-proteins leaves the discs more vulnerable to the effects of pressure than they would otherwise be. The initiation of lumbar disc lesions is soon after adolescence, with prolapse commonest in the 20 to 40 year age group. Later, in the elderly, lesions may also be caused by inadequacy of the bone or interspinous ligaments. In the lumbar spine the greatest mobility is at the levels L4 to L5 and L5 to S1, and it is these two discs which are most commonly affected.

Lindblom (1957) has provided evidence to show that the start of the lesion is an abnormal pressure unevenly distributed and sufficiently great to cause cell death. This pressure atrophy is basically the same mechanism as is found in arthritic lesions in the cartilage in weight-bearing areas. Some cells die in the nucleus pulposus and Diamant, Karlsson and Nachenson (1968) have shown that the lowered pH of degenerated discs is related to the presence of lactate. Under some circumstances lactic acid can help to stimulate cell division (Mottram, 1927). There is also a tendency for the discs to rupture, on the concave side of the spinal curvature. Lindblom has shown that both men and women now have a higher tendency to disc degeneration in the lumbar spine than primitive people had. Modern women have a higher frequency of degeneration of the lumbosacral disc than have modern men, this difference being absent in primitive men and women. He has provided evidence that the height of the heel is a relevant factor. Radiographs have shown that elevation of the heels by a support is followed by a compensatory change in the equilibrium of the spine. The forced angulation in the lumbosacral region produces an increased pressure on the posterior portion of the lower lumbar intervertebral discs.

In the course of development of a lumbar disc prolapse breakdown of the intercellular matrix takes place around dead cells. Usually only a portion of the nucleus pulposus is involved. Lactate is present, but so are the polysaccharide degradation products which favour cell proliferation. Prolapse of the lumbar disc is not simply an extrusion of necrotic tissue, but is accompanied by active cell proliferation in sequestrated fragments lying in the vertebral canal. In the midst of the prolapsed tissue there is often an abundant formation of the mature beta-protein (Fig. 5.16). The periphery of the prolapsed tissue is usually occupied by elongated fibroblasts, that may subsequently change to rounded cells Figure 8.40 shows a section of prolapsed tissue, taken at operation and then placed in a tissue culture medium containing tritiated uridine. The isotope has been taken up in cells which were active at the time the tissue was taken. The cell on the left was mature and inactive and therefore unlabelled. Cell activity is not continuous, but occurs in phases, one demonstration of this being successive layers of protein around some cells (Fig. 5.14).

Thoracic disc lesions

The thoracic vertebrae are held by the ribs in a more rigid position than the lumbar vertebrae. As a result, although the thoracic discs do not contain so large a proportion of the beta-proteins as do the lumbar

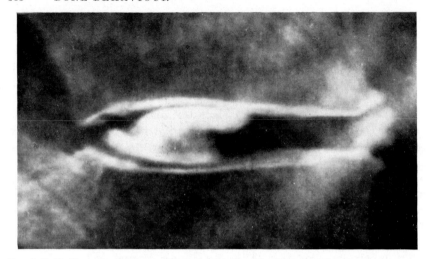

Fɪɢ. 8.41. Radiograph showing calcified thoracic intervertebral disc. The cartilage end plate is uncalcified, so that gaps show between the calcified nucleus pulposus and vertebral bodies. The annulus is also intact. The author thanks Prof. T. K. F. Taylor for this figure.

discs, they are better protected from accidental trauma, so that trouble-some lesions are comparatively rare, whereas lumbar disc lesions are common. Taylor (1964) has collected data from the Oxford region for the period 1943–1961, and in an area with an average population of approximately 284,000 there were only 17 patients with a calcified thoracic disc proceeding to prolapse and spinal cord compression.

In this rarer thoracic disc lesion there is again a failure of the gel structure of the intercellular matrix, and as with other conditions that develop after a breakdown of the gel most lesions develop in the 35–55 year age group. At this site almost twice as many men are affected as women. The level most frequently affected is T9 to T10, followed by T8 to T9. Unlike the smaller areas affected in the lumbar disc, if a thoracic lesion does occur the greater part of the nucleus pulposus is liable to become necrotic and then calcify. The mineral phase consists of the large and irregular hydroxyapatite crystallites, with sometimes magnesian whitlockite and calcite crystals, that are characteristic of necrotic tissue. The consistency of the mixture of mineral crystallites and necrotic fibro-cartilage is rather like that of toothpaste. With these necrotic changes in the matrix, together with widespread cell death, there is little tendency for stimulation of cell division.

The cartilage end plate remains uncalcified, and a gap between the calcified nucleus pulposus and bone can be seen clearly on radio-graphs such as that shown in Fig. 8.41. Frequently the annulus also remains intact. It is, however, thinner than the annulus of a lumbar disc,

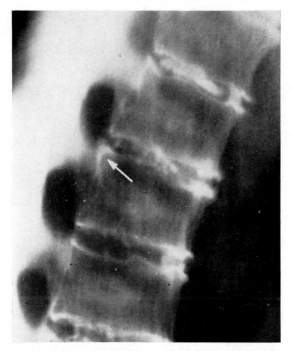

FIG. 8.42. Radiograph showing calcified thoracic disc of 60-year-old woman. At the place arrowed the calcified material has been extruded into the spinal canal. The junctions between the vertebral bodies and discs are rough and uneven. The author thanks Prof. T. K. F. Taylor for this figure.

so that when prolapse does occur it is by a process of the creamy calcified material squeezing through a rupture of the annulus into the vertebral canal (Fig. 8.42). When this happens a calcified shell is left behind where the mineral was deposited in the transitional area between annulus and nucleus. One cell reaction that may occur occasionally in a calcified disc or very frequently in the prolapsed calcified tissue is a slow vascular penetration, with a gradual ossification of the material. In this way it is possible in some thoracic lesions for the greater part of the disc space to be replaced by bone. Prolapsed material in the vertebral canal is usually gradually replaced by bone (Taylor, 1964).

Interactions between vertebrae and discs

Frequently there is a temptation to think in terms of either the intervertebral disc or the vertebral body, but appearances such as the irregular junction of these two tissues seen in Fig. 8.42 are a reminder that events in one may affect the other. Changes are particularly common in the central part of the junction where the nucleus pulposus is

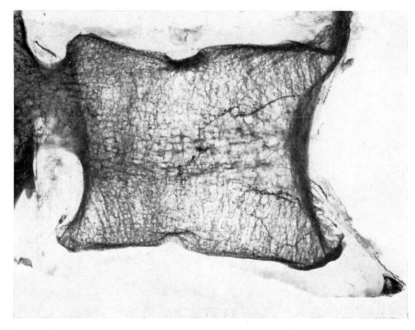

Fig. 8.43. Section through vertebral body. The cartilaginous protrusions into the bone in the central region are known as Schmorl's nodes. In this instance they have probably been caused by faulty enchondral ossification.

directly behind the cartilage end plate. It is here that cartilaginous "protrusions" into the bone are most frequently seen (e.g. Fig. 8.43). They are often called Schmorl's nodes, after the pathologist who first carried out an extensive and detailed survey of the various types of spinal pathology (Schmorl and Junghanns, 1932). Some are caused by faulty enchondral ossification during the period of growth, while others are the result of minor fractures.

The irregular bony ingrowth seen in places in Fig. 8.42 was the result of defects in the cartilage. Conversely, osteoporosis is character-ized by a ballooning of the intervertebral disc (Fig. 5.27). In a porotic vertebra, too great a pressure can result in a crush fracture such as that shown in Fig. 5.30, where the whole width of the bone is affected, or a minor one such as that shown in Fig. 8.44 where only a small part of the junction between bone and cartilage is affected.

On the vertebral side of the border one finds the normal processes of fracture repair, with woven bone formation (Fig. 4.18), followed by remodelling to ordinary bone. Sometimes, as was the case with osteo-arthritic cysts, cells mature before there has been adequate vascular penetration or before a sufficient quantity of the osteogenic factor has

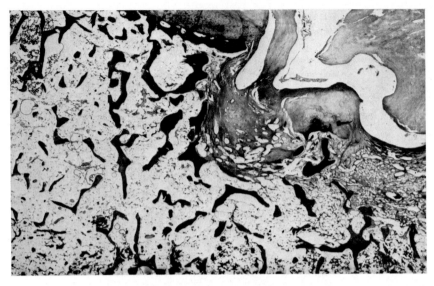

FIG. 8.44. Site in a case of osteoporosis where a portion of the vertebral body has collapsed. Fracture repair has resulted in the formation of larger trabeculae than in the surrounding bone, but the tear in the disc tissue is as yet unhealed. ×35.

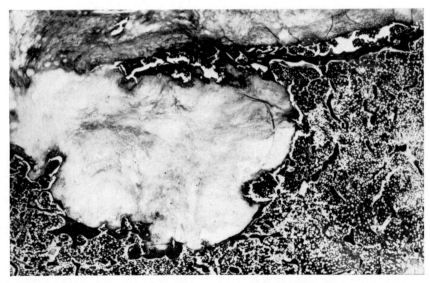

FIG. 8.45. Osteoporotic vertebral body. Repair tissue adjoining a damaged part of the cartilage end plate remains as an island of fibrocartilage. ×35.

diffused into the defect. A mass of fibrous tissue results which, because of the applied forces in the vertebral column, rapidly differentiates to cartilage. Figure 8.45 shows a typical island of cartilage adjoining a

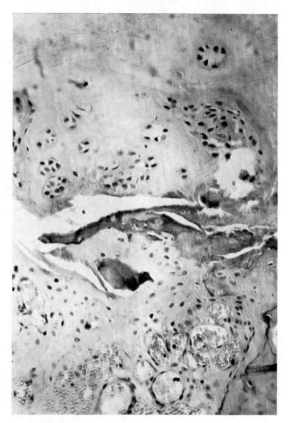

FIG. 8.46. Tear in intervertebral disc tissue near crush fracture in osteoporotic vertebra. There is cell nest formation on either side of the crack. Vessels proliferating from the bone can be seen at bottom of figure. ×100.

damaged part of the end plate. Sometimes in an active phase of osteoporosis the proliferation of granulation tissue is sparse, and a rather sparse fibrous tissue is formed from this.

As the bone collapses tears are formed in the cartilage of the disc (Fig. 8.46). Sometimes the cartilage end plate is torn away from the nucleus pulposus, and sometimes its cells die and the tissue is resorbed. The type of repair tissue found in the disc depends partly on the nature of the damage and partly on the forces acting on the area. Sometimes the repair tissue very closely resembles the tissue previously present at the site of damage. Figure 1.3 was an example of this. Sometimes it is

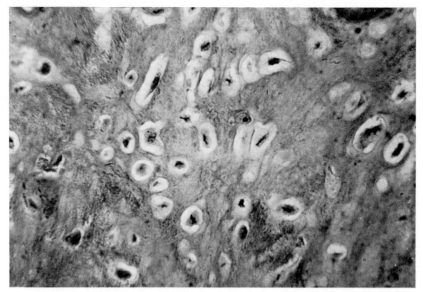

FIG. 8.47. An active stage in the formation of extra disc material in a ballooned intervertebral disc. Cartilage cells have finished proliferating, and are now producing a matrix containing fibrous tissue and beta-proteins.

very irregular. Figure 8.46 shows cell nest formation around a crack that is still present. Farther into the nucleus pulposus the tissue is dead, while some vascular invasion can be seen at the bottom of the figure In a typical ballooned disc in the lumbar regions cells proliferate and then differentiate into isolated cartilage cells. Figure 8.47 shows quite uniform tissue at a fairly early stage of the process, while Fig. 5.31 is the appearance when the process of ballooning is complete.

In the normal intervertebral disc the mature and dense beta-proteins are present to provide resilience and strength, but elastic tissue is absent. In the new tissue of ballooned discs both the dense beta-protein and elastic tissue are commonly present. Figure 5.31 showed an area in which the elastic tissue dominated. These tissues are characterized by their X-ray diffraction patterns, but may also be recognized in histological sections.

Pathological Calcification

Pathological calcifications can occur in almost any part of the body. The greater part of the available information had already been collected when H. G. Wells (Chicago) wrote his review in 1910. In this he concluded, correctly, that calcification was a physio-chemical process, the nature of the mineral deposited depending upon the composition of the under-lying matrix. That statement has since been amplified, but not modified. Types of mineralization were mentioned in Chapter 1: very small complex crystallites (Fig. 1.50) are found in calcifiable matrix, while larger crystallites (hydroxyapatite, whitlockite and calcite) are found on necrotic tissues.

There are several ways in which pathological calcifications might be classified. An early approach was to consider which remain as calcifications and which go on to ossification (Thoma, 1894). It was observed that the first change is frequently to cartilage, which then calcifies (e.g. Andral, 1827, 1837). This change is often followed by ossification. Sometimes fibrous tissue turns to cartilage which then calcifies, while at other times normally occurring cartilage is modified and then calcifies. A review of the early literature on this type of pathological calcification was given by Hasse in 1841. Examples of possible sites for such a lesion are the intervertebral discs, costal cartilage, cartilage in lungs and trachea.

It seemed that ossification might follow on after calcification when, as Paul (1886) described it, "irritation leads to inflammatory proliferation". The proportion of lesions to go on to ossification varies according to the tissue. Poscharisky (1905) and Harvey (1907) found that the ossification process might occur in almost any tissue, but that it is by no means inevitable. It is now known that a necessary predisposing condition for ossification is either the prior presence of cartilage in an environment where it can produce the calcifiable matrix, as in the lungs, or occasional metaplastic cartilage production, as in the aorta.

Pathological calcifications of cartilaginous tissue are usually of little clinical importance. They may start soon after maturity, and they predominate in the female. The phenomenon has been investigated in some detail for the larynx (O'Bannon and Grunow, 1954) and the costal cartilages (Elkeles, 1966a). Figure 8.48 shows the costal cartilage of a girl of 16, and the appearance by the age of 20 is shown in Fig. 8.49. These radiographs are from Elkeles' work. He found that the rise in incidence and severity with age is fairly steady, with the female predominating, until there is a further sharp rise in women over 70. Thoma (1894) remarked that the calcification in the costal and laryngeal cartilages selects "the finely fibrillated split-up parts of the intercellular substance", and it seems that this type of calcification is limited to non-viable parts of the cartilage. X-ray diffraction of the mineral has confirmed that it is essentially a calcification on necrotic tissue and not on the calcifiable matrix which cartilage cells can produce.

A similar type of patchy calcification is sometimes found in place of an organized secondary bone nucleus in the epiphysis of a developing

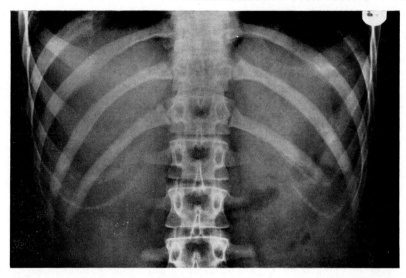

Fig. 8.48. Radiograph of girl, aged 16, showing calcified costal cartilage. The author thanks Dr. A. Elkeles for this figure.

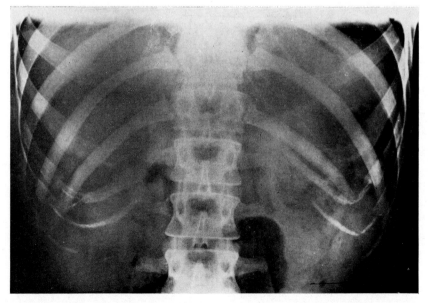

Fig. 8.49. Same girl, aged 20. The calcification in the costal cartilage has increased. The author thanks Dr. A. Elkeles for this figure.

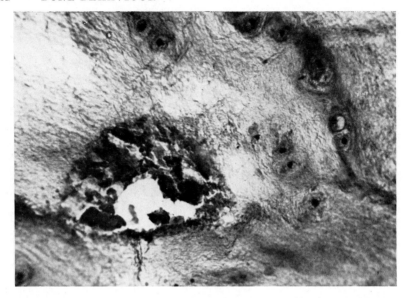

Fɪɢ. 8.50. Adult nucleus pulposus. A very small localized patch of dead cartilage, in which magnesian whitlockite crystals are deposited. × 100.

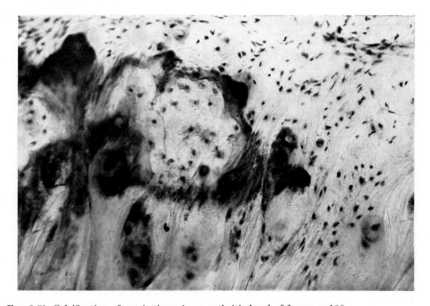

Fɪɢ. 8.51. Calcification of repair tissue in an arthritic head of femur. × 100.

bone if for any reason the blood supply to the epiphysis is hindered. Chemical analysis of such pathological "calcification" in a developing epiphysis may show a high proportion of magnesium as compared with other pathological calcifications. Where the blood supply is seriously affected periosteal calcification has also been observed. A very small and localized patch of dead cartilage with magnesian whitlockite deposition in an adult nucleus pulposus is shown in Fig. 8.50. Here the small mineralized patch is surrounded by viable cells. This histological appearance may be contrasted with the early stages of calcification of the calcifiable matrix in repair tissue from an arthritic head of femur shown in Fig. 8.51.

With the exception of cartilage calcifying after the production of the calcifiable matrix, most pathological calcification is on non-viable cartilage or on necrotic tissue. Lick (1908) came to the conclusion that whether or not necrotic tissue calcified depended on the blood supply. With too free a circulation there was no calcification, and with too little there was a slow calcification. This was undoubtedly one of the factors, but there are other considerations. With too complete a tissue breakdown there may also be no calcification and the whole area may liquefy; while with a rather slower, but still extensive, breakdown one may get the toothpaste consistency described for the calcified thoracic disc lesions. This type of calcification is also found in tendons (Fig. 8.52). For a less complete degradation the anabolic and catabolic levels are important. This was illustrated in Chapter 6 where the fate of necrotic patches caused by the deposition of thrombi was described. At the catabolic end of the scale calcification was found, and at the anti-catabolic end there was a fibrous replacement. Figure 6.32 showed the liver from a rabbit that was being given both cortisone and nore-thynodrel. A large thrombus lodged in the liver, and tissue surrounding the affected vessels had begun to calcify.

The tissues which have been most carefully examined are the arteries, and here the incidence and distribution with sex is more complicated, since overlying the greater tendency for calcification to occur in the female, there is the greater tendency for the sequelae of stress to produce necrotic tissue in the male. In the abdominal aorta calcification begins in the media in the 3rd decade, although it is already evident in coronary arteries in the second decade (Lansing, Blumenthal and Gray, 1948). The incidence and severity of calcified arterial lesions is greater in males than in females before the age of 60. Beyond 70 the incidence and severity of calcified lesions is significantly higher in females than in males (Elkeles, 1957, 1966b). Blumenthal, Lansing and Wheeler (1944) found that medial calcification of the aorta was primarily a function of age, and precedes the formation of fibrous intimal

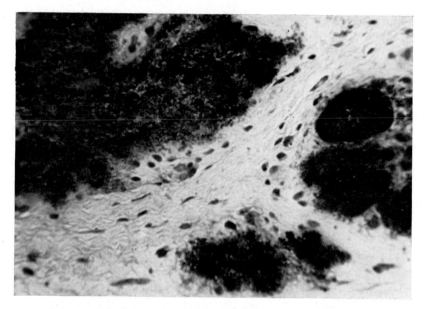

Fig. 8.52 Patches of calcified necrotic tissue in inner part of tendon sheath. ×100.

plaques. These plaques appeared to be associated with an appreciable amount of calcification of the media, and are not observed unless calcification is already present. Many vessels in the body may show symptomless medial calcification.

Calcification of the abdominal aorta is particularly easy to distinguish radiographically (Fig. 8.53), and is frequently used in comparative surveys. It has been found that it is associated with most conditions that are thought to be caused by stress: post-menopausal and senile osteoporosis (Elkeles, 1957), gastric ulcer (Elkeles, 1953, 1964), disease (Price, 1962). A close relationship also exists between Pagets' the extent of coronary artery calcification and the occurrence rate of myocardial infarction (Elkeles, 1966b). This type of calcification is not associated with other pathological changes which are not stress-induced, as for example carcinoma of the stomach (Elkeles, 1966b).

Histological observations and X-ray diffraction evidence demonstrate that pathological calcifications are on dead or partially necrotic tissue. These observations on the incidence of calcification of the arteries show that it tends to occur when the individual has been subjected to stress, since there is a correlation with known stress-induced conditions. The detailed effects of stress on the tissue still

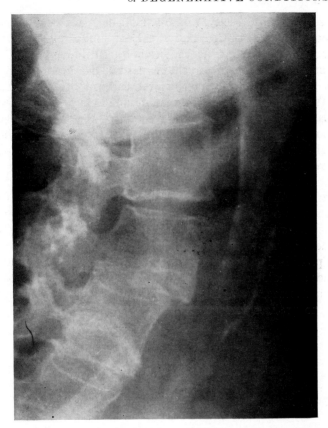

FIG. 8.53. Clinical radiograph of osteoporotic subject. Calcification can be seen in the walls of the abdominal aorta. The author thanks Dr. A. Elkeles for this figure.

require to be worked out. One might speculate that a hindering of the diffusion of fluid through vessel walls, if the supply of nutrients is already scanty, could lower it below danger level, and also hinder the removal of acid waste products from the vicinity of cells. The actual blocking of minor vessels, or lowering the flow through other vessels could be another contributory factor. Cells in the media of arteries would then be at risk for the same reason that cells in articular cartilage are at risk in the early stages of osteoarthritis.

The distribution of vascular lesions tends to be in those sites where turbulence might be expected in the flow of blood. In Paget's disease, where the abnormal vasculature and arteriovenous shunts cause disturbances in blood flow, including the flow through the heart the interventricular septum may calcify, and cardiac calcification is about 5 times more frequent than in other individuals of similar age (Harrison and Lennox, 1948). Where cell death does not occur immediately, although the gel structure of the intercellular matrix has been damaged, cells attempt to repair the damage by producing more polysaccharide for the gel. Where there is long-continued minor damage this polysaccharide accumulates. It is quite frequently seen in the articular cartilage of older people, and also in the media of arteries. It calcifies readily. If the conditions are such that the cause of the trauma is removed it is often slowly resorbed.

When calcification in the soft tissue is on cartilage, whether present normally as in the lung, or as a result of metaplasia of tendons or fibrous tissue, there is a possibility of vascular invasion, followed by ossification. Once a centre of ossification has been produced in the soft tissues, the sequel depends upon its vascular surroundings and blood supply. A small pathological bone may be formed (e.g. Scapinelli, 1963), while sometimes a whole muscle may be replaced by bone, particularly when there is a decreased blood flow to an otherwise normal muscle. More usually the pathological bone would remain as a small focus or be resorbed.

Summary

1. Differences between degenerative conditions of the teeth—usually dental caries—and other hard tissues are due to the fact that teeth protrude through the mucous membrane, so that it is not possible for those parts of a tooth without access to a blood supply to be repaired by natural means. Vessels penetrate through dental pulp to the inner dentine surface, and chemicals necessary to maintain the dentine reach it by diffusion processes.

2. The texture of dentine is similar to that of bone, and its gel structure is necessary to maintain resilience. The gel can be destroyed slowly by interruption of the diffusion processes, or more rapidly when odontoblasts on the inner surface of the dentine are activated by corticosteroids to produce proteolytic enzymes.

3. The resilience of dental enamel is also due to its organic matrix. This consists of two rubber-like beta-proteins, one of these being resistant to the proteolytic enzymes. Both require to be wet to maintain their resilience. The more stable protein completely covers the surface layers of teeth formed in the presence of adequate supplies of vitamin D, fluoride and other essential chemicals. Where there are defects in the structure the less stable protein beneath can be attacked by acids and bacteria from the mouth. This chemical attack is considerably accelerated if the protein has been partly degraded by proteolytic enzymes. Teeth are most susceptible to rapidly developing caries when there is a raised level of blood cortisol—at adolescence, during pregnancy and when the individual is under stress.

4. The most prevalent causes of osteoporosis are a lowered blood flow (disuse), a hormonal imbalance (post-menopausal) and the deposition of platelet thrombi in minor vessels (senile). Vitamin C deficiency also causes osteoporosis, and an excess of parathyroid hormone stimulates an excessive removal of bone by the osteoclasts derived from phagocytic cells.

5. Disuse osteoporosis arises when there is a lack of adequate muscle activity, so that the flow of blood through the bone is hindered. This causes excess pressure within the bone, which can damage membranes covering osseous surfaces in the cortex so stimulating the formation of phagocytic osteoclasts. When sufficient bone has been removed for a pressure equilibrium to be established the decreased rate of flow prevents the replacement of lost bone tissue.

6. In the post-menopausal type of osteoporosis episodes of stress, or sometimes the use of catabolic steroids, or steroids which interfere with the function of the pituitary gland, result in an excess of corticosteroids in the blood. These stimulate osteogenic cells to coalesce and form osteoclasts. When catabolic and anabolic conditions alternate, with the catabolic dominating, a considerable amount of bone may be removed. In active phases the resorbing bone is frequently surrounded by haemopoietic tissue. In passive phases this is replaced by fatty marrow. Changes in activity show as "arrest" lines in the bone tissue, which stain strongly with haematoxylin. Some widely used contraceptive steroids produce a diminution in the quality of bone.

7. Senile osteoporosis, so called because it is most prevalent in elderly people, is also due to stress. Comparatively prolonged and severe stress (and also many progestational steroids) stimulate the formation of multiple small platelet thrombi. Many of these are deposited on the walls of minor blood vessels, and then invaded by fibrous tissue, and so partly block the vessels and contribute to the diminished rate of flow of blood. This is followed by bone removal, often with the same mechanisms as operate in disuse osteoporosis.

8. Small vessels may be completely blocked by thrombi, and when this happens in compact bone patches of bone tissue die. Diffusion of nutrients from vessels may also be hindered by the excess cortisol present so that more bone, both compact and cancellous, may become moribund and die. Cortisol hinders the maturation of macrophages to osteoclasts, and also decreases the amount of bone tissue laid down by osteoblasts. Sometimes dead or moribund trabeculae may be covered by a layer of viable bone. When the cause of stress is removed, dead bone is then removed by phagocytic osteoclasts.

9. Pathological fractures are a fairly frequent complication of osteoporosis. Common sites are the vertebrae, head and neck of femur, and the wrist. The severity varies from the fracture of isolated trabeculae to displaced fractures of the bone. Crush fractures of the vertebrae cause a shortening of the spine of osteoporotic subjects.

10. The frequency of these pathological fractures shows sex and racial variations.

11. Fractures of the head of femur due to post-menopausal osteoporosis are frequently intracapsular, and result from a loss of bone tissue. Fractures due to senile osteoporosis are frequently extra-capsular, and result from a loss of strength of dead bone tissue.

12. Decompression sickness is caused by the release of small bubbles of gas in the blood stream. Pain (the bends) is due to a temporary obstruction of the venous outflow through cortical bone. Larger obstructions can cause areas of avascular necrosis. The rate of healing and detailed histological appearances vary according

to the degree of stress also present and the relative proportion of fibrous repair tissue and woven bone that are formed.

13. In Paget's disease there are areas of excessive remodelling in the bone, and sometimes a consequent disturbance of blood flow. The excessive remodelling causes the affected bone to assume an irregular shape.

14. A dominant characteristic of Paget's disease is the exuberant proliferation of blood vessels and of cells from the vessel walls. This is only triggered off after a certain level of ordinary cell proliferation has been exceeded.

15. Paget's disease is racially specific, and occurs in the age group in which stress diseases are prevalent. There are indications that it might be a result of stress, mediated by effects in the thyroid gland.

16. Osteoarthritis is caused by an imbalance of the forces acting across joints. The sites which cause most problems are the hip, because it is an important main weight-bearing joint, and the forefeet, because of the prevalence of ill-fitting shoes and the high proportion of the population affected.

17. The initial lesion is an excessive breakdown of the gel structure in articular cartilage. Subsequently, even minor trauma can cause a complete breakdown of structure and cell death.

18. Cartilage breakdown products often include chemicals which stimulate cell proliferation and activity. This enables local repair to take place within the cartilage where it is needed.

19. Where a more complete mechanical breakdown occurs, so that minor vessels in the underlying bone are damaged there is a proliferation of granulation tissue. When repair tissue proliferates over cartilage suitable mechanical forces exerted across the joint allow it to be converted to cartilage, so that if these forces revert to normal repair and restoration of the function of the joint is rendered possible.

20. Forces are also exerted by tendons and ligaments surrounding a joint. When there is an imbalance of forces across the joint these may exert too great a tension, and the subsequent remodelling of cartilage and bone leads to osteophyte formation.

21. In weight-bearing joints bone changes are often those associated with repeated minor fracture and repair processes.

22. In lumbar disc lesions degeneration of previously weakened patches of the intervertebral disc material, following after excess pressure, stimulates cell proliferation. The increase of intra-disc pressure causes rupture through the annulas. There is evidence that disc lesions are more likely to develop if inadequate quantities of beta-protein are formed during adolescence, while uneven pressure distribution as a result of unsuitable height of shoe heels is also a factor.

23. Acute thoracic disc lesions are rare, while limited movement as a result of being held in place by the rib cage leads to a different type of pathology. Cartilage in the disc degenerates, and then calcifies to form a material with the consistency of toothpaste. Very rarely this is extruded into the canal to result in spinal cord compression. Sometimes vessels penetrate into the calcified material and it is then gradually replaced by bone.

24. When osteoporosis leads to damage of vertebral bodies, there is also trauma to the disc material. When this repairs, often with the production of elastic tissue as well as beta-protein, the result contributes to a resilient "ballooned" disc.

25. Pathological calcification followed by ossification is found when the surrounding mechanical forces are such that cartilage cells enlarge to form the calcifiable matrix. Sometimes these cartilage cells have been formed metaplastically from fibrous tissue.

26. Other pathological calcifications are found on dead cartilage or partly necrotic tissue. Occasionally vascular penetration of these calcifications is followed in due course by ossification.

27. When patches of necrotic tissue are formed, the prevailing level of catabolic and anabolic steroids is a factor in deciding whether the result is calcification or fibrous tissue replacement.

28. Calcification of the media of arteries is a usual accompaniment of the various stress diseases.

9. CELL PROLIFERATION

Although a separate chapter is being devoted to this topic, no attempt
will be made to provide a comprehensive survey of the subject. Instead,
a few aspects that are relevant to the main theme of the book will be
discussed, and in particular the effects of various stimuli on cell division
in bone.

An important practical application of a knowledge of the mechanisms
involved is the choice of suitable conditions for the preparation of tissues
for grafts. Here an understanding of the inflammatory and rejection
mechanisms is useful, and also a knowledge of the effects of radiation,
since the more widespread use of tissue banks may well lead to an
increasing use of radiation techniques for the preparation of these
tissues.

A condition which is characterized by an abnormality in the mechanism of cell division is osteosarcoma, and any understanding of this
requires not only a strict application of the rules for proceeding with a
scientific investigation, but also a knowledge of the various cell processes
that are possible and the stimuli required for each.

Cell Division

The pre-mitotic phase

Accounts of cell division frequently start with the stage at which
chromatin is organized and ready to form chromosomes, but the stage
which is in many ways the most important is the predivision phase. It
has also been given names such as the antephase (Bullough, 1952) or
the synthesis phase. In connective tissues its duration is about 8 h,
although the precise time depends upon the prevailing anabolic or
catabolic climate.

At the beginning of the predivision process direct connections between
the nucleus and the extra-cellular regions become apparent. A conducting pore mechanism was first suggested on theoretical grounds by
Danielli (1954). Dawson, Hocsack and Wyburn (1955) were the first
to show that the number of "pores" in the cell nucleus varied according
to the stage in the cell's life cycle. The formation of channels between

the nucleus and the extra-cellular regions is the first event to be recorded and there is evidence of an increase of phospholipid in the cytoplasm early in antephase (Clayton, 1959). Channels in a cell in anlage cartilage are shown in Fig. 9.1. This is a section with the embedding medium

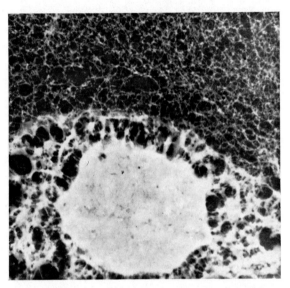

FIG. 9.1. Anlage cartilage cell in the predivision phase, or antephase. The nucleus is near the cell wall, and there are channels joining it to the exterior of the cell. ×5000.

removed, and of sufficient thickness to include the whole of some of the tubes. Figure 9.2 shows a cell in its predivision stage in a section of articular cartilage from a scorbutic guinea-pig. An absence of vitamin C does not affect the membranes of the cell surface and nucleus, nor the membranes of which these channels are composed, but it does hinder the production of endoplasmic reticulum and other cytoplasmic components. In this instance the tissue was not fixed immediately, so that all the cytoplasmic components have been lost except for the connections between the nucleus and the outer cell membrane (Rigal and Little, 1962).

Studies using tritiated thymidine in culture media have shown that the extra chromatin precursors necessary for the production of chromosomes and the two daughter nuclei are taken in within 10 min of the connections being established, and probably within the first 2 min. In the early stages the nuclei show a uniform density (Fig. 9.1), while later an increasing degree of organization is seen (Fig. 9.3). In this figure the contrast in density of nuclei in the resting phase and in the predivision stage is demonstrated. As with other electron microscope illustrations in this book, the tissue was unstained.

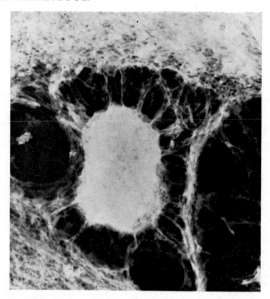

Fig. 9.2. A cell in the predivision stage in the articular cartilage of a young scorbutic guinea-pig. During processing cytoplasmic contents have been lost, so that the nuclear and cell membranes and the channels joining them can be clearly distinguished. ×5000.

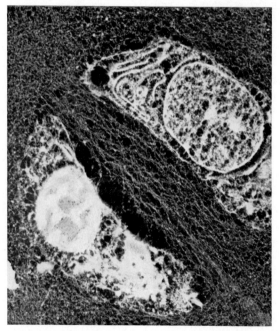

Fig. 9.3. Rabbit anlage cartilage. The cell, upper right, is in a resting phase, and the other, lower left, is in the predivision phase. Extra chromatin makes the nucleus denser. ×3500.

Rigal (1961a) took fresh tissue slices, placed them in a culture medium containing tritiated thymidine, and then removed them at intervals for examination. He found that for cartilage cells the level of activity in each nucleus rose rapidly, and then remained at the same level during the 8 h preceding division. When the tissue slices were treated with acid before histological preparations were made, the curve depicting the level of activity in each nucleus was of the exponential type familiar to students of reaction kinetics (Fig. 9.4). The acid had removed un-

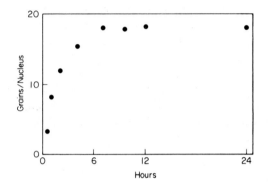

FIG. 9.4. Tritiated thymidine is rapidly taken up into nuclei at the beginning of the predivision phase, and then polymerized more slowly. Before polymerization it can be removed from tissue slices by acid treatment. This curve shows the results obtained from a slice of cartilage. The number of grains per nucleus gives a measure of the amount of polymerized thymidine retained, and this is plotted against time. It is found that all the thymidine is polymerized in 8 h. The author thanks Dr. W. M. Rigal for this graph.

polymerized thymidine, and it became apparent that mitosis must take place very soon after polymerization is complete.

In a review of the energy requirements for mitosis Bullough (1952) has pointed out that it is during the predivision stage that energy is used. Once prophase is reached cell division carries on to completion without additional energy requirements. Presumably energy is required primarily to reorganize cell membranes and to polymerize the extra chromatin. To provide this energy carbohydrates are oxidized, so that there is a rise in oxygen consumption during the predivision phase. The number of cells entering division at any one time has been found to be related to both the oxygen tension and the concentration of available carbohydrate. Adult tissues require more oxygen than their embryonic counterparts, presumably because the saccharides and polysaccharides in the embryo are less polymerized.

Carrel and Baker (1926) when investigating the essential nutritional requirements for cell division found that the higher cleavage products of the protein molecule were necessary. With the optimum digestion of fibrin, the growth of tissues in culture exceeded that produced by embryo juice. They found that a suitable level of degradation could be achieved by pepsin, but that trypsin broke the proteins down into fragments that were too small for utilization. They further found (Baker and Carrel, 1928) that the essential nutritional requirements were the higher cleavage products of proteins, nucleic acid and glycocoll.

Since the first stage of cell division is the formation of channels between the exterior of the cell and the nucleus, through which essential precursors of the daughter cell constituents can pass, it follows that in any study of the regulating mechanisms of cell division the conditions under which these cell membrane changes take place are the most important factor. So far as the initiation of cell division is concerned, chromosome formation and properties are of secondary importance—and are therefore outside the scope of this book. It may be noted that some so-called mitotic inhibitors and poisons act by cutting the membrane connections between the nucleus and cytoplasm or exterior environment of the cell (see Fig. 3.8).

Cell membranes

Cells contain two main groups of membranes, which may be described as the rough and the smooth. Rough membranes, commonly known as the endoplasmic reticulum, are covered by an array of ribonucleic acid: protein particles, the ribosomes. One of their functions is as a part of the protein synthesizing mechanism. Cell surfaces, nuclear membranes, and the membranes formed during the predivision phase that are primarily concerned with ion transport are in the group of smooth membranes. Clayton (1959) has shown that when various lipid stains are applied to histological sections the pre-treatment required to unmask the lipid in rough and smooth membranes differs. Another difference between the two types of membrane is that their synthesis is hindered by different chemicals. Thus, an absence of vitamin C does not affect the production of the smooth membranes, but hinders the production of endoplasmic reticulum. Conversely, colchicine destroys those smooth membranes which serve as channels between the nucleus and its surroundings. On a less drastic scale there are differences in the effect of steroids on the membranes, such as those described in Chapter 6. The anabolic and anti-anabolic properties are concerned with their effects on endoplasmic reticulum, while anti-catabolic and catabolic actions affect the properties of smooth membranes. When placed in order of potency the steroids which have been examined have shown generally parallel behaviour, but there are differences. For example,

Ba 36644 is the most anabolic steroid yet examined, while stanozolol is the most anti-catabolic. It is the smooth membranes with which we are concerned in the consideration of cell division and cell proliferation.

That cells are able to divide suggests that at least during certain phases of their existence the smooth membranes are labile, and there are various lines of observational evidence which support this hypothesis. In 1955 Dawson *et al.* realized that the variations in the number of pores in the nuclear membrane meant that it must be labile, although it normally appears intact except for the actual period of cell division. Particularly in cells of the connective tissue series, the behaviour of the membranes may be influenced by the physical state of the cytoplasm. Usually the contents of a cell are present in the form of a gel, but there are occasions, such as during cell division or when the cell assumes phagocytic activity, when those contents become fluid. During the phagocytic process some cell types are able to coalesce, to form multinucleated cells. Again, fibroblasts moving over a solid substrate leave behind a mucous trail, which may include quite large fragments of cytoplasm (Little and Edwards, 1962). This implies immediate repair and joining up of cell surfaces. Not all cell types show the same degree of mobility of their surfaces. An extreme example is the mature erythrocyte—a cell which does not divide. Any rupture of its surface membrane causes irreversible damage and haemolysis. Experimentally, erthrocyte membranes are easy to handle, but care needs to be taken in extrapolating observations on their properties to other cell types.

Cell membranes are approximately half lipid and half protein, and it is generally believed that they are phospholipids sandwiched between protein, though many properties can be explained if they are packed miscelles of lipids and proteins (Cameron, 1952). In the case of the gram negative bacteria the cell envelopes contain complex lipo-polysaccharides which are responsible for their antigen specificity (Weiser and Rothfield, 1968), but there does not seem to be equally specific evidence concerning the cell membrane components responsible for tissue rejection reactions. The main structural components, however, are phospholipid and protein. The lipid composition and content varies with the organism and the membrane. The proteins have plenty of hydrophobic amino acids (alanine, leucine, phenylalanine, methionine and valine); they contain no sulfhydroxyl (cystein) or disulphide groups, thus ensuring flexibility; and their high glutamic and aspartic content prevents extensive ionic binding between phospholipids and the membrane proteins (Benson, 1968). The available active groups are responsible for the ion transport which is one of the primary functions of the membranes. The lipid component would seem to be responsible for diffusion processes. That hormone action requires an intact cell provides evidence that their target is a part of the cell structure and not a part of the cell contents (Berliner, 1965).

Chapman (1968) has provided evidence about the physical state of phospholipid membranes. He has found that some molecular motion occurs even in the solid, but when membranes are warmed there is a phase transition to a "melt" with a high degree of molecular motion. This phase transition involves hydrocarbon chains of the phospholipid. Shorter chain lengths, unsaturated bonds and higher water content lead to a lower transition temperature. At room temperature many possible membrane systems are solid, but at body temperature phospholipids which contain highly unsaturated chains are usually mobile and fluid. This means that some material with an inhibitory action, such as a steroid or protein, is needed to suppress the mobility. Cholesterol has been found to affect the mobility of experimentally produced phospholipid membranes. It would seem from considerations such as these that the stability of the erythrocyte membrane is due to a coherent protein layer, while the more mobile connective tissue cells probably do not have a continuous protein layer. This is a speculation that might be worth investigating.

Regulating mechanisms

The requirements for controlling membrane properties of different cell types vary, and so do the chemicals which regulate their activity (Willmer, 1970). Some regulating mechanisms are the same for all cell types, while others vary from one cell type to another. In this section the mechanisms which regulate cell division of connective tissue and bone cells will be considered.

Supply of raw materials. If a cell is to divide and form two new cells it must have the essential raw materials to form the new cells. In a series of experiments with fibroblasts in different culture media Carrel and Baker (1926; Baker and Carrel, 1928) showed that the minimum requirements for cell proliferation were glycocoll (glycine, $NH_2.CH_2.COOH$, the simplest of the amino acids), nucleic acid and protein cleavage fragments. Enzymic degradation of intercellular matrices by phagocytic cells produces such cleavage compounds.

Supply of energy producing materials. Bullough (1952) has reviewed the energy requirements for cell division, which are that active mitosis can develop only when a carbohydrate substrate is efficiently oxidized. The number of cells entering division at any given time is related both to the oxygen tension and to the glucose concentration.

Other factors are involved. Thus, in epidermis, *in vivo,* mitoses were found to occur only during rest when glucose is deposited from the blood, a fact which accounts for the form of the diurnal mitotic cycle. (Tissues such as the epidermis which show clear mitotic cycles have a naturally low glucose intake, while tissues such as lymph node centres which show mitotic activity at all times have a high glucose intake.) But blood sugar is high during exercise and low during rest, which is the opposite of the mitotic cycle. Since lowering the blood sugar lowers the mitotic rate other factors need to be considered. One possibility is that other cell activities intervene, and another is that some regulating factors also vary. Thus, there is a diurnal rhythm for cortisol levels and for haemopoiesis. There is also a diurnal rhythm in the production of intercellular matrices, which Okado (1943) has shown leads to the production of lamellae in bone and striae in teeth. Of the variables he investigated, he found a direct correlation with the carbon dioxide combining power of the blood plasma. Factors such as adding insulin, heavy exercise or extreme cold also reduce mitosis. This last is probably because the temperature falls below the transition point of the phospholipids of the cell membranes and solidifies them.

The need for an adequate source of energy and supply of raw materials is straightforward, and areas of tissue formation and turnover in cartilage, bone and marrow correspond closely with their availability. A fairly general statement is that cell proliferation occurs wherever either chemical or mechanical factors or cell activity have resulted in the breakdown of existing proteins and intercellular matrices, or the production of inadequately polymerized material. Incomplete polymerization is one reason for the prolific cell division in foetuses and young children. In tissue culture media these products encourage active cell division when used under conditions in which any growth hormone present would have been inactivated.

During growth there is a steady breakdown of cartilage matrix at the bottom of the epiphyseal growth cartilage, and in this region there is the most active bone formation and turnover. In remodelling of the cortex there is first osteoclast activity with the breakdown of matrix and then proliferation of new cells and osteoblast activity. Cell proliferation occurs in mature cartilage after a breakdown of the gel structure, followed by an interval in which one may presume there is also chemical degradation, resulting in either the penetration of vessels from the epiphysis or a proliferation of existing cells to form cell nests. The distribution of haemopoietic tissue in the marrow is also related to the availability of protein and polysaccharide fragments, and proliferating red marrow is found near areas of active bone resorption. Where the bone is stable and static, as in the midshaft in an adult long bone, fatty marrow is normally found.

Some observations by Jellinek (1909) have helped to confirm that without a breakdown of dead tissue vascular proliferation, cell proliferation and inflammation do not occur. Among his patients he found quite different clinical reactions to burns caused by heat, and to electrical injuries. In the former case the heat accelerated breakdown of tissue components with consequent cellular activity. In the latter case the mechanism of the process was such that cell death occurred without any significant breakdown of the tissue components. These electrical injuries (including lightning burns) are caused by high frequency oscillating currents which have the property of liberating energy in materials with a high dielectric constant. Consequently, when the water contained in the tissues (which has a high dielectric constant) is heated and evaporated the release of energy ceases and the temperature promptly drops, so that the solid components of the tissues (with a low dielectric constant) are not degraded. Degradation of tissue components is a comparatively slow reaction which has not time to start during the short period the electric current is flowing. So in patients with electrical injuries only, there was little or no cell activity and inflammation around the injury. Instead, the drying process helps to preserve tissue components from subsequent molecular cleavage.

Partial pressure of oxygen. Oxygen is the other essential factor required to provide energy for both cell division and the specialized activities of cells. Since proteins and polysaccharides in embryos are less highly polymerized, adult tissues require more oxygen than their embryonic counterparts. Although cartilage is often described as an anaerobic tissue, a high proportion of dividing cells are near vessels. It does require some oxygen, but a lower tension is required than for most other tissues. When the vessels supplying the epiphyseal side of the epiphyseal growth cartilage are blocked, cell proliferation in that cartilage ceases. In bone too, the location of osteoblast activity is partly dictated by the available blood supply. Where there is a good flow of blood osteoblasts are active, but where the flow is diminished osteoblasts are unable to make good the loss of bone tissue caused by osteoclast activity.

When Bond *et al.* (1967) introduced a high local concentration of oxygen into monkey's jaws, by perfusing hydrogen peroxide and then irradiating, the added oxygen, although transient, caused profuse osteoblastic activity, with new bone filling both pulp cavities in teeth and the marrow spaces in the jaw bone. Similarly, the introduction of oxygen locally during the treatment of both sarcoma and carcinoma has resulted in a considerably accelerated rate of healing. By contrast, tissue culture experiments and clinical observations have both suggested that the effect of oxygen on damaged or unhealthy cells is to accelerate their death and removal by macrophages.

Partial pressure of carbon dioxide. Okado's observations (1943) showed that there is a direct relation between the partial pressure of carbon dioxide and the activity of connective tissue cells. Facts which have since emerged have shown that the concentration of carbon dioxide within a cell need not parallel the acid/base measurement of the blood, but that there is a parallel between the acidity of the blood and adrenal cortex activity. It is a corticosteroid which produces the physiological action that could easily have been ascribed to carbon dioxide. *Thus, there was a direct correlation, but not a causative relationship. Correlations of this type should never be taken to imply a causative relationship,* unless there is *adequate* evidence for the biological mechanisms concerned.

The available information about the effects of carbon dioxide on cells has been collected together by A. Joseph (1965, pers. comm.). Many of the fundamental facts were known by 1927 (Mottram, 1927). The mechanism of action of carbon dioxide involves a sol/gel equilibrium in the cytoplasm, which is necessary for the membranes in the cell to reorganize themselves. It affects the viscosity of cell contents. Carbon dioxide is more soluble in body fat than in water or serum, and it is likely that it diffuses as a gas across the lipid of the cell membranes. In so doing it increases their permeability, so that oxidation is increased and the metabolic rate raised; but, since it is a metabolic end product its rate of removal will control the velocity of cellular oxidation. There is therefore an optimum partial pressure of carbon dioxide for cell division, and above or below this cell activity is depressed. A local excess of carbon dioxide causes capillaries to dilate.

Peptide hormones. One of the factors which regulate cell division, particularly during growth, is the peptide hormone known as growth hormone. In cartilage Rigal (1964) has demonstrated that it initiates the predivision stage in stem cells, and there is reason to think that it activates stem cells in other tissues.

In the experiment of Baker and Carrel (1928) which was mentioned earlier, normal fibroblasts grown in their artificial medium ceased proliferating and died after 8 to 10 days, even though the medium was changed every two days. Similarly, when Rigal (1961*b*) attempted to grow slices of epiphyseal and metaphyseal bone in a culture medium consisting of a mixture of a synthetic medium and plasma the marrow cells died after a few days. But when growth hormone was added to the medium the marrow remained in a healthy condition until the end of the experiment. Many questions still remain to be answered about the direct effect of growth hormone on cells.

BB

Insulin. In addition to its more general effects, in which there is a close relationship between insulin, plasma glucose levels and growth hormone (see Chapter 7), insulin has a direct effect on cells. It stimulates cell growth in tissue culture (Latta and Bucholz, 1939; Leslie and Davidson, 1951), and its presence is necessary before many hormones can act on cell surfaces (Prop, 1961). Woods, Hunter and Burk (1955) have collected evidence which strongly suggests that its site of action is the cell membrane, and that it acts by causing some change in the membrane which allows a more rapid entrance of glucose into the cell. That is, it relieves some inhibiting mechanism. When the intact body is considered, insulin lowers the concentration of glucose in the blood. In any attempt to speculate on these effects it must be remembered that Gey and Thalhimer (1924) showed that when identical cultures were prepared, except that some contained insulin while the remainder acted as controls, insulin increased the utilization of sugar in a manner which did not depend upon the concentration of glucose in the culture medium.

Steroids. The influence of the steroids was discussed in some detail in Chapter 6. Those with high anti-catabolic activity increase the flexibility of the cell surfaces and membranes in connective tissues, even to the extent of increasing the actual speed of mitoses. All the activities of the cell are intensified. Conversely, with steroids of high catabolic activity flexibility and motion of the cell surfaces decreases, until activity is almost at a stand-still. Even when there is an adequate amount of carbohydrate cell division remains at a very low level.

Dougherty, Berliner and Berliner have studied biotransformations at the surfaces of cells of several types—lymphocytes, fibroblasts, reticulo-endothelial cells and hepatocytes—and found that the behaviour of the cells can be modified by the changes that they themselves induce (Dougherty *et al.*, 1961; Berliner and Dougherty, 1961; Berliner, 1965). The term "biotransformation" is used to designate molecular changes produced by non-endocrine cells, these changes being characterized by a series of oxidations and reductions in the steroid molecules. *In vitro* the action on the cell is a fast one, occurring within a minute or two of adding either cortisol or cortisone (Frank and Dougherty, 1953). Since cortisol is the active compound (Dougherty, Berliner and Berliner, 1960) the biotransformation must also have occurred exceedingly rapidly. As well as inhibiting cell division the action of cortisol on fibroblasts leads to a retraction of the cell processes and a rounding of the cells (Dougherty and Schneebeli, 1955; Ruhmann and Berliner, 1965). This is one anti-inflammatory effect, and all the anti-inflammatory effects of the corticosteroids can be similarly explained by this stabilizing of membranes.

Protein and amino acid levels. Since steroid transformations take place at cell surfaces, properties of both steroids and cells are, to a certain extent, modified by local factors. Thus, serum proteins have been shown to compete with cells for the available steroids, while cells metabolize the steroids in different ways according to the medium in which they are acting (Berliner, 1965). The type of activity, whether cell division or matrix formation, is influenced by protein and amino acid levels in the surrounding tissue fluids.

In a similar manner, chondroitin-B when taken up by fibroblasts inhibits the transformation of cortisone to cortisol, but not cortisol to cortisone. (Chondroitin sulphate itself requires the presence of thyroid hormone for its formation.)

Cell Differentiation

The reactions of cells to different media helps to explain how cell differentiation comes about. The processes which take place in wound healing are among the most important examples. Some of the basic principles have been worked out, but many details, and particularly the precise nature of the stimulating agents, still await elucidation.

One of the earliest accounts of the mechanism of wound healing was by Meyer (1852) who described the processes of sprouting of new vascular buds from damaged pre-existing vessels, followed by capillary formation and differentiation of vessels into arteries and veins, followed by the regression of many vessels as the tissues were stabilized. In the 1930s more detailed observations became possible with the use of the rabbits ear chamber (Clark and Clark, 1935), and the fragility of the newly formed vessels was observed. More recently Schoefl (1963) has carried detailed observations a stage further, and reviewed previous work on the subject.

The picture which emerges is that in the clot macrophages soon congregate, accompanied by leucocytes, mast cells and eosinophils. In the zone of tissue breakdown there are more leucocytes and macrophages. All these show considerable membrane movement and the cells themselves are mobile. Fibroblast-like cells in the zone of tissue breakdown are also very active, moving around and dividing at intervals. Cells proliferating from vessels in or near this zone lead out from the vascular endothelium, form vascular loops and clusters, and when the growing sprouts meet they fuse, giving rise to loops and networks. As the scar tissue matures a few vessels remain and take on the characteristics of arteries or veins, while most of the capillaries regress.

Carrel (1924) carried out tissue culture experiments designed to sort out some of these observations. Initially he established that in attempts to grow fibroblasts in plasma they did not feed on any serum constituents, but only on the remains of tissue (if any). Next he considered the macrophages, and found that when they were cultivated in embryonic tissue juices they displayed great activity at first, but died after a short time. When the medium was diluted with serum they remained alive and spread. That meant they could build-up their protoplasm from constituents of serum. Neither fibroblasts nor epithelial cells shared this property. Lymphocytes cultured in plasma increased in size and became transformed into macrophages.

Another observation was that aqueous extracts of inflamed connective tissue, which contains lymphocytes, had the power to increase the rate of fibroblast proliferation. Since lymphocytes are capable of proliferating in serum it would seem that they can produce cleavage products of serum proteins of a suitable size for assimilation. In an experiment to simulate wound healing colonies of lymphocytes and fibroblasts were embedded in plasma and cultured in serum. After a few days the fibroblasts seemed moribund, but as they were reached by the actively proliferating macrophages, they became rejuvenated. This experiment demonstrated that lymphocytes could transport to fixed cells the substances required for their proliferation.

Some tissue culture experiments on bone (W. M. Rigal, 1963, pers. comm.) have provided more relevant observations. In serum, cell activity was suppressed and marrow cells rapidly died, but granulation tissue cells were able to proliferate. They came from the cells of sinusoid vessel walls, at the upper end of the metaphysis and in the epiphysis, which normally proliferate to osteogenic precursor cells. Labelling with tritiated thymidine showed that both for normal bone proliferation and for the proliferation of granulation tissue all the vascular endothelial cells of the vascular loops in the metaphysis were involved. When the serum was diluted by a third, by the addition of Hank's solution or a synthetic culture medium, marrow cells survived for a time but did not proliferate. Growth cartilage and bone cells survived and could form new matrix, and in some instances quite large quantities of the calcifiable matrix were produced (Fig. 1.33). They were able also to enter the predivision stage, but not more than one mitosis was completed.

In vivo, wherever conditions are such that plasma diffuses through the marrow, the proliferation of red cells ceases and the cells in the red marrow die. Figure 9.5 shows the edge of the affected region near a fractured trabecula in the head of the femur. Figure 9.6 shows another damaged trabecula, surrounded by new bone, but with haemopoietic activity in the vicinity still suppressed.

One facet of the problem investigated by A. Carrel, and later by

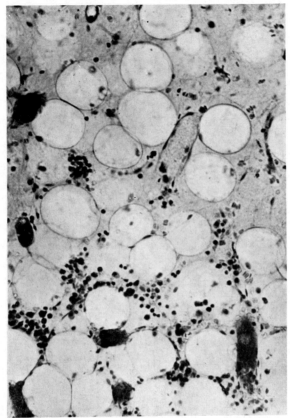

FIG. 9.5. When plasma diffuses from a damaged vessel in bone haemopoietic activity is suppressed. This figure shows the edge of an affected region near a fractured trabecula in the head of femur. The plasma has spread between cells, so that fat cells are separated. The layer of fat cells (top of figure) is unaffected. × 200.

W. M. Rigal, was the stimulation of granulation tissue and fibroblasts. Another very interesting facet is the elucidation of the factors which stimulate vascular proliferation. Many facts are known, but there is no clear hypothesis as yet which covers a sufficient number of observations to point to any specific stimulant for the differentiation of vascular endothelium and vessels. The endothelium gives rise to buds, in wound healing, at the time when macrophages have provided sufficient protein in a form in which it can be utilized. Dead tissue and dead cells are also in the vicinity. Vessels invade damaged cartilage, and here the possibilities are rather more restricted. When the gel in the matrix has broken down and cartilage cells have died, this is frequently followed by a vascular invasion. The vessels themselves, however, can provide serum.

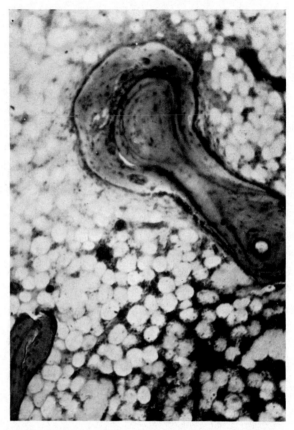

Fig. 9.6. Another damaged trabecula in the head of femur is surrounded by new bone, which has itself cracked and damaged a neighbouring vessel. Where the plasma has diffused all haemopoietic tissue has been destroyed. Marrow, bottom right of figure is unaffected. ×60.

Newly formed proliferating vessels have an increased fragility and increased permeability, as also do blood vessels in sarcomata, and both serum and proteins leave the vessels at their growing tips (Brånemark, 1964). The cells at the growing tip proliferate, are motile, and are very active. Their membranes also show great activity, and it has been postulated (Schoefl, 1963) that in the course of this activity and while wriggling about gaps appear at intervals between the cells. An impermeable basement membrane over the whole of the vessel wall does not seem to form until after sprouting vessels have fused. When the stimulus is less there is a tendency for vascular loops to elongate by proliferation. This situation is analogous to that in the metaphysis of a young rapidly growing animal, where vascular loops extend to the base of each column of cells, and in contact with the last cell of the column have been observed to be open ended so that blood is in contact with the dead cell and surrounding capsule wall (Fig. 3.13). In these budding and developing vessels there is no organized blood flow, and in places the blood may be stagnant. This gives rise to a situation where there is likely to be a low partial pressure of oxygen and a higher content of carbon dioxide than normal. Carbon dioxide dilates capillaries, and also renders lipid membranes more permeable.

The conditions for the differentiation of vessels, granulation tissue and later fibrous tissue are general ones. Other types of cell differentiation are quite specific. The osteogenic factor has already been discussed. In its presence ordinary cells that differentiate from sinusoid vessel walls become osteogenic precursor cells and many of them proceed to function as osteoblasts. Usually the granulation tissue that proliferates from damaged vessels forms a labile fibrous tissue that remodels to a small quantity of mature fibrous tissue. In the presence of the osteogenic factor it forms a labile woven bone that remodels to ordinary bone. When conditions are slightly different the cells that differentiate around sinusoid vessels are not connective tissue cells but haematopoietic tissue cells. Haemopoietic tissue is only formed in those tissues where sinusoid vessels are present. In addition to bone marrow it is often found in the spleen or liver. Bone is not formed in those two sites.

The other cell type that is formed in quantity in marrow is fat. Here more information is available. General observation shows that where matrix breakdown products are present there is either bone or haemopoietic tissue. In the quiescent parts of the marrow there are fat cells. Tissue culture experiments by von Haam and Cappel (1940) showed that under their experimental conditions the cultures treated with insulin showed an early appearance of fat droplets in the fibroblasts, with a later conversion of these cells to ones with the appearance of fat cells.

Tissue Grafts

Living tissues or organs used to replace missing or diseased tissue are known as *transplants*; dead tissues are known as *grafts*; while other materials are called *implants*. When tissues for grafting are taken from the same individual they are called *autografts*; when from immunologically identical individuals, e.g. a twin, they are called *isografts*; when from another individual of the same species they are called *homografts*; and from individuals of another species they are called *heterografts*. These terms are unambiguous, and are the terms most frequently used. In the last 10 years a variety of other terms have been introduced, none of which is completely unambiguous and none widely used, so that it would seem wisest to keep to accepted words whose meaning is clear.

The mechanisms of incorporation of autografts are basically the same as for fracture healing, and the primary need is for an adequate blood supply to be established as soon as possible. In the absence of an intact blood supply bone cells can only survive for a short time, so that in practice the living bone tissue taken for the graft usually dies, as does the bone tissue involved in Perthes disease or an infarct, and in due course is resorbed and replaced by host tissue. This importance of the blood supply has been recognized for many years, both for bone grafts and for fracture healing. Groves (1913–14) described how non-union and delayed union of fractures was due to interference with the circulation in the ends of bone fragments, and how with a decrease in the already meagre circulation of the periosteum callus formation was prevented. Fifty years later Lima (1963) replaced pieces of cortical bone in different positions, and demonstrated that re-incorporation was dependent on the availability of channels for vascular proliferation.

The sequence of events is similar to that observed in fracture healing. A blood clot is formed, new vessels sprout from the damaged vessels around the site, and granulation tissue proliferates. Macrophages arrive to remove the remains of the clot, dead cells, and dead tissue. Where the osteogenic factor is available woven bone is formed, and during subsequent remodelling is replaced by normal bone tissue. Without a blood supply there can be no granulation tissue, and too few macrophages for adequate cleaning-up operations, The grafted bone acts as a scaffold, but it needs to degrade gradually, to form the protein and polysaccharide cleavage products necessary as sources of food and energy for the proliferating cells. Marrow adhering to the bone also acts as a source of raw materials (Burwell, 1966).

Siffert and Barash (1961) have investigated some of the conditions which can lead to failure of a graft. If transplanted into a fresh haematoma it may be isolated for too long in a proteolytic medium and become necrotic, while if there is not a reasonably quick vascular penetration, with accompanying granulation tissue, a barrier of mature fibrous tissue forms between the graft and the vessels which should be advancing to incorporate it. It is also necessary for the osteogenic factor to survive and be in a position where it can function. It has a limited range around each bone chip (Fig. 9.7) and so its distribution needs to be adequate.

So far we have considered the use of grafts to fill osseous defects in bone, where their primary functions are to act as a scaffolding while repair tissue enters and fills the gap, and to act as a source of the essential raw materials. About three months are required for adequate consolidation. When both shaft and marrow need to be replaced the time required is considerably longer. Eyre-Brook, Bailey and Price

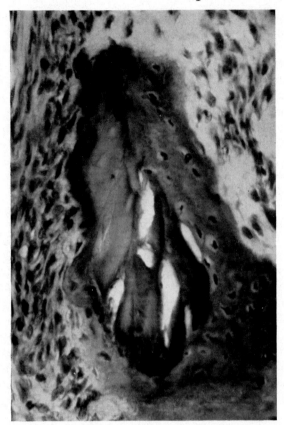

FIG. 9.7. Bone chip in proliferating granulation tissue. Cells in the vicinity of the chip have differentiated to osteoblasts and woven bone. ×200.

(1969), for example have described the repair of infantile pseudarthrosis. They used a delayed autogenous graft, separated and then left 8 weeks for callus to be formed on all surfaces. After placing the graft in position it then took five years before a medullary canal was properly formed and vascularization complete.

The use of autografts is limited, since the bone tissue has to be taken from other parts of the body, and in many instances it is better to use homografts or heterografts. All the factors already mentioned apply and have to be allowed for, but additionally fresh bone homografts or heterografts provoke an immune response. The first stage observed is an effect on the proliferating blood vessels. Whatever the type of graft there is an initial proliferation of vessels, which can last for 4 to 5 days. Subsequently the vascular supply continues to increase for autografts and isografts, but it decreases for homografts and heterografts (Sabet,

Hidvegi and Ray, 1961). For rats, Hammack and Enneking (1960) found the change occurred after 8 or 9 days. In the case of established organ transplants the initial stages of rejection are also vascular, with subsequent ischaemic changes (Woodruff, Nolan, Robson and MacDonald, 1969; Dempster 1969). There has been localized cellular destruction, and a hindrance to the flow of the blood. This is followed by increased permeability of vessels with oedema in their surroundings and round cell infiltration, and the typical appearances of an inflammatory reaction. Antibodies are taken into macrophages and lymphocytes. There is fibrous proliferation in the oedema fluid, so that the graft becomes isolated by a fibrous capsule and then degenerates. It is finally either completely resorbed or rejected.

In the preparation of homograft and heterograft bone for grafts it is therefore necessary to destroy or immobilize those tissue components responsible for provoking the rejection reaction. Freezing diminishes the response, and in some cases frozen bone can be used satisfactorily. Consistently better results, however, are obtained when freeze-dried bone grafts are used (Berkin et al., 1957; Burwell et al., 1963). although stable union takes rather longer than for autogenous grafts. Freeze-drying renders the polymeric matrix components more stable, the result being similar to that described for the drying action in electrical injuries (see p. 368). This has been demonstrated particularly clearly in the use of freeze-dried homologous aortic valves for grafting. Even after a lapse of years there has been no indication of penetration by host vessels into the graft. In bone, however, remodelling does take place, after the lapse of several months.

More recently sterilizing doses of radiation (2·5 megarad) have been used to prepare tissue for grafting. The method was introduced because sterilization of tissue stored in bone banks reduces the possibility of accidental contamination and infection (Marmor, 1960). This treatment with radiation has another effect. The radiation causes molecular changes in the intercellular matrices which under the conditions that have been used allows more rapid penetration by host vessels and cells (Little, 1970 c, d). In animal experiments Tarsoly et al. (1969) have demonstrated a rapid resorption and substitution by new bone, and they showed that for cortical bone this process is accelerated if small holes are drilled to facilitate the ingrowth of vessels. Radiation also destroys the chemicals responsible for the rejection reaction, so that with suitable conditions of preparation it is almost as satisfactory as autograft material (L. Marmor, 1967, pers. comm.; Malawski and Serafin, 1969). The effects of radiation on bone matrix are complex. The polymeric molecules are degraded, but the broken ends may reform to provide a more resistant material than the original, and the end result depends on the conditions of treatment and radiation. Campbell, Bassett and Luzio (1970) used irradiated skull grafts in which the remodelling process was sufficiently controlled for the bone to provide adequate protection for underlying structures throughout the time taken for incorporation.

Osteosarcoma

The purpose of this book is to describe the behaviour of cells in bone, and the various cell mechanisms which produce pathological states. This discussion on osteosarcoma is therefore limited to a consideration of the mechanism of production of osteosarcoma and the properties of cells in tumours, and is not concerned with the problems of diagnosis and treatment. For an account of tumour pathology "Tumors of Bone and Cartilage" by Ackerman and Spjut (1971) should be consulted. There is an enormous literature on the subject of carcinogenesis, and most of the relevant facts are known. The main problem is to see the wood for the trees. To do this it is necessary to approach the subject logically, assemble facts, consider hypotheses, and ruthlessly discard all hypotheses that fail to conform with the facts. In this way the problem can be brought down to manageable proportions, and the gaps in our knowledge which still remain can be more easily recognized.

The premalignant state

Early observations were collected and summarized by Virchow and his school. In 1863 he formulated his "non-specific chronic irritation" theory, which has recently been restated more precisely by Smithers (1960). In the intervening years an impressive amount of evidence had accumulated to support the theory that a common factor in all types of cancer is that the malignant change is preceded by a period when the tissue in question is stimulated to over-activity. In all the examples which have been adequately assessed so far, with all types of malignancy included, the observed sequence of events starts with a stimulation of cell proliferation in circumstances in which such stimulation persists. The continuation may be steady, or possibly intermittent, but in due course a number of the cells in the tissue change to the malignant form. Once this has happened, cell proliferation is independent of the initial stimulus, and the cells acquire the power to proliferate and grow in sites away from their origin.

This theory is one that can be tested experimentally, and a number of workers have overstimulated cells in culture and produced a malignant change in those cultures. Sandford, Likely and Earle (1954), for example, obtained normal and malignant strains from a single cell by varying the culture conditions.

Willis (1960) has given the definition

"A tumour is an abnormal mass of tissue, the growth of which exceeds and is unco-ordinated with that of the normal tissues, and persists in the same excessive manner after cessation of the stimuli which evoked the change".

He has assembled sufficient evidence to establish as a fact that tumours do not arise from a single minute focus, but from considerable fields of prepared tissue.

Overstimulation is a consistent finding, but the causes which lead to this overstimulation vary. Some stimulate prolific cell division immediately, while others initiate a series of changes which only culminate in excessive cell division after several years. Sometimes the malignant change is precipitated by injury to the precancerous tissue (Ewing, 1940). One perennial cause of confusion in the literature on cancer is the fact that many research workers have mistaken the various causative agents for the real initiating state, and have worked on the assumption that one particular causative agent, of the many that have been observed, must be the initiator of all types of cancer. There is a very great deal of evidence that the initial cause is a stimulation of cell proliferation in circumstances in which this increased cell proliferation continues, but there is no evidence to support any of the series of hypotheses which suggests that some particular cause of over-proliferation is the cause of all types of cancer. One of the latest of these untenable hypotheses is the suggestion that viruses cause cancer. They do—but only in a limited number of rare conditions. There are one or two human tumours, a few in mice and other laboratory animals, and a number of bird tumours that are caused by the reaction to virus infections, and that is all. Far more important is the reaction to carcinogenic chemicals, and there are a wide range of possible chemicals (Clayson, 1962) which vary from one tissue to another. Over reaction to repeated trauma is another important cause. Neoplasia due to asbestos is among the best-known examples.

Various predisposing causes for bone tumours have been described. Among these are:

(a) An aberration of the remodelling of bone. This is sometimes thought to be a consequence of some form of embryonic derangement, and there may be a genetic factor. The very rare chordoma arises from vestiges of the notocord (Fig. 9.8). Figures 9.9., 9.10 show typical appearances in this tumour.

It is possible for mechanically induced sarcoma to arise as a reaction to trauma, with a subsequent over-stimulation of the remodelling process. This type of sarcoma formation has been induced by Gardner

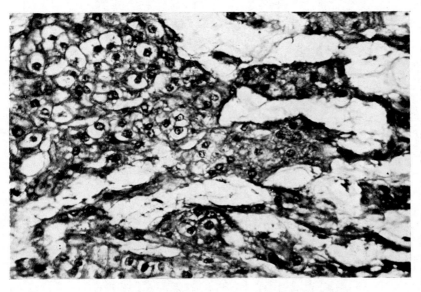

FIG. 9.9. Proliferating notocordal cells in a malignant chordoma. Cells are of variable size and appearance. × 200.

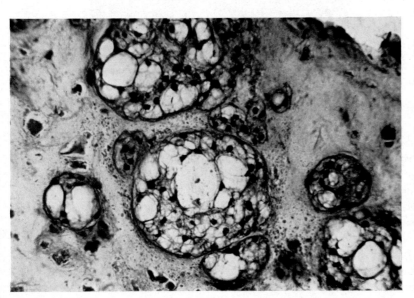

FIG. 9.8. Notocordal cells, still proliferating, in pockets of the nucleus pulposus in an adult intervertebral disc. × 200.

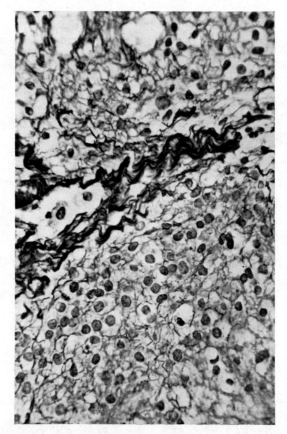

FIG. 9.10. Another typical field in a chordoma. Here the cells are of more uniform appearance. ×200. The author thanks Dr. C. H. G. Price for the material from which these three figures were taken.

and Heslington (1946) and others by injecting beryllia particles into the blood stream of rabbits, where they are trapped in the marrow sinusoids. Many beryllia particles have little or no effect but some, like that depicted in Fig. 9.11, have sharp edges and corners which can snag the walls of blood vessels. Repeated rupture and attempted healing results in the proliferation of vascular endothelial cells, with the possibility of formation of a reticulum or round cell sarcoma, or in this case an osteosarcoma (Fig. 9.12).

A straightforward overstimulation has sometimes resulted from the forced growth of broiler chickens. A variety of tumours, including osteosarcomas, have been observed (Campbell and Appleby, 1966). These metastasizing osteosarcomas were of rapid development, since they were present before the age of 10 weeks.

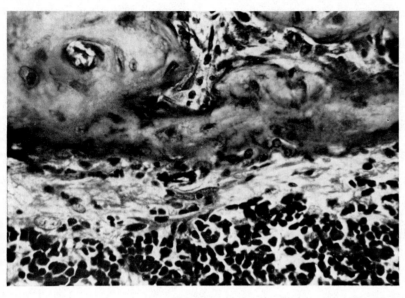

Fig. 9.12. Osteosarcoma, in marrow space of rabbit with beryllia particles trapped in vessels in the marrow. The marrow (left) is filled with actively proliferating cells, while the bone to the right contains typical sarcoma cells. ×200. The author thanks Prof. W. F. Enneking for the material from which these two figures were taken.

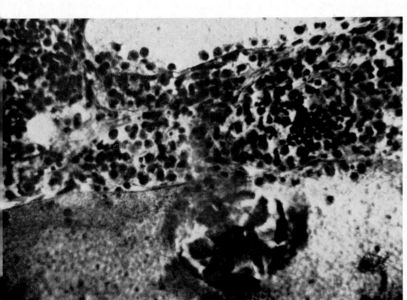

Fig. 9.11. Beryllia particle in sinusoid vessel in bone marrow in rabbit. This particle is of a grade which breaks up into fragments with sharp corners and edges. These can snag the vessel wall repeatedly, thus giving rise to the conditions necessary for a malignant change to take place. ×200.

(b) Any lesion in bone which leads to continued and vigorous cell proliferation may in due course lead to a sarcoma. There is a wide range in the relative incidence. Fibrous dysplasia, for example, reaches the malignant stage comparatively frequently, while it is only rarely that sarcomas arise in the walls of bone cysts. These latter have been described by Johnson, Vettner and Putschar (1962). A case of fibrosarcoma arising from a bone infarction in decompression sickness has also been reported (Dorfman, Norman and Wolff, 1966).

Paget's disease involves a considerable over-proliferation of cells, and a proportion of cases progress to either osteogenic or fibrogenic osteosarcoma. The majority of cases where there is a malignant development are men, with their higher anabolic level, and it has been observed that the usual sites where malignant lesions develop are in the bones most actively used. The right femur is involved more often than the left; while the humerus, although less often involved in Paget's disease, has a higher risk of malignancy (Price and Goldie, 1969).

Some congenital and hereditary bone dystrophies can lead to sarcoma formation. Commonest examples are the exostoses which give rise to chondrosarcoma. Dyschondroplasias and on occasion osteogenesis imperfecta, have also given rise to sarcoma.

Benign tumours in bone, such as the giant cell tumour and cartilage tumours may also in due course progress to their malignant counterparts. (c) Radiation of a benign lesion, or ingestion of bone-seeking isotopes, can result in the delayed formation of an osteosarcoma. The effects of radiation on bone will be discussed further in Chapter 10.

The behaviour of malignant cells

Having established that the necessary prerequisite for malignancy is an overstimulation of cell division, the next stage is to consider the behaviour of the malignant cells. Bone is a very good tissue to choose for this exercise, because of the variety of pathways along which precursor cells can differentiate, according to surrounding applied stimuli, and the wide variation in behaviour of individual cells. Osteogenic cells, for example, can function as osteoblasts, osteocytes and osteoclasts, and if they were formed in sites removed from a supply of the osteogenic factor they can proliferate as fibroblasts.

Bone and cartilage tumours assume an equally wide variety of forms, and various attempts have been made to classify them. Ackerman and Spjut's book (1971) is one such attempt. The problems are caused by the diversity of appearance and behaviour of these tumours, and the need for classification arises because of the differences in prognosis, and sometimes in treatment.

Willis (1960) on the basis of observation of tumours of many different types has shown that there is evidence that the degree of malignancy of tumours is roughly proportional to the degree to which they fail to attain histological differentiation: that is, the most anaplastic tumours are the most malignant. This hypothesis is fully supported by observations on bone and cartilage. The histological fields in different parts of an osteosarcoma tend to vary in appearance, but according to the dominant type of cell behaviour they may be described as chondroblastic, fibroblastic or osteoblastic osteosarcomas, and it is observed that the chondroblastic are more malignant than the fibroblastic which are more malignant than the osteoblastic osteosarcomas (Price, 1961). The chondroblastic osteosarcomas are composed of those cells which normally proliferate to fracture cartilage, and they produce very little intercellular matrix (Figs 9.13, 9.14). In this they differ from the osteo-

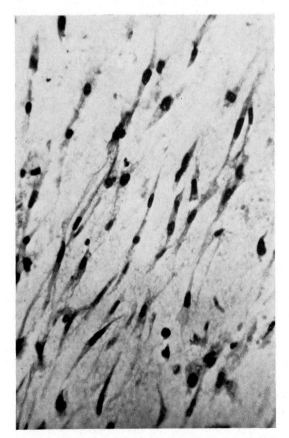

Fig. 9.13. Chondroblastic osteosarcoma. Longitudinal section through cartilage cells. ×200.

CC

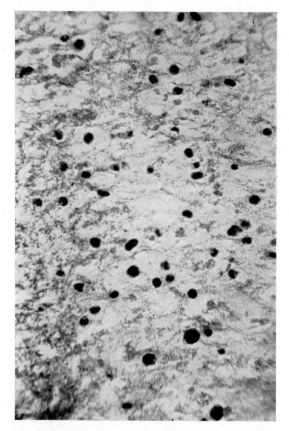

FIG. 9.14. Transverse section through cartilage cells. The nuclei are of variable sizes, and there is very little intercellular material. × 200.

blastic osteosarcomas (Figs 9.15, 9.16), and even more from those chondrosarcoma derived from hyaline cartilage (Fig. 9.17). Chondrosarcoma usually have a very low malignancy, metastasize late, and can kill by a local extension of the tumour (Barnes and Catto, 1966). There are similar variations with fibrosarcoma of bone, fibroblastic osteosarcoma and periosteal fibrosarcoma. Periosteal fibrosarcoma is slow to metastasize and has a similar prognosis to that of fibrosarcoma of soft tissues (Eyre-Brook and Price, 1969). Paget's sarcoma has the added initial stimulus associated with Paget's disease itself, and the survival time is less than for osteosarcoma which is less than for fibrosarcoma (Price and Goldie, 1969).

Another possible way of stating the hypothesis would be that cells that proliferate rapidly in the normal state, proliferate rapidly when malignant, while cells that proliferate slowly in the normal state also

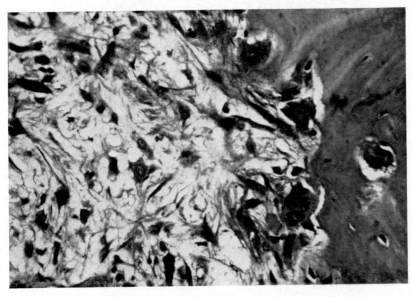

Fig. 9.16. Osteoblastic osteosarcoma. Cells in this field are functioning as osteoclasts. The cytoplasm of the cells has a higher fluid content than normal, so that on drying spaces are left in the cell cavities. ×200.

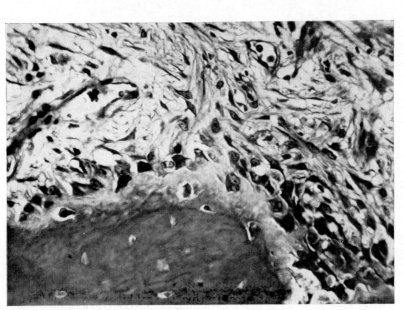

Fig. 9.15. Osteoblastic osteosarcoma. Cells are of variable size and shape. Those on the bone surface are functioning as osteoblasts, and in this field have an appearace which resembles that of woven bone formation. ×200.

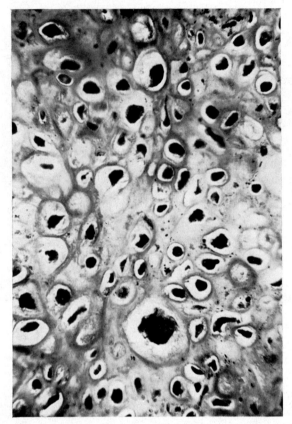

Fig. 9.17. Quiescent region in chondrosarcoma. After matrix formation cell proliferation ceases. The cytoplasm of these cells was abnormally fluid, so that spaces are left on drying. ×200.

continue to proliferate slowly when malignant. This strongly suggests that malignant cells are not completely removed from the influence of their regulating mechanisms. The treatment of conditions such as breast cancer depends upon this fact.

For bone, this concept has been placed on a wider and unifying basis by Johnson's field theory of bone tumours (1953). It was based on a large number of observations, and while more evidence has accumulated none has been found to invalidate the theory. He has shown that once a sarcoma is present in bone it behaves in the manner that might be expected from its location in the bone. Although sarcomas in children tend to be osteogenic and alike, in older individuals a tumour may show different characteristics in different areas, while different types of tumours originate in different sites. In this, the rabbit tumour shown in Fig. 9.12 showed the characteristic of a tumour in a child.

This same tendency to conform with normal tissue behaviour, within the limits imposed by indiscriminate cell proliferation, is seen on the microscopic level. On the whole the malignant cells do the same as their non-malignant counterparts. Thus the intercellular matrices found are those usual for the cell types concerned. Price (1961) has observed that, as in normal tissues, the tumours of older people show relatively less matrix formation than those typically seen in juveniles. This same type of functional conformity with normal tissues is seen in other types of secretory activity. For example, tumours of the adrenal medulla often continue to produce adrenalin. Schajowicz (1961) has investigated the giant cell tumours, or osteoclastomas, in some detail. He demonstrated that their origins are the undifferentiated stromal cells of the marrow or "reticulo-histiocyte elements". These are the cells which are the precursors of one type of osteoclast. As in the case of other tumours he has found them to be rich in newly formed blood vessels, and has commented that because of the comparatively normal appearance of individual cells the degree of malignancy is difficult to be sure of, so that attempts at grading are not always reliable. His detailed histochemical studies showed that the multinucleated cells of these tumours give identical results as those obtained from normal osteoclasts and chondroclasts.

Many highly malignant cells have an almost normal appearance. The experimental tumour shown in Figs 9.11, 9.12 was one example of this. Figures 9.18, 9.19 show the tissue reaction to a somewhat toxic implant and a typical area of a fibrosarcoma. The main difference is in the greater vascularity of the sarcoma. In other aspects the behaviour of the cells, apart from their greater proliferative capacity, is almost normal, and they produce cancellous bone, woven bone (Fig. 9.15) or function as osteoclasts (Fig. 9.16) according to the local circumstances.

Many patients with a sarcoma are under stress, and so there may be local deposition of platelet thrombi or fibrin. When these deposits are within a sarcoma, invasion of the deposit is by malignant cells instead of the usual fibroblasts which invade and organize them. Two examples are shown in Figs 9.20, 9.21. That in Fig. 9.20 is indisputably an invasion of a deposit, but it is still debatable whether accumulations of cells blocking the vessels are always derived from the invasion of such deposits, or whether sometimes they are proliferating cells from malignant linings of vessels. The aetiology of the deposit shown in Fig. 9.21 could, therefore, be in doubt. These deposits can break away as emboli, and in Fig. 9.22 one has been trapped in a vessel in the lung. Cell proliferation has continued and neighbouring lung tissue invaded, with bone formation. In fact, Fig. 9.22 is a photograph of an early metastasis.

In Figs 9.20, 9.21, 9.22, and also Figs 9.15, 9.16, 9.17 the cells,

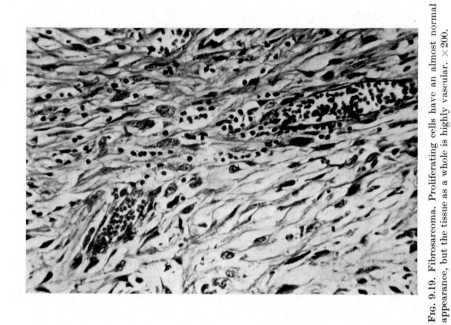

Fig. 9.19. Fibrosarcoma. Proliferating cells have an almost normal appearance, but the tissue as a whole is highly vascular. ×200.

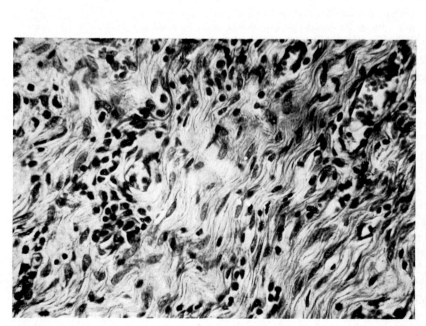

Fig. 9.18. Tissue reaction to a mildly toxic implant. Vascular proliferation was accompanied by an infusion into the tissue, in which fibrous tissue has proliferated. × 200.

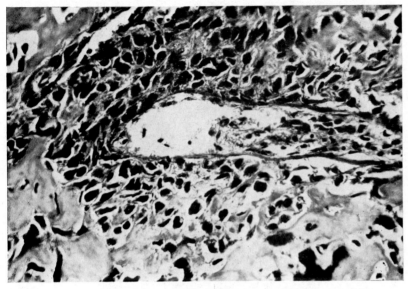

Fig. 9.21. Malignant cells in lumen of vessel. It is not possible to tell from their appearance whether they were also derived from an invasion of a deposit from the blood, or whether they have proliferated from malignant vascular endothelium. ×200.

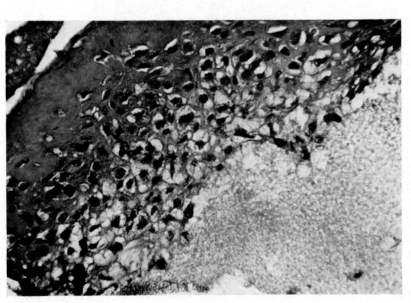

Fig. 9.20. Fibrin deposit in blood vessel, being invaded by neighbouring malignant granulation tissue. ×400.

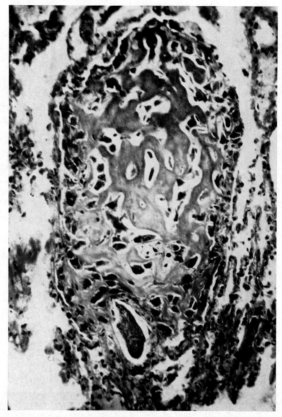

Fig. 9.22. A malignant embolus is trapped in a vessel in the lung (near bottom of figure). Cell proliferation has continued, and neighbouring lung tissue invaded, with bone formation. Spaces left on drying indicate that the cytoplasm of osteocytes was abnormally fluid. ×100.

although behaving comparatively normally, have an unusual appearance, being large, more irregularly shaped and with a more fluid cytoplasm than normal. It is the investigation of differences such as these, together with the extra vascularity and the uninhibited cell division which can give an indication of the nature of the malignant change. In a discussion of bone pathology as a whole Johnson (1964) has stated that:

"Disease processes never involve any strange or new reactions, but only altered relationships in normal reactions. The alteration may, however, separate out and focus attention upon stages in reactions that are otherwise overlooked".

This is equally as true of osteosarcomas as it is of osteoporosis or osteoarthritis, and so attention must be paid to those stages of cell proliferation and activity where a difference in cell behaviour has been observed.

The malignant change

During the last century and a half investigations into the cause and nature of the malignant change have been numerous, but not all productive. The need in an investigation of this kind is to assemble observations, form hypotheses, test those hypotheses, make new observations and so on, until there is sufficient information for the mechanism of the change to be described in detail. All too often, however, hypotheses have been confused with facts, and a considerable volume of work has been abortive because based on incorrect hypotheses.

Observations that have so far been mentioned are that when a tissue is overstimulated in circumstances in which such stimulation persists a neoplastic change takes place (Smithers, 1960), and that once this change has occurred cell proliferation continues in an excessive manner even when the stimulus is withdrawn. Further, tumours do not arise from single minute foci, but from considerable fields of prepared tissue (Willis, 1960). Once the malignant state has been established the cells behave in the same way as normal cells in the majority of their activities (Johnson, 1953), while the degree of malignancy of tumours is roughly proportional to their degree of histological differentiation (Willis, 1960). Abnormal appearances of nuclei and cytoplasm, in some but by no means all cells, has been commented on, together with an abundant vascular proliferation.

These and other facts and observations need to be considered in more detail, and the various mechanisms involved established. Some possible hypotheses have been easily rejected. Thus, Cameron (1952) has reviewed evidence concerning enzyme action, and found that there is no fundamental divergence from normal tissues. Tumour cells, too, are subject to the same degenerative changes as normal cells. If anything, they seem to be more susceptible to the effects of vascular disturbance and overcrowding.

In 1886 Bard reported that neoplastic cells were derived from proliferative elements of the same nature, and since then these observations have been amplified. The statement implies, for example, that factors responsible for ordinary cell differentiation are not involved. This has been verified (some of the evidence for osteosarcomas was discussed in the last section). One possibility suggested was that some of the possible stimuli might remain involved with the changed tissue. Lewis (1935) considered the available evidence and found that this hypothesis was untenable.

"Although one might explain the multiplication of malignant cells by the presence of a virus which increases with cell increases it is difficult to understand, if a virus is always present, why after tumours are once started no additional cells of the host are converted into malignant ones".

He then proceeded to show that the continued presence of some chemical agent could be eliminated, and so arrived at the conclusion that malignant cells are permanently altered cells derived from normal cells.

Although the nuclei of many tumour cells, particularly the more malignant, look almost normal, many other tumour cells show obvious abnormalities in their chromosomes and nuclei. This fact soon led to the hypothesis that the primary change was in the nucleus. Various other facts were inexplicable on this hypothesis, and as Mohr pointed out in 1934

"The pronounced uniformity of tumour tissue as regards phenotypical characteristics is just the opposite of what one would expect from the exceedingly variable chromosome relations of the tumour cells".

A year later, on the evidence then generally available Lewis (1935) concluded that the variable distribution of chromosomes in malignant cells was probably secondary to alterations of other parts of the cell, possibly the cytoplasm or the centrosomal system. As he put it

"Malignant cells are notoriously afflicted with chromosome troubles", but "the chromosome abnormalities are only the manifestation of a more subtle trouble of the cell. A boil, a fever and leucocytosis are manifestations of an infection, not the cause of it".

One cannot be sure until the precise mechanisms have been elucidated, and in this case the mechanism which leads to chromatin abnormalities, variable nuclear sizes and a somewhat watery cytoplasm had been found several years earlier. By no means the least problem in a field with a very large literature is the adequate dissemination of facts.

Mottram (1928) compared cells in tissue cultures so arranged that the tension of carbon dioxide could be varied up to 200 mm as compared with the normal of 40 mm for the experimental conditions used. With high levels of carbon dioxide abnormal mitoses and abnormal configurations of chromatin were observed. There was an irregular migration of chromatin towards the centrosomes which was frequently asymmetric. The sizes of nuclei of undividing cells under high tensions of carbon dioxide increased, while they were reduced at lower tension than normal. If one postulates, therefore, that the permeability of cell membranes for carbon dioxide is increased during the malignant change, there is an explanation of the nuclear irregularities and also the evidence of a decreased viscosity of cytoplasm. The differing degrees of cell abnormality observed in different parts of a tumour will tend to reflect differences in local carbon dioxide concentration.

Other less important hypotheses have been similarly considered, so that by 1960 Willis was in a position to state:

> "The first steps in this elucidation have been taken; when it has been completed it will be found that neither embryonic cell-rests nor their reverse— senescent cells, neither ultra-microscopic parasites nor disordered chromosomes nor mutant genes, are concerned in the change from normal to neoplastic cells".

Two of the differences so far established remain, both of which involve changed characteristics of the cell membranes. The increased ease of permeability of carbon dioxide was one, and the other the evidence of uninhibited cell division which is the dominant clinical problem. The first stage of cell division is the rearrangement of membranes in the antephase, and the rest follows on from this. Cell membranes, therefore, were subjected to a more detailed investigation.

As well as their increased permeability to carbon dioxide, the cell membrane permeability for a number of other chemicals has been shown to increase after the malignant change. Various physical and mechanical properties are also affected, with greater mobility and less adhesiveness. Pitot (1966) has reviewed the biochemical properties which change with malignancy, and again it can be seen that it is those properties which in one way or another are controlled by the cell membranes which are affected. Among the most important are:

Cell nutrition. Baker and Carrel (1928) have shown that whereas glycocoll, nucleic acid and protein cleavage fragments are sufficient for tumour cells, normal fibroblasts cease to proliferate and die in this artificial medium after 8 to 10 days, even though the culture medium is changed every 2 days. The cells accumulate dark granules in their cytoplasm. The mechanism of this change is not known, but it would seem probable that normal cells have more difficulty disposing of waste products than do malignant cells. There is a possibility, too, that the action of growth hormone on the cell membranes affects the process, and this would seem to be a potentially profitable line of investigation.

Supply of energy producing materials. In tumours there is a high rate of glycolysis, which is associated with the high rate of cell division. Mottram (1927) demonstrated that sarcoma cells were active in much lower concentrations of oxygen than normal cells, but that their activity was reduced at low tensions and absent under completely anaerobic conditions. It seems that insulin is no longer required to facilitate the entrance of glucose into cells, and Woods *et al.* (1965) have commented on evidence of an imbalance in the insulin:anti-insulin system.

Steroids. Dougherty, Berliner and their colleagues have studied a number of biotransformations at the surfaces of malignant cells, and found that a characteristic feature of malignancy is the capacity of the cells to metabolize biologically active compounds which normally help control their proliferation to metabolites which have no such function. Cell types they have investigated include lymphocytes from lymphatic leukaemia and lymphosarcoma, fibroblasts and osteosarcoma cells (Dougherty *et al.*, 1961; Berliner and Dougherty, 1961). Metabolism by malignant lymphocytes (Dougherty *et al.*, 1962) and other malignant cells (Berliner, Berliner and Dougherty, 1956; van Dooren and Dougherty, 1957) results in several different compounds only found in minute amounts in the normal. Malignant fibroblasts in *in vitro* culture were 250 times as resistant to the growth inhibiting action of cortisol as normal, and metabolized it at least twice as fast (Grosser, Sweat, Berliner and Dougherty, 1962). Similarly, although immature lymphocytes can transform cortisol (active) to cortisone (inactive) to a greater extent than mature cells (Dougherty *et al.*, 1960), this cortisol to cortisone reaction is helped by malignant cells to a considerably greater extent (Dougherty, Berliner, Schneebeli and Berliner, 1964).

All these various observations—the increased permeability to carbon dioxide and other materials, the uninhibited changes to the premitotic configuration, increased ease of penetration of glycol, with a lowered requirement for oxygen, together with alterations in the action of insulin and steroids at cell surfaces—are consistent with the removal of an inhibiting mechanism.

Sobel has, therefore, conducted a search for materials which might be consistently present in normal tissues, and consistently absent in malignant tissues. He found two such compounds (A. E. Sobel, 1963, pers. comm.)

"In 62 different cases of cancer which included all varieties there was an absence of two positively charged substances related to mucopolysaccharides. (Probably containing anywhere from di- to tetra-amino sugars.) All cases of normal were high, and pregnancy showed the same as normals. In other diseases the positively charged substance was present but migrated in a continuous pattern rather than as two discrete steps". A few months later he wrote "The work on the macromolecules P_1 and P_2 is progressing well. We know that other diseases behave like the normal".

He also found that rats, whose tissues become malignant very easily, contained only small quantities of the two compounds in their tissues; while guinea-pigs, which are far more resistant, have large quantities present. This was an interesting observation, because it has been found that malignant cells metabolize steroids differently from normal cells, and one of the characteristics of rats which makes them unsuitable for use as experimental animals when one wishes to compare metabolic activities with the human is that they have different hormones present and acting.

There is fragmentary evidence that the inhibiting agents in the cell membranes are the same as, or associated with, the compounds responsible for homograft and heterograft rejection reactions. Investigations along these lines are still in their infancy, but there are a number of suggestive observations. On several occasions with kidney transplants there have been neoplasms in the transplanted kidney which have spread, and it has seemed that patients on immunosuppressive drugs have an impaired ability to prevent or restrict the growth of neoplastic cells. At the present stage of knowledge alternative hypotheses could be advanced.

Ewing (1940) in discussing the mechanisms involved in tumour regression and apparently inactive phases has pointed out that one of the body's defence mechanisms is an inflammatory reaction to meet the invasion of tumour cells. The reason prednisone is used as an immunosuppressive agent is that it suppresses the inflammatory reaction which is the second stage of the rejection reaction. This is one possible hypothesis. Observations which would not seem to support it are those of clinicians who have suggested that adversity and worry can, in some individuals, cause an enhanced reaction of the body to carcinogenic agents (e.g. Harper, 1962). This type of stress causes a raised blood cortisol, which has the same type of corticosteroid activity as does prednisone. Another hypotheses concerns the action of the other widely used compound, azathioprine. This has a different action, which is thought to be on the first stage of the rejection reaction, the vascular change. It has been hoped that it would inactivate the compounds responsible for rejection. There would seem to be at least a possibility that it inactivates the compounds responsible for the control of cell membranes in the reticulo-endothelial system. After only a few years' clinical use, a number of cases of reticulum cell sarcoma had been reported by 1969 (Woodruff et al., 1969; Doak, Montgomerie, North and Smith, 1968), which seemed to have been caused by the azothioprine. Should this hypothesis be substantiated, it will mean that any efficient immunosuppressive drug will also be a carcinogenic agent. This leaves accurate tissue matching as an essential prerequisite for successful transplantation surgery, in the same way that blood is matched for transfusions.

It is usually thought that carcinogenesis is a unique phenomenon. One might speculate that this is not necessarily the case. The various observations which have been recorded all suggest an abrupt change in membrane properties with the onset of malignancy. There is at least

398   BONE BEHAVIOUR

one other situation where an abrupt change in properties of cell membranes has been observed, and that is in the emergence of strains of bacteria with a resistance to antibiotics to which they had previously been susceptible.

Summary

1. The first stage of cell division is the antephase or pre-mitotic phase. Some time before mitosis commences, about 8 h in the case of the connective tissue cells, direct channels are formed between the cell nucleus and the exterior of the cell. Chromatin precursors enter, are then slowly polymerized, and when this polymerization is complete mitosis takes place. A supply of energy is only required during the antephase.

2. The factors which control cell division are those factors which control membrane changes at the beginning of antephase.

3. The main structural components for cell membranes are protein and phospholipids. A number of other chemicals are present which modify their properties. The cell wall, the nuclear envelope and the channels which form during antephase are smooth membranes. The membranes of the endoplasmic reticulum are known as rough membranes. There are chemical differences between the two groups of membranes.

4. The phospholipids in the smooth membranes are labile, or fluid, and are stabilized by proteins and steroids.

5. The regulating mechanisms which control membrane properties and cell division include:

(a) The supply of raw materials for formation of a new cell. Most important are glycine, nucleic acid and protein cleavage fragments.

(b) A supply of energy producing carbohydrates. During growth and tissue turnover cell division takes place where these cleavage products of protein and polysaccharide are available. The presence of haemopoietic tissue in the marrow is also dependent on their availability.

(c) The partial pressure of oxygen. Oxidation of carbohydrate is necessary for both cell division and the specialized activities of cells. This means that blood flow is important. A high oxygen level favours anabolic activity.

(d) The partial pressure of carbon dioxide. There is an optimum level for cell division, and above or below this cell activity is depressed. A local excess of carbon dioxide causes capillaries to dilate.

(e) Peptide hormones. Growth hormone activates stem cells. It also affects the properties of cell membranes.

(f) Insulin. Insulin regulates glucose uptake by cells, and its presence is also necessary before many hormones are able to act on cell surfaces.

(g) Steroids. These compounds regulate the flexibility of cell membranes. The cell membranes are responsible for a series of biotransformations of steroids. In turn they are themselves controlled by the steroid whose production they have catalysed. Corticosteroids exert their anti-inflammatory action by stabilizing phospholipid membranes.

(h) Protein and amino acid levels. The levels of these compounds in surrounding tissue fluids influences the type of cell activity, whether cell division or matrix formation.

6. In wound healing macrophages congregate in the clot, and in the zone of

tissue breakdown. Connective tissue cells in this latter zone are also active, moving around and dividing. Cells proliferate from vessels to form vascular sprouts or buds, the vascular loops and clusters. As they meet they fuse. Later, as the scar tissue matures a few vessels remain, while the rest regress.

7. Fibroblasts cannot feed on serum constituents, but macrophages do. The macrophages cleave serum proteins into fragments which can then act as a source of food for fibroblasts and proliferating endothelial cells. Fibroblasts and granulation tissue cells can also feed on dead tissue. Bone and cartilage cells are unable to divide in the presence of diluted serum, but they can produce the calcifiable matrix.

8. Newly formed proliferating vessels are fragile, and permeable to serum and blood constituents. The endothelial cells are motile and very active. The more impermeable basement membrane of the vessel walls does not form until after sprouting vessels have fused.

9. Fat cells are formed metaplastically from fibroblasts and connective tissue cells. Insulin is one of the factors involved in this conversion.

10. Bone grafts are used as a scaffolding and source of raw materials to assist in the replacement of substantial quantities of bone. The sequence of events is similar to that in fracture healing, and an adequate vascular ingrowth is essential. If delayed, degradation of the graft may proceed too far, with the production of necrotic tissue, or a barrier of dense fibrous tissue may prevent further vascular penetration. When the conditions are correct adequate incorporation takes about three months.

11. The replacement of a segment of bone to form a new medullary canal with adequate vascularization takes about 5 years in children.

12. Whatever the type of graft there is an initial proliferation of vessels for 4 to 5 days. Subsequently the vascular supply continues to increase for autografts and isografts, but it decreases for fresh homografts and heterografts. This is because of the immune response. (The initial stages of rejection of an established transplant are also vascular.) The ischaemic changes are followed by an inflammatory reaction around the graft.

13. To prepare homografts and heterografts it is necessary to immobilize or destroy the components responsible for provoking the rejection reaction. Freezing diminishes the response; freeze drying gives satisfactory results; but a sterilizing dose of radiation (2·5 megarad) is even more satisfactory, with the rejection factor destroyed and, under suitable conditions of irradiation, enhanced remodelling.

14. A common factor in all types of cancer is that the malignant change is preceded by a period when the tissue in question is stimulated to overactivity. In due course a number of cells in the tissue change to the malignant form and cell proliferation is then independent of the initial stimulus.

15. The various "causes" of cancer—chemical carcinogens, radiation, repeated trauma, viruses, and so on—are causes of overstimulation of cells, and none in itself is an initiator of the malignant change.

16. Predisposing causes for bone tumours include over-stimulation of growth or an aberration of the remodelling of bone; lesions in bone which lead to continued and vigorous cell proliferation, such as fibrous dysplasia, Paget's disease, exostoses and benign tumours such as the giant cell tumours and cartilage tumours; and radiation.

17. In many of their activities malignant cells behave in the same manner as normal cells, perform the same activities, differentiate as a result of the same

stimuli, and show the same degree of reproductive activity. One difference is the diminution or lack of a restraint on proliferation. Otherwise, once a sarcoma is present in bone, it usually behaves in the manner that might be expected from its location in the bone.

18. In addition to the tendency to go into the predivision state, other properties which characterize the malignant state are properties associated with cell membranes:

(a) They are permeable to carbon dioxide and other diffusable compounds. Where there is excess carbon dioxide in the surroundings an excess can also build-up within cells. The result of an excess of carbon dioxide within cells is to cause abnormal mitoses, abnormal configurations of chromatin and an increased size of nuclei.

(b) Various physical and mechanical properties of cell surfaces are altered, there is greater mobility and less adhesiveness.

(c) Controls for cell nutrition are less exacting.

(d) Lower concentrations of oxygen are needed for glycolysis, there is an imbalance in the insulin: anti-insulin system, and probably insulin is no longer required to facilitate the entrance of glucose into cells.

(e) The action of steroids on cells are modified, together with the biotransformations of steroids that take place at cell surfaces.

19. All these changes are consistent with the removal of an inhibiting mechanism, and A. E. Sobel has found that two substances related to mucopolysaccharides that are present in both the normal and in other diseases are absent in all types of malignancy.

20. There is fragmentary evidence that these inhibiting agents in cell membrane are the same as, or associated with, the compounds responsible for homograft and heterograft rejection reactions.

10. EFFECTS OF IRRADIATION
ON BONE

Because of the increasing use of radioactive isotopes, not only in teaching and research laboratories, but also as an essential source of power and as explosives, there is a need to understand the mechanisms of the biological changes they produce. Many of the industrial isotopes concerned are bone seekers, and are either heavy atoms or fission products of medium atomic weight. Many of the isotopes of heavy elements emit short range alpha particles, while the medium atomic weight elements of importance are mostly beta-emitters. In general the effects on bone of these beta-emitters and of external radiation are similar.

A considerable amount of information about the biological effects of the bone-seeking isotopes, and of radiation on bones, has now been obtained. In the case of changes induced in bone and bone marrow there have been accidental isotope assimilation, accidental injury from external radiation, the sequelae of the atom bombs in Japan, and a large number of cases resulting from the administration of radioactive isotopes by doctors who failed to realize the dangers to which they were exposing their patients. Detailed mechanisms have been sought by irradiating or administering isotopes to beagles and pigs, together with a number of other species.

Acute radiation effects stem from damage to blood vessels, particularly in the bone marrow; and the long-term effects, osteosarcomas or marrow disorders, are also the result of damage to vessels in the bone or marrow.

Physical and Metabolic Variables

When one considers the biological effects of irradiation a number of separate mechanisms have to be taken into account. The wide range of lethal doses is one indication of this. Doses of the order of 1–2·5 megarads are required to kill bacteria and their spores, and a few spores with low water content may need up to 4 megarad before they are all destroyed, although their reproductive capacity is blocked before these doses are reached. The lethal dose for insects and other creatures without a circulation or lymphatic drainage is considerably lower, being of the order of several thousand rad. For the furniture beetle, for example, it is 10,000–20,000 rad. But for humans death of the individual follows after a whole body dose of only a few hundred rad. When the radiation is localized to a portion of a limb doses of a few thousand rad cause local tissue death, but not the death of the person—except possibly from a malignant lesion some considerable time later. Radiation doses as low as 10 rad have been shown to produce detectable effects in mammals when the radiation is directed towards the adrenal gland (Dougherty and White, 1944). The cells of the adrenal cortex are stimulated to produce higher levels of corticosteroid than normal. Before considering the mechanisms of action of radiation in more detail, there are a number of other types of variable that need to be considered.

External radiation, usually X-rays or gamma radiation, can have variable wavelength, dose rate and patterns of administration of the dose. Isotopes deposited internally emit alpha particles or electrons (beta rays), and sometimes gamma radiation. The energy of these radiations, and hence their range of action, is variable, while the half-life of activity also varies over a very wide range. Thus, ^{87}Sr has a half-life of 2·7 h; ^{89}Sr, 53 days; ^{85}Sr, 65 days; and ^{90}Sr, 28 years. Some isotopes have half-lives that are only a fraction of a second, while at the other end of the scale some of the isotopes of heavy elements have half-lives of the order of thousands of years. For two isotopes of the same element, with identical metabolism, different half-lives can result in different effects. ^{226}Ra, with a half-life of 1600 years was ingested by a number of dial painters during the 1914–18 war, and was also administered "therapeutically" in the 1920s. The lowest average skeletal dose at death was 1200 rad for one of these individuals who later developed a radiation-induced osteosarcoma (Evans et al., 1969). In the period 1946 to 1951 ^{224}Ra was administered "therapeutically", and among these patients osteosarcomas developed after a much lower average skeletal dose. The lowest, in an adult, was only 90 rads (Spiess and Mays, 1970). This difference was mainly due to the short 3·62 day half-life of ^{224}Ra, which resulted in a large fraction of the skeletal ^{224}Ra decaying while still on the bone surfaces. The occasional very low dose is an indication of the fact that isotopes are not distributed uniformly through the skeleton. A substantial proportion is concentrated in "hot spots" where some remodelling was in progress at the time of ingestion. A tumour could be initiated in the vicinity of a cluster of hot spots. In some of these same patients further primary osteosarcomas have developed three and four years after the first sarcoma (Spiess, 1969). This again is an indication of the uneven distribution of the isotope.

An important variable is introduced by differences in metabolism. Many isotopes are held selectively in specific organs; iodine in the thyroid, strontium in bone, plutonium in bone and liver, and so on. Their mode and rates of excretion are also highly variable. Even among the bone-seeking isotopes their manner of association with the mineral and organic phases of bone vary so that, for example, Jowsey and Orvis (1967) demonstrated that although ^{45}Ca and ^{91}Y are both associated with the mineral phase, the precise manner is different. These variations mean that there are differences in the subsequent biological effects. Jee (1962) has compared four bone-seeking alpha-emitters, radium (^{226}Ra), plutonium (^{239}Pu), mesothorium (^{228}Ra) and radiothorium (^{228}Th) in beagles, and found different histological appearances resulting from their different distribution. He has found abundant evidence of local variations (Jee et al., 1962b). These bone-seeking alpha emitters cause osteosarcomas, but they can also produce neoplasms in tissues closely adjacent to the bone. Thus, in 46 cases of radium-induced malignant tumours in man, Finkel, Miller and Hasterlik (1969) found that 16 were carcinomas of tissues close to the skull—principally mastoid and paranasal air cell carcinomas.

Again, the changes may or may not be cumulative. In the case of beagles which were given plutonium, Jee (1962) found that the appearances after 760 rad for 1711 days were virtually identical with those after 1645 rad for 1178 days. For ingested radium Rowland (1963a, b) found the final pattern after 10 to 30 years different according to whether it had been ingested chronically over a period of time, as in the radium dial painters, or administered "therapeutically" in a series of weekly injections. Using these criteria he was able to deduce the approximate time and manner of ingestion of radium in a woman who died from a radium-induced sarcoma, but with the radium "therapy" not included in her medical records.

There are also variations as between the effects on one tissue or another. Plutonium is taken up in bone and in the liver. It damages both, but death occurs from osteosarcoma before liver tumours show neoplastic changes (Cochran, Jee, Stover and Taylor, 1962). In a few instances where the ^{239}Pu level has been low death has been from bile duct tumours (Taylor, Dougherty, Shabestai and Dougherty, 1969). The most likely hypothesis, on present evidence, to account for these is that they arise from toxic products of irradiated hepatic cells. That is, they arise from a secondary mechanism. A further complication in the case of comparatively short-lived isotopes is the effect of radioactive decay products. The ^{224}Ra given to patients in Germany has ^{212}Pb as one decay product. This is taken up in erythrocytes, and is found in organs well supplied with blood, such as the liver. Another decay product is ^{212}Bi which is concentrated in the kidney. So, as well as the bone lesions, some of those patients have died from liver and kidney disorders.

Alpha emitters have a limited range, while electrons from beta-emitters travel farther. Dyson (1966) has collected evidence to show that the effects of ^{32}P, with a range of 0·72 cm for the electrons it emits, are similar to those produced by external X-rays and gamma rays, while for ^{90}Sr and ^{90}Y also the effects on the marrow tend to dominate over those on the bone. For all types of radiation the effect on the marrow tends to be greatest in sites near bone tissue. This observation was first recorded in 1926 by Ewing.

Evidence which has so far accumulated has suggested that the range of radiation end results which are observed in practice follows from a limited number of biological mechanisms, and that the variations observed result from variations in the type of radiation, its range and intensity, its distribution, and the metabolic state of the individual. Dark people, for example, are more resistant to high radiation doses than are fair people. An interesting experiment by Cater, Basergar and Lisco (1959) has shown that when rat bones were irradiated with 3000 rad gamma radiation from ^{102}Ir osteosarcomas were produced in some but not all cases. Eighty days after the radiation a ten week course of growth hormone had the effect of almost doubling the proportion of lesions which progressed to osteosarcomas, while administration of thyroxine for a similar time reduced the latent period for sarcoma formation. (It may be remembered that thyroid hormone is suspected as a possibly causative agent in the aetiology of Paget's disease.) An indication of the biological mechanisms concerned may be gained by considering the main types of bone involvement: from external radiation, from bone-seeking beta-emitters, and from bone-seeking alpha-emitters. Some typical examples of each will be discussed.

Biological Mechanisms

Effects on bone tissue

Because of the importance of the subject, the United States Atomic Energy Commission set up a number of large scale research projects in the years after the 1939–45 war to investigate the effects of isotopes. The main project on the bone-seeking isotopes, and the alpha emitters in particular, is at Salt Lake City, in the Anatomy Department of the University of Utah, where beagles are the main experimental animal. External radiation and the beta-emitting isotopes are being studied at the University of California, Davis, where beagles are also used; while at Handford, Washington, swine are the principal experimental animals. Somewhat less comprehensive investigations have been carried out in other parts of the United States and elsewhere.

The alpha-emitting bone-seeking isotopes are the most potent carcinogenic agents, and will be discussed first. They have a short range of action: 35 microns in soft tissues for ^{239}Pu, which has a half-life of 24,000 years; 38 to 82 microns for ^{228}Th (half-life 1·9 years) and its decay products; 40 microns for ^{226}Ra, and so on. Whether these isotopes remain on the bone surface or are buried within the bone tissue therefore affects their biological action (Mays et al., 1969). The range of beta rays is far greater. In soft tissue it is 1800 microns for ^{90}Sr, and 10,700 microns for ^{90}Y, the corresponding range in bone tissue being about half of these values.

Rowland (1963b) and others have investigated the mode of uptake of ^{226}Ra into bone. This element has a chemical action similar to that of calcium. After injection the concentration in plasma falls exponentially and it is incorporated into newly formed bone in the same Ra:Ca ratio as it exists in the blood. Some is distributed in the bone in a diffuse manner as a result of ion exchange processes, while secondary mineralization of remodelling bone results in higher concentrations of diffusely distributed isotope. Local "hot spots" are found in places where there was active bone deposition. Because of the short range of alpha particles it is only those close to a vulnerable target that are biologically effective. Figures 10.1, 10.2 (Figs 26, 27 from Jee et al., 1962b) show detailed autoradiograms of two regions of bone containing radium. Where there is a hot spot neighbouring osteocytes have died, but in the vicinity of the diffusely distributed isotope osteocytes remain viable.

Plutonium remains on bone surfaces, and so is available to irradiate adjacent structures. When remodelling takes place in plutonium-laden bone these active areas are frequently buried. In Fig. 10.3 the lines of heavy activity represent the deposition at the original trabecular border, the bone deposited before injection of plutonium is free of activity, while the bone deposited later during the remodelling process contains a diffuse distribution of alpha activity. During the process of remodelling some bone containing high concentrations of plutonium is taken up by macrophages. When killed, these cells remain in the marrow as small centres of activity (Figs 10.4, 10.5).

Jee and Arnold (1961) have carefully described the sequence of events when a comparatively large dose of ^{239}Pu is ingested (2·7 μc/kg). A detailed consideration of these shows which of the various consequences of the ingestion of alpha-emitters are the most important for the formation of osteosarcomas.

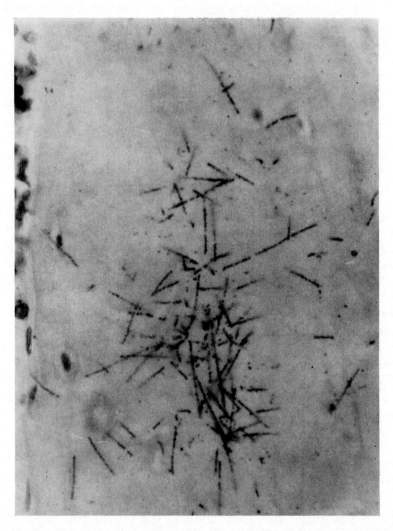

Fɪɢ. 10.1. Autoradiogram of bone containing radium. In the vicinity of this "hot spot" osteocytes have died, and so do not take up stain. ×320 The author thanks Prof. W. S. S. Jee for this figure.

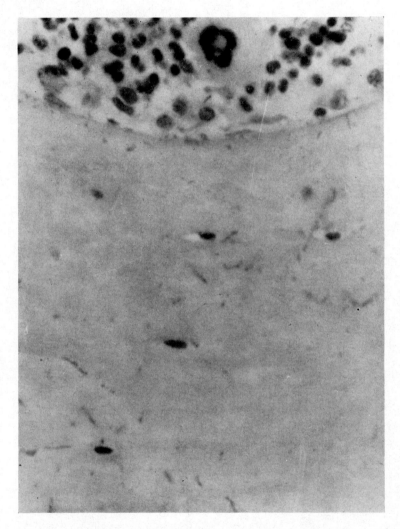

FIG. 10.2. Autoradiogram of bone containing radium. The isotope is diffusely distributed, and the osteocytes are unaffected. In the marrow at the top of the photograph is a megakaryocyte. ×320. The author thanks Prof. W. S. S. Jee for this figure.

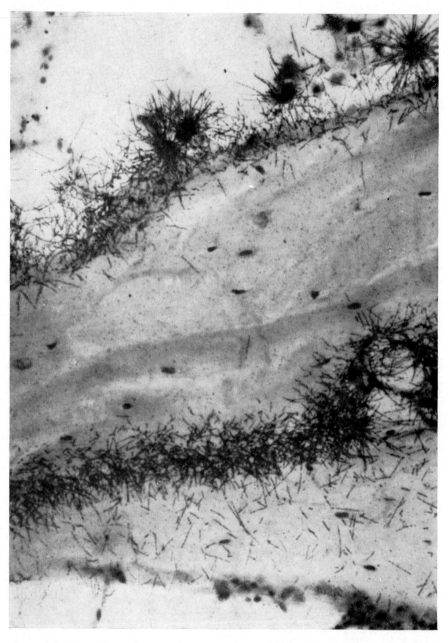

FIG. 10.3. Autoradiogram of bone containing plutonium. The lines of heavy activity show the deposit on the original trabecular border. Bone deposited since injection contains a diffuse distribution of alpha activity. The author thanks Prof. W. S. S. Jee for this figure.

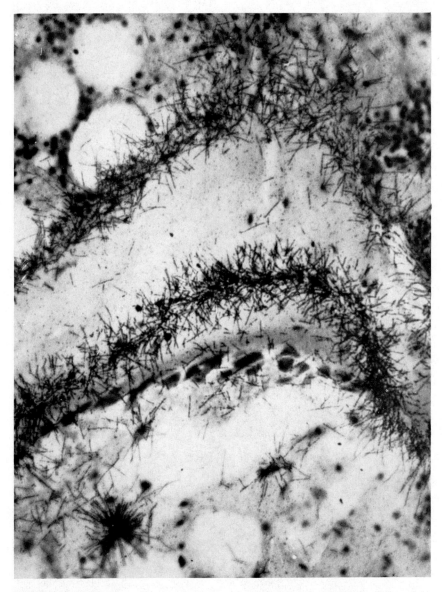

FIG. 10.4. Autoradiogram of bone containing plutonium. New bone, showing a diffuse alpha activity, is being deposited on the original heavily labelled trabecular surface. Macrophages containing plutonium are present in the marrow. The author thanks Prof. W. S. S. Jee for this figure.

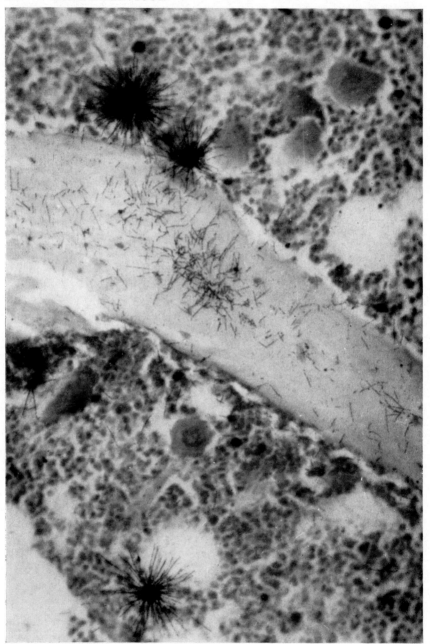

FIG. 10.5. Autoradiogram of bone containing plutonium. Dead macrophages, containing high concentrations of plutonium taken up during remodelling, remain in the marrow as small centres of activity. The marrow in this dog contains a high proportion of megakaryocytes. The author thanks Prof. W. S. S. Jee for this figure.

*A disturbance of enchondral bone formation which results in the form-
ation of transverse cartilage plates in the ribs* (1–28 days). See Fig. 3.27.
This is almost certainly a secondary effect caused by the release of
corticosteroids as a result of the effect of ^{239}Pu on the pituitary or
adrenal glands, or both. It could not be irradiation rendering the
cartilage matrix more stable, since plutonium does not penetrate into
growth cartilage. This stress effect would tend to delay cell activity in
the pre-sarcoma stages, so that it is unlikely that it would make a
positive contribution to the metaplastic change.

Disturbances at endosteal surfaces of trabecular and cortical bone.

(a) *Destruction of endosteal cells* (1 week).
(b) *Pathological remodelling of trabeculae—apposition of a typical post-
injection bone and inhibition of resorption* (1 month).
(c) *Death of osteocytes near bone surfaces within range of alpha particles*
(2 months).
(d) *Formation of peritrabecular fibrosis* (2–3 months).
(e) *Occurrence of abnormal resorption* (3 months).

The destruction of the endothelial cells and the death of the osteocytes within range of the alpha particles would both seem to be direct
effects of radiation on cells, and the difference in the time taken a reflection of the degree of sensitivity of the cells concerned. (There is already
abundant evidence that dividing cells are the most vulnerable and resting cells the least vulnerable for any given cell type.)

Cell death releases chemicals which stimulate and provide raw
materials for vascular proliferation. Since dead endosteal cells are close
to the bone surface one can therefore expect vascular proliferation close
to the affected surfaces. Further, osteoblasts are formed from osteogenic precursor cells which differentiate from vessel walls, so that these
vessels may also be sufficiently close to the surface to be at risk. Irradiation of blood vessels is therefore a factor to be taken into account.

During the last few years there have been a number of investigations
into the effect of irradiation on vessels. Mount and Bruce (1964), for
example, have irradiated rabbit skin, and found that a single dose of
800 rads of X-rays caused the walls of vessels to relax, so that the volume of fluid they contained doubled within a day. Five to ten days after
irradiation their permeability had increased by a factor of 10. The
sensitivity of vessels varies, and it has been a frequently observed fact
that tissues where sinusoids are present react to considerably smaller
radiation doses than do other tissues. Dividing and recently formed
vessels are particularly sensitive—no doubt because their basement
membrane is absent or only imperfectly formed.

With higher doses there is immediate damage to vessels. Song and Levitt (1970) investigating tumours in rats, found that after single exposures with 3000 and 6000 rad X-rays, the vascular volume in tumours decreased, whereas it increased in the skin and muscle. Within an hour the permeability of vessels in the tumours was 20 to 30 times that of vessels in skin or muscle. Lymphatic vessels have walls similar to those of sinusoids, and Wells (1963) showed that if these vessels were perfused immediately after irradiation (this time of the skin of mouse ears) weakened patches in the vessel walls burst. This happened above doses of 2000 to 4000 rad. His method of perfusing lymphatics had the advantage that it was a procedure that could be carried out on living animals. Subsequent observation showed that it was those mice which had been found to have damaged vessels that later developed sarcomas or carcinomas.

There would seem to be a connection between the immediate damage and the increased permeability several days later, but detailed information about this mechanism awaits further investigations. Hurley, Ham and Ryan (1969) have made a start by providing evidence that there might be a weakening of the bond between epithelium and basement membrane that takes several days to develop, and they have also shown that after this same period there is histological evidence of damage to cells in the vessel wall. The local dose required varies from one individual to the next, and between capillaries and sinusoids of different degrees of maturity. When one considers late results in the human, mention has already been made of the variations observed in the action of ^{224}Ra (Spiess, 1969). There have been many similar observations on the undesired late effects of therapeutic irradiation. Children's bone is particularly susceptible. Katzman, Waugh and Berdon (1969) have reported considerable damage to bone structure and remodelling after doses ranging from 1400 rad to 4284 rad, while in a general series Sabanas, Dahlin, Childs and Ivins (1956) have reported sarcomas developing after doses ranging from 1400 to 10,000 rad, and with latent periods in the range 32 months to 30 years.

Returning to Jee and Arnold's observations (1961). They found that peritrabecular fibrosis (Fig. 10.6) occurred within a month of the accumulated dose having killed osteocytes in the vicinity. This suggests that the dose required to kill the cells is approximately the same as the dose required to increase the permeability of the vessel walls. When that happens, if sufficient protein diffuses out and is suitably degraded cells proliferate (see Figs 4.8, 4.9, 4.10) and produce an intercellular matrix. In Fig. 4.10 these perivascular cells were exhibiting osteoblastic activity at the bone surface, but in the peritrabecular fibrosis in isotope-laden

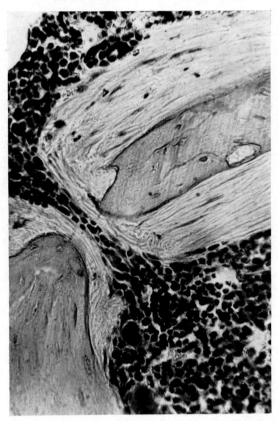

FIG. 10.6. Fibrous tissue around trabeculae in cancellous bone of beagle which had been given plutonium. ×200. The author thanks Prof. W. S. S. Jee for the material from which this figure was taken.

bone no such differentiation occurs. There would seem to be two possible explanations for this. One is that the local radiation dose has been sufficient to deactivate the osteogenic factor. The other is that radicles and ions produced by the effect of radiation on the surrounding water might be present in sufficient quantity to produce a chemical effect.

That this is a possibility has been clearly demonstrated in some cases where a metal pin containing a gamma source was inserted into the head of the femur for approximately 4 h. Figure 10.7 shows the state of affairs a year later. The blood which replaced the nail in the hole clotted, but then remained inert, without necrotic changes, resorption or tissue ingrowth. Broken and dead trabeculae, damaged during insertion and removal of the nail showed further calcification (Fig. 10.8) but were not resorbed. Apparently similar additional calcification has

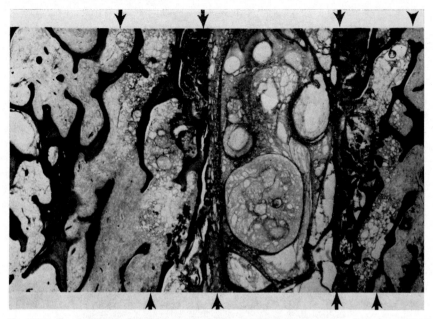

Fig. 10.7. Track of nail containing gamma source, which had been inserted in the head of femur for 4 h a year previously. The blood which replaced the nail clotted, and then remained inert. Broken and dead trabeculae, damaged during insertion and removal of the nail, have not been resorbed. Some differentiation of granulation tissue cells occurred after removal of the radiation source. In the region closest to the cavity a comparatively small amount of intercellular matrix was formed (between the arrows). Farther away more fibrous matrix was formed, and farther out still there has been some vascular penetration (extreme left). ×35.

been observed in patches of bone which have been irradiated during therapy (Goodman and Sherman, 1963) but is not found in ordinary bone. Some differentiation of granulation tissue cells occurred around the cavity after removal of the radiation source. In the region closest to the cavity a comparatively small amount of intercellular matrix was formed (between the arrows in Fig. 10.7). A similar sparse inert matrix can be found near hot spots in isotope-containing bone. Figure 10.9 is from a vertebra in a spot adjacent to the intervertebral disc. The local dose was high, cell death has occurred with the intercellular matrix only partly formed, and the bone deprived of its source of nutrition has died. Because of the short range of the alpha particles the neighbouring disc tissue is viable and unaffected.

In the femoral head (Fig. 10.7), farther away from the radiation source a higher proportion of fibrous matrix was formed. In an intermediate zone the fibroblasts were still viable at the end of the year, but the bone tissue dead (Fig. 10.10), and between this zone and the normal marrow and trabeculae was a zone containing fibrous tissue with pene-

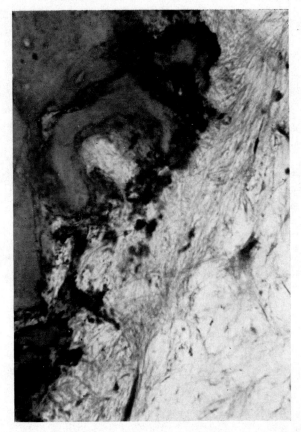

Fig. 10.8. Detail of broken trabecula. There has been further calcification (more darkly staining) in the dead bone. Some fibrous tissue, formed in the 5 days after irradiation remains inert and unresorbable. ×200.

trating vessels. The border between these two zones is shown arrowed in Fig. 10.11. The inertness of the coagulated blood and of the matrix in the fibrous tissue around the track of the nail is abnormal. Since all this repair tissue was formed after removal of the radiation source it follows that the modified properties must be due to chemical chain reaction, continuing for several days.

A related phenomenon, apparently depending on a series of slow chemical reactions, has been described by Kaplan (1959). Experimenting with mice he found lymphoid tumours which arose from thymic cells that, though residing in irradiated hosts, had never themselves been exposed to radiation. This change could only have been due to a series of slow chemical chain reactions in the thymus.

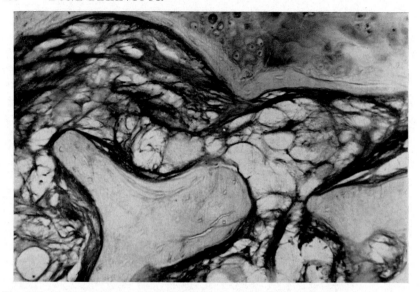

Fig. 10.9. Vertebra of beagle which had been given plutonium, near a hot spot. Osteocytes deprived of their source of nutrition are dead. A sparse inert matrix fills this portion of the marrow cavity. Neighbouring disc tissue is unaffected. × 100. The author thanks Prof. W. S. S. Jee for the material from which this figure was taken.

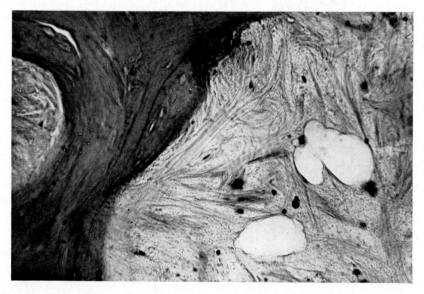

Fig. 10.10. Area of femoral head, near track where the gamma source had been inserted. In this zone there is a more profuse intercellular matrix, but it is chemically inert and cannot be resorbed. Osteocytes in the trabecula it surrounds are dead, but cells in the inert fibrous tissue still take up stain and would appear to be viable. × 200.

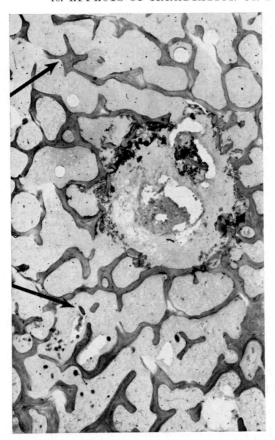

Fig. 10.11. Transverse section through another femoral head which had received gamma radiation a year previously. The track of the nail is filled with inert clotted blood, and in this case there has been a little fibrous replacement. Parts of the broken trabeculae are more heavily calcified. The border of the region in which the fibrous matrix is too inert for vascular penetration is indicated by the arrows. At a similar distance again from the nail track (off the figure) there were signs of some normal remodelling. ×35.

Disturbances in Haversian bone.

(a) *Formation of Haversian canal plugs* (1 year).

(b) *Death of osteocytes in affected osteones and adjacent interstitial lamellae* (2 years).

(c) *Formation of large resorption cavities* ($2\frac{1}{2}$ years).

(d) *Formation of abnormal osteones* ($2\frac{1}{2}$ years).

(e) *Occurrence of periosteal bone resorption and fibrosis* ($2\frac{1}{2}$ years).

(f) *Occurrence of spontaneous fractures in ribs and spinous processes* ($2\frac{1}{2}$ years).

EE

These changes in Haversian bone did not take place until 1 year and more after the administration of the isotopes. One explanation of this greater time interval, as compared with the change at the endosteal surfaces in that there are fewer hot spots, so that it takes longer for an effective dose to be reached.

In this sequence the most important stage is the formation of the Haversian canal plugs. The authors have shown that most of the other disturbances are secondary effects resulting from the interruption of the blood supply. Once a bone cell is cut off from its source of nutrition, whether by canal plugs, overlying bone or fibrous tissue, it dies. This, together with osteocyte death caused directly by the radiation, results in large masses of dead bone. When the resorption process is stimulated the available marrow spaces are frequently filled with haemopoietic tissue (see Fig. 10.6). Jee (1962) has found that once the consequences of radiation have led to altered circulation and partial ischemia in the bone there is massive resorption and endosteal and periosteal bone rare-faction. This provides a large store of nutrients for bone formation, so that in other areas there is deposition of endosteal bone which on occasion can fill the entire marrow cavity, and a considerable periosteal thickening. On radiographs the cortical bone can present a very patchy appearance.

Massive resorption of trabecular and cortical bone, and apposition of atypical bone (3 years).

Formation of osteogenic sarcoma (3½ years).

The time lag between administration of the isotope and initiation of the neoplastic lesion depends on when the massive resorption takes place, and for very high doses this was sooner than for lower doses. An interesting observation is that although the majority of tumours arise in cancellous bone (Jee, Stover, Taylor and Christensen, 1962a) the malignant change requires the massive resorption of pre-existing Haversian bone to provide the necessary energy and nutrients for overstimulated proliferation. In spite of the high carcinogenic potential of these alpha-emitting isotopes, the somewhat more stable matrix produced as a result of radiation-induced chain reactions hinders resorption (Arnold and Jee, 1959), and thus slows down the remodelling, that is initiated by vascular damage, of bone laid down in the presence of the isotope.

The essential cause for the production of osteosarcomas by bone-seeking isotopes is thus the damage done to blood vessels and the plug-ging of Haversian canals. This follows logically from the observed evidence, and is not dependent on the confirmatory evidence that it is in accord with what is already known about the initiation of neoplastic lesions. Jee and his co-workers have therefore investigated this vascular aspect of the problem further.

An initial assessment showed that most of the damage in Haversian bone is due to vascular occlusion, and not to any direct effect on the devitalized bone. Appearances were consistent with the secretion of a "matrix-like" material in Haversian canals (Jee and Arnold, 1960). This could fill the spaces between vessel walls and the inner surface of the canal (see the normal appearance in Fig. 4.14) and then proceed to vascular occlusion. More recently a direct correlation has been found between the dose level above which sarcoma formation as a result of the action of the alpha-emitters is probable (Dougherty and Mays, 1969) and the dose level at which there is a significant interference with blood flow in compact bone (Jee et al., 1969). Vessels in spongy bone are more sensitive, but the greater stability of the irradiated trabecular bone counteracts this.

There are several possible mechanisms for the plugging of Haversian canals, each of which would involve the deposition of an amorphous protein: polysaccharide complex that would calcify when surrounding tissue ceased to be viable. A high proportion of polysaccharide in the complex is usually responsible when the calcification is heavier than normal. Jee et al. (1969) have found that the mechanism which dominates is the secretion of an abnormal matrix by the cells of the vessel walls. There would seem to be a similarity between this and the abnormal matrix formed by the vascular endothelial cells in osteogenesis imperfecta in that in both instances the matrix may be deposited either outside or inside the vessel (see Chapter 4). Osteogenesis imperfecta is known to be due to a biochemical block in the matrix-producing cells, so that one might speculate that in the present instance ions or radicles formed by the radiation interfere with chemical processes in the endothelial cells.

So far the effects of bone-seeking alpha-emitters have been considered. When beta-emitters such as ^{90}Sr are present in bone there are other complications, because the range of radiation in the bone tissue is about a millimetre instead of about 40 microns. McClellan and Jones (1969) have summarized the various findings and shown that they lead to the conclusion that ^{90}Sr is most likely to cause osteosarcomas after a large single dose, and most likely to cause haematopoietic neoplasms with a high continuous intake started early in life. The dose to the marrow is only a half to three-quarters that to the bone tissue, but at a level of radiation at which, say, ^{226}Ra would be showing spontaneous fractures and osteosarcomas, ^{90}Sr-containing bone shows only a little endosteal and periosteal thickening in those experiments where

[90]Sr is fed to beagles daily from mid-gestation to young adulthood (Goldman, Della Rosa and McKelvie, 1969; Bustad, 1969). The bone has been described as "flint-like" and resisted breaking, while resorption and hence remodelling was almost completely prevented in the adult. The hardening of the intercellular matrix is an effect which is frequently found in polymeric materials which have been irradiated. The effect of the radiation is to break bonds in the long chain molecules. According to the chemical nature of the bonds (Little, 1954) and their flexibility and range of movement (Little, 1957) they may either remain apart or reform or join up with another free end. Cross-linking may occur, and chemical stability is increased whenever there is not an undue amount of degradation. In the present instance the proteolytic enzymes from osteoclasts are powerless to degrade the altered protein.

Effects on marrow

The dominant effect of radiation on the marrow, whether from beta-emitters or external radiation, is almost identical with that on bone. A few dividing cells may be killed, but the important action is the damage done to vessel walls, and particularly sinusoid vessels. The mechanism of this is only imperfectly understood, but from then onwards the sequence of events is reasonably clear. The main difficulties in describing it are the variety of terms used for the same or similar happenings in different papers. Thus, the malignant tumours from the marrow of beagles fed with ^{90}Sr have at different times been called lymphoblastic or primitive lymphosarcoma or reticulum cell sarcoma (Andersen and Goldman, 1962) or myelogenous leukaemia (Bustad et al., 1969) or haemopoietic neoplasm (McClellan and Jones, 1969). The real problem is that the same basic lesion can show a whole spectrum of appearances. Vessels are damaged, and after 4 or 5 days their contents leak out, and it is another 2 to 4 weeks before they completely recover (if they are not too damaged for that to be possible). What happens after the escape of vessel contents depends on a variety of factors: whether or not the irradiation is a single event or repeated, the local availability of proteins and polysaccharides that favour fibroblastic activity, the hormonal state, the rate of blood flow and the level of oxidation of the blood.

The effects of a single acute radiation dose may be considered first. In whole body irradiation other organs may be affected, but the changes initiated in the bone were demonstrated by Edington, Ward, Judd and Mole (1956) who killed monkeys with a single large dose of [90]Sr. Little apparently happened for 4 to 5 days, then first the circulating lymphocyte and then leucocyte and platelet counts fell. Erythrocyte levels began to drop at the 10th day, and animals died of aplastic anaemia between 2 and 4 weeks. Loss of serum into the marrow causes immediate destruction of haemopoietic tissue (see Figs 9.5, 9.6) so that in these animals the marrow contained fat and reticulum cells. The authors noted that in the marrow of the longest-lived animal (4 weeks) regeneration of the haemopoietic tissue had commenced. In this acute injury that leads to death in 2 to 4 weeks there is further damage to the vessels, not only in the bone, but also in other parts of the body, as a result of which erythrocytes also leave the vessels, and there are widespread small haemorrhages. The straying erythrocytes were phagocytosed, and iron was found in the liver, spleen and lymph nodes. The spleen in particular, with its high proportion of sinusoids, was found to be badly damaged. This second type of vascular injury seems to be caused indirectly, but the precise mechanism awaits elucidation. Winchell, Anderson and Pollycove (1964) have found that a polysaccharide deposit is associated with the local haemorrhage, which suggests damage to cells of the vessel wall, possibly related to that postulated by Jee et al. (1969) after a sufficient cumulative dose to vessels in the Haversian canals. Similar acute damage to capillaries is caused by external radiation, whether by X-rays (Ross, Furth and Bigelow, 1952) or from a nuclear weapon (De Courcey, 1948).

Damage to vessels results from the action of ions and radicles produced by the effect of radiation on water, and there have been several reports of decreased damage when ion scavengers have been administered to experimental animals (Dogherty, Congdon, Makinodan and Hollaender 1958). These investigations have thrown light on the mechanism of the changes, but have not led to the discovery of compounds which could be used with advantage therapeutically. The development of techniques of marrow grafting for severely irradiated cases has been more successful.

When the radiation dose is lower, so that secondary damage to the vessels does not appear as a complication, changes occur whenever the dose is sufficient to cause sinusoids and possibly other vessels to become permeable. This means that there is a theoretical threshold dose. This was an almost self-evident conclusion, since we normally contain radioactive isotopes. Naturally occurring active carbon and potassium account for approximately 10,000 disintegrations per person per minute. The threshold value for biological damage, however, depends on the state of the vessels, and so will vary from one individual to another, and will not be the same for any individual over a prolonged period. In practice, the International Committee on Radiological Protection have based their recommendations on observed signs, and given 3 rad/year as the maximum permissible dose for the whole skeleton for the general population, and 30 rad/year as the maximum permissible dose for the adult working population.

A description of the effects of the lower doses can only be a general one relating to mechanisms, since there are detailed variations from isotope to isotope and from species to species (Dougherty, 1962). In the living animal the earliest change noted tends to be a depression of leucocytes, followed by lymphocytes (Bustad, 1969; Bustad *et al.*, 1969; Dungworth, Goldman, Switzer and McKelvie, 1969). Erthrocytes tend to be unaffected until what has been described as myeloproliferative disease develops. This disease presents "a morphological spectrum varying from myelofibrosis and myeloid metaplasia to granulocytic leukaemia". Another term used has been myelogenous leukaemia, to denote an extreme granulopoietic stimulation superimposed on radiation damaged bone marrow. Until the terminal stages there is little effect on the erythrocyte level, because myelofibrosis is commonly accompanied by extramedullary erythropoiesis, particularly in the spleen (Erf and Herbert, 1944), but if a neoplasm does not intervene erythrocyte failure and anaemia tends to be the eventual cause of death (Dougherty and Taylor, 1968).

When serum diffuses into the extra-vascular regions haemopoietic cells in the surrounding marrow are killed. Should there be a sufficient protein level in the serum some fibrous tissue proliferation occurs. Ions and radicles cause a more inert fibrous tissue to be formed than normal, so that once formed it remains. In experiments on ^{90}Sr-fed swine, Clarke, Howard and Hackett (1969) have found that more fibrous tissue is formed in the marrow of adult than of young animals. They also found proliferating cell types to be different, with myeloproliferative disorders in parents and lymphoproliferative disorders in their offspring. Even with a single exposure to radiation inert fibrous tissue tends to be formed. Goodman and Sherman (1963) described the marrow changes produced locally after radiation therapy of neighbouring tissues to be fibrotic and edematous. In these cases the dose was below that needed to produce cell death. Describing the myelofibrosis found in survivors of the atomic bomb in Hiroshima, Anderson, Hoshino and Yamamoto (1964) found the frequency of the conditions inversely proportional to the distance from the hypocentre. (It is possibly the only serious late sequel of the bomb.) Clinically the presenting symptoms were anaemia and a massive splenomegaly. They found a hyperplasia of megakaryocytes and the fibrous tissue was generally loose and reticular in character, often in coarse bands separating small islands of hyperplastic haematopoietic elements. In some cases the bone marrow space was occupied almost exclusively by dense fibrous tissue and hyperplastic megakaryocytes.

The marrow changes tend to prevent not only normal regeneration of haemopoietic tissue, but also the normal distribution of blood vessels and blood flow that is necessary for both healthy marrow and healthy bone. Hindered attempts at proliferation, spreading to lymphatic tissue and the spleen, with repeated stimulation, presents a classic premalignant situation. The spleen is also a site of erythrocyte destruction, so that whereas white cells can reach the neoplastic stage, over-stressing of the erythropoietic system produces a severe anaemia.

Inert products from the effect of ions and radicles on initial repair tissue can delay healing after radiation therapy. The presence of oxygen in excess inactivates many ions, so that healing after therapy is enhanced by the presence of excess oxygen during the irradiation process. In the experiments of Bond *et al.* (1967) mentioned in an earlier chapter, irradiation after hydrogen peroxide perfusion, instead of rendering the marrow spaces inert, resulted in a greatly stimulated osteogenic activity.

Summary

1. The resistance of cells, tissues and organisms towards ionizing radiations varies. Bacterial spores, with a low water content, are the most resistant, then bacteria. Insects without a circulation and lymphatic drainage have a medium resistance, while mammals and men who possess a circulation have a low resistance to whole body radiation. Their limbs have a somewhat higher resistance to local doses. The adrenal cortex is affected by doses as low as 10 rad.

2. The main categories of radiation are alpha particles, with a range of the order of 40 microns, and beta rays, with a range of the order of 10,000 microns, these being from unstable isotopes, and external radiation with variable energy and dose-rate. Half-lives of isotopes have a very wide range, so that two isotopes of the same element can have different effects according to their rate of emission of energy. Thus ^{224}Ra with a 3·62 day half-life is more lethal than ^{226}Ra with a half-life of 1600 years.

3. Differences in end results arise from differences in metabolism and excretion of the isotope concerned, and the vulnerability of the target organs may be partly dependent on the dose pattern and rate. The metabolic state of the individual is also relevant.

4. In the case of the bone-seeking alpha-emitters pathological effects are produced by radiation emitted at the bone surfaces. In trabecular bone, cells that proliferate near the bone surface form an inert fibrous tissue in sites where new bone formation might be expected. Its formation can be accounted for in terms of damage to sinusoid vessels, followed by reactions involving ions and radicles.

5. When vessels are irradiated there is a threshold dose, that varies according to the type of vessel and stability of the vessel wall, above which the vessel wall is damaged by the ionizing radiation. This is followed after a period of 5 to 10 days by a phase in which there is a considerable increase in the permeability of the vessel wall to plasma and proteins, and often there is also evidence of damage to the endothelial cells. Subsequent pathological changes are dependent upon the location of the damaged vessels.

6. When the head of femur was irradiated by a gamma source which was withdrawn after a few hours, the appearances a year later were investigated. Blood which filled the hole left by the source clotted, then remained inert. Fibrous repair tissue formed around the site of damage was similarly inert. The outer parts of this repair tissue were penetrated by blood vessels, but in those regions where the dose had been highest the matrix of the repair tissue was abnormally chemically resistant. These observations provide evidence that the tissues are affected by ions and the products of slow chain reactions for several days after the irradiation has ceased. That is, many effects of ionizing radiations are indirect and are caused by the products of ionization of water and solutions.

7.   The main effect of alpha emitters in Haversian bone is on the vessels in the Haversian canals. Cells of the vessel walls in these canals secrete an abnormal matrix, and in due course the vessels are occluded and plugs form in the canals. Changes secondary to the presence of these plugs result in massive resorption, followed by exuberant proliferation and the over-stimulation of cell activity which is a pre-requisite condition for sarcoma formation.

8. The action on bone tissue of beta-emitters is different from that of alpha-emitters. Because of its greater range the radiation acts on the protein of the matrix and converts it to a less soluble polymer that is resistant to proteolytic enzymes. With a single large dose conditions may be suitable for sarcoma production, but with continuous administration the bone becomes hard and resists resorption and remodelling.

9. With both beta-emitters and external radiation the dominant effect is on vessels in the marrow. They are damaged and rendered permeable to serum and proteins, and in severe cases erythrocytes. Little apparently happens for 4 to 5 days, then lymphocyte, leucocyte and platelet counts fall. Should the more severe damage be present the erythrocyte counts begin to fall at about the 10th day, and death from aplastic anaemia occurs in 2 to 4 weeks.

10. When the damage is less leucocyte and lymphocyte counts drop, as haemopoietic tissue is killed. In the continued presence of isotope there are repeated attempts at new proliferation, which if carried too far can lead to a neoplastic change. The erythrocyte levels tend to remain undisturbed, because extramedullary sites of erythropoiesis develop, particularly in the spleen. When effusions in the marrow have a high protein level inert fibrous tissue is formed. When this happens, since the spleen is also a site of erythropoietic destruction, the final result is anaemia. Excessive fibrous tissue tends to form in the adult and disorders of haemopoietic proliferation in the young.

REFERENCES AND AUTHOR INDEX

The numbers in the square brackets refer to the page or pages in the text where mention of the reference is made

Ackerman, L. V. and Spjut, H. J. (1971). *Tumors of Bone and Cartilage*. Armed Forces Institute of Pathology, Washington D.C.   [379, 384]

Adams, P. and Jowsey, J. (1967). "Bone and mineral metabolism in hyperthyroidism: an experimental study." *Endocrinology*, **81**, 735.   [173]

Aegineta, Paulus (sixth to seventh century AD). *The seven books of Paulus Aegineta* Trans. from the Greek by Francis Adams. 3 vols. London Sydenham Soc., London, 1844–7.   [17, 301, 304]

Albright, F. (1941). "Therapy in Cushing Syndrome." *Clin. Endocr. Metab.*, **1**, 75.   [305]

Albright, F. (1947). "Osteoporosis." *Ann. intern. Med.*, **27**, 861.   [302, 304]

Albright, F., Bloomberg, E. and Smith, P. H. (1940). "Postmenopausal osteoporosis." *Trans. Ass. Am. Physns*, **55**, 298.   [18, 302, 304]

Albright, F., Smith, P. H. and Richardson, A. M. (1941). "Postmenopausal osteoporosis: its clinical features." *J. Am. med. Ass.*, **116**, 2465.   [18, 302, 303]

Alffram, P. A. (1964). "An epidemiologic study of cervical and trochanteric fractures of the femur in an urban population. Analysis of 1664 cases with special reference to etiologic factors." *Acta. orthop. scand. Suppl.*, **65**, 1.   [278]

Alffram, P. A. and Bauer, G. C. (1962). "Epidemiology of fractures of the forearm." *J. Bone Jt Surg.*, **44A**, 105.   [314]

Alexander, P. and Horning, E. S. (1959). *Observations on the Oppenheimer method of inducing tumours by subcutaneous implantation of plastic films, in Carcinogenesis—Mechanism of Action*, p. 12. Publ. Churchill for the CIBA Foundation.   [198]

Altes, A. J. K. (1966). Cholesterol granuloma in the tympanic cavity. *J. Lar. Otol.*, **80**, 691.   [280]

Andersen, A. C. and Goldman, M. (1962). "Pathologic sequelae in beagles following continuous feeding of ^{90}Sr at a toxic level." *Some Aspects of Internal Irradiation*, p. 319. Pergamon Press, Oxford.   [420]

Anderson, D. J. and Naylor, M. N. (1961). "Chemical exitants of pain in human dentine and dental pulp." *J. dent. Res.*, **40**, 1275.   [339]

Anderson, D. J., Curwen, M. P. and Howard, L. V. (1958) "The sensitivity of human dentine " *J dent Res*, **37**, 669   [339]

Anderson, R. E., Hoshino, T. and Yamamoto, T. (1964). "Myelofibrosis with myeloid metaplasia in survivors of the atomic bomb in Hiroshima." *Ann. intern. Med.* **60**, 1   [60, 149, 350, 422]

Andral, G. (1827, 1837). "Precis D'Anatomie pathologique." Paris. Vol. 2, 1827, p. 38: 1837, p. 52.   [60, 350]

Appleby, J. F. and Norymberski, J. K. (1957). "The urinary excretion of 17-hydroxy-corticosteroids in human pregnancy." *J. Endocr.*, **15**, 310.
[113, 240, 291]

Aretaeus, (B.C.). *The Extant Works of Aretaeus, the Cappadocian.* Translated by Francis Adams. London Sydenham Soc., London.   [15]

Arnold, J. S. and Jee, W. S. S. (1957). "Bone growth and osteoclastic activity as indicated by radioautographic distribution of plutonium." *Am. J. Anat.*, **101**, 367.   [170, 171, 172, 173, 174]

Arnold, J. S. and Jee, W. S. S. (1959). "Autoradiography in the localization and radiation dosage of ^{226}Ra and ^{239}Pu in the bones of dogs." *Lab. Invest.*, **8**, 194.
[418]

Arnold, J. S. and Jee, W. S. S. (1962). "Patterns of long term skeletal remodelling." *Hlth Phys.*, **8**, 705.

Aslander, A. (1963). "The theory of complete tooth nutrition." Report from the Division of Agriculture, Royal Institute of Technology. Stockholm. No. 4. [299]

d'Aubigne, R. M. (1964). "Idiopathic necrosis of the femoral head in adults." *Ann. Roy. Coll. Surg.*, **34**, 143.   [285]

Baker, L. E. and Carrel, A. (1928). "The effect of digests of pure proteins on cell proliferation." *J. exp. Med.*, **47**, 353.   [364, 366, 369, 395]

Baker, S. L. (1939) "The General Pathology of Bone," in *A Textbook of X-ray Diagnosis* (S. C. Shanks and P. Kirby, eds) 3rd Ed., Vol. 4. p. 55. H. K. Lewis & Co., London.

Bard, L., (1886). "La specificite cellulaire et l'histogenese chez l'embryon." *Archs. Physiol.* Ser. 3, **7**, 406.   [393]

Barnes, R. and Catto, M. (1966). "Chondrosarcoma of bone." *J. Bone Jt Surg.*, 48B, 729.   [386]

Barns, J. W. (1964). "The Hippocratic Oath. An early text." *Br. Med. J.*, **3**, 567.
[13]

Bassoe, H. H., Aarskoy, D., Thomsen, T. and Stoe, K. F. (1965). "Cortisol production rate in patients with acute bacterial infections." *Acta. med. scand.*, **177**, 701.   [113, 276]

Beaumont, G. D. (1965). "The effects of surgical exclusion of air from pneumatized bone." M.S. Thesis, University of Adelaide.   [84]

Beaumont, G. D. (1967a). "The intraosseous vasculature of the ulna of *Gallus domesticus.*" *J. Anat.*, **101**, 543.   [84]

Beaumont, G. D. (1967b). "Cholesterol granuloma." *J. oto-lar. Soc. Aust.*, **2**, 28.   [280]

Beck, J. C. and McGarry, E. E. (1962). "Physiological importance of cortisol." *Br. med. Bull.*, **18**, 134.   [234]

Belchier, J. (1735–36a). "An account of the bones of animals being changed to a red colour by Aliment only." *Phil. Trans. R. Soc.*, **39**, 286.   [16]

Belchier, J. (1735–36b). "II. A further account of the bones of animals being made red by Aliment only." *Phil. Trans. R. Soc.*, **39**, 299.   [16]

Bell, B. (1824). "Remarks on Interstitial Absorption of the Neck of the Thighbone." Maclachlan and Stewart, Edinburgh.   [17]

Benson, A. A. (1968). "The cell membrane: a lipoportein monolayer." *Membrane Models and the Formation of Biological Membranes* (L. Bolis and B. A. Pethica, eds), p 190 North-Holland, Amsterdam.

Berkin, C. R., Yeoman, P. M., Williamson, G. M., Zinneman, K. and Dexter, F. (1957). "Freeze-dried bone grafts." *Lancet*, **1**, 730.   [378]

Berliner, D. L. (1965). "Studies of the mechanisms by which cells become resistant to corticosteroids." *Cancer Res.*, **25**, 1085.   [28, 150, 234, 366, 370, 371]

Berliner, D. L. and Dougherty, T. F. (1958). "Metabolism of cortisol by loose connective tissue *in vitro*." *Proc. Soc. exp. Biol. Med.*, **98**, 3.   [239]

Berliner, D. L. and Dougherty, T. F. (1960). "Influence of reticuloendothelial and other cells on the metabolic fate of steroids." *Ann. N.Y. Acad. Sci.*, **88**, 14.   [234]

Berliner, D. L. and Dougherty, T. F. (1961). "Hepatic and extrahepatic regulation of corticosteroids." *Pharmac. Rev.*, **13**, 329.   [233, 234, 270, 370, 396]

Berliner, D. L. and Ruhmann, A. G. (1966). "Comparison of the growth of fibroblasts under the influence of 11B hydroxy- and 11 keto- corticosteroids." *Endocrinology*, **78**, 373.   [29, 30]

Berliner, M. L., Berliner, D. L. and Dougherty, T. F. (1956). "Chemical transformation of cortisol-4-C¹⁴ by lymphatic leukemia cells *in vitro*." *Proc. Am. Ass. Cancer Res.*, **2**, 94.   [396]

Berzelius, J. J. (1835). *Lehrbuch der Chemie*, 3rd Ed. Vol. 4. Arnold, Dresden. [60]

Berzelius, J. J. (1845). "Om basisk fosforsyrad Kalkjord." *Ann. chem. pharm.*, **53**, 286.   [60]

Bjerrum, N. (1936). "Investigations in the solubility of calcium phosphates." Report of Nordic (19th. Scand.) Scientist Meeting. p. 344.   [60, 61]

Bjerrum, N. (1949). "Solubilities of calcium phosphates, in Selected papers." p. 245. Einer Munksgaard, Copenhagen.   [60, 61]

Bjerrum, N. (1958). Calcium orthophosphates: 1. The solid calcium orthophosphates. 2. Complex formation in solutions of calcium and phosphate ions. *Mat. Fys. Medd. Dan. Vid. Selsk.*, **31**, No. 7. (English Translation: *AERE Trans.* 941/1959. HMSO London).   [60, 72]

Bliss, E. L., Mijeon, C. J., Branch, C. H. N. and Samuels, L. T. (1956). "Reaction of the adrenal cortex to emotional stress." *Psychosom. Med.*, **18**, 56.
[113, 280, 281]

Blumenthal, H. T., Lansing, A. I. and Wheeler, P. A. (1944). "Calcification of the media of the human aorta and its relation to intimal ateriosclerosis, ageing and disease." *Am. J. Path.*, **20**, 665.   [353]

Boldero, J. L. and Kemp, H. S. (1966). "Radiological changes in Perthe's disease." *Br. J. Radiol.*, **39**, 744.   [96]

Bolton, C. H., Hampton, J. R. and Mitchell, J. R. A. (1967). "Nature of the transferable factor which causes abnormal platelet behaviour in vascular disease." *Lancet*, **ii**, 1101.   [114, 295]

Bolton, C. H., Hampton, J. R. and Mitchell, J. R. A. (1968). "Effect of oral contraceptive agents on platelets and plasma phospholipids." *Lancet*, **i**, 1336.
[286]

Bond, W. R., Matthews, J. L. and Finney, J. W. (1967). "The influence of regional oxygenation on osteoradionecrosis." *Oral Surg.*, **23**, 99.   [181, 368, 423]

Boyle, P. E., Bessey, O. A. and Howe, P. R. (1940). "Rate of dentine formation in incisor teeth of guineapigs on normal and on ascorbic acid deficient diets." *Archs Path.*, **30**, 90.   [183]

Bragg, W. H. and Bragg, W. L. (1913). "The reflection of X-rays by crystals." *Proc. R. Soc.*, **88A**, 428.   [37]

Brånemark, P-I. (1964). "Capillary form and function: The microcirculation of granulation tissue." 3rd. Europe Conf. Microcirculation (Jerusalem), **7**, 9.
[374]

Brånemark, P-I., Breine, U., Johansson, B., Roylance, P. J., Rockert, H. and Yoffey, J. M. (1964). "Regeneration of bone marrow: A clinical and experimental study following removal of bone marrow by curettage." *Acta anat.*, **59**, 1.   [259]

428   REFERENCES AND AUTHOR INDEX

Bredig, M. A. (1933). "The apatite structure of the inorganic substance of bone and tooth." *Hoppe. Seyler's Z. physiol. Chem.*, **216**, 239.   [76]
Br. Med. J. (1969). "Oral contraception and depression." Leading Article. **4**, 380.   [285]
Buhr, A. J. and Cooke, A. M. (1959). "Fracture patterns." *Lancet,* i, 531.
                                                              [278, 314]
Bullock, G., White, A. M. and Worthington, J. (1968). "The effects of catabolic and anabolic steroids on amino acid incorporation by skeletal muscle ribosomes." *Biochem. J.*, **108**, 417.   [235, 248]
Bullough, W. S. (1952). "The energy relations of mitotic activity." *Biol. Rev.*, **27**, 133.   [180, 182, 360, 363, 366]
Bunney, W. E., Mason, J. W. and Hamburg, D. A. (1965). "Correlations between behaviourable variables and urinary 17-hydroxycorticosteroids." *Psychosom. Med.*, **27**, 299.   [113, 280]
Bunting, C. H. (1906). "Formation of true bone with cellular red marrow in a sclerotic aorta." *J. exp. Med.*, **8**, 365.   [149]
Burkhart, J. M. and Jowsey, J. (1967). "Parathyroid and thyroid hormones in the development of immobilization osteoporosis." *Endocrinology*, **81**, 1053.
                                                         [173, 180, 233]
Burrows, F. G. O. (1965). "Avascular necrosis of bone complicating steroid therapy." *Br. J. Radiol.*, **38**, 309.   [285]
Bursten, B. and Russ, J. J. (1965). "Pre-operative psychological state and corticosteroid levels of surgical patients." *Psychosom. Med.*, **27**, 309
                                                              [113, 277]
Burwell, R. G. (1966). "Studies in the transplantation of bone. VIII. Treated composite homograft—autografts of cancellous bone: an analysis of induction mechanisms in bone transplantation." *J. Bone Jt. Surg.*, **48B**, 532.   [376]
Burwell, R. G., Gowland, G. and Dexter, F. (1963). "Studies in the transplantation of bone: VI. Further observations concerning the antigenicity of homologous cortical and cancellous bone." *J. Bone Jt. Surg.*, **45B**, 597.   [378]
Bustad, L. K. (1969). "Effects of single or fractionated X-irradiation and of bone-seeking radionuclides on mammals. A Review." (California Univ. Davis Radiobiology Lab.). CONF-690303, pp. 231–53. Abstract in Nuclear Science Abstracts.   [420, 422]
Bustad, L. K., Goldman, M., Rosenblatt, L. S., McKelvie, D. H. and Hertzendorf, I. I. (1969). "Hematopoietic changes in beagles fed ^{90}Sr." *Delayed Effects of Bone-seeking Radionuclides* (C. W. Mays, ed.), p 279 University of Utah Press, Salt Lake City.   [420, 422]
Cameron, G. R. (1952). "Pathology of the Cell." Oliver and Boyd, Edinburgh.
                                                              [365, 393]
Campbell, J. and Rastogi, K. S. (1966). "Growth hormone induced diabetes and high levels of serum insulin in dogs." *Diabetes*, **15**, 30.   [230]
Campbell, J. and Rastogi, K. S. (1967). "Effects of growth hormone on the rate of disappearance of insulin from blood in depancreatized dogs." *Metabolism*, **16**, 562.   [230, 293]
Campbell, J. B., Bassett, C. A. L. and Luzio, J. (1970). "Replacement of deficits in peripheral nerves and skull bone with frozen irradiated homografts. IAEA-PL-333/8." *Sterilization and Preservation of Biological Tissues by Ionizing Radiation*, p. 59. IAEA, Vienna.   [379]
Campbell, J. G. and Appleby, E. C. (1966). "Tumours in young chickens bred for rapid body growth (Broiler Chickens). A study of 351 cases." *J. Path. Bact.*, **92**, 77.   [382]

Caniggia, A., Gennari, C., Bianchi, V. and Guideri, R. (1963). "Intestinal absorption of ^{45}Ca in senile osteoporosis." *Acta. med. scand.*, **173**, 613.   [184, 308]

Cannon, W. B. and Mendenhal, W. (1914). "Factors affecting the coagulation time of the blood." *Am. J. Physiol.*, **34**, 232.   [114]

Carlson, L. A. and Ostman, J. (1961). "Effect of salicylates on plasma free fatty acid in normal and diabetic subjects." *Metabolism*, **10**, 781.   [291]

Carlström, D. (1955), "X-ray crystallographic studies on apatites and calcified structures." *Acta. radiol.*, Suppl. 121.   [74]

Carrel, A. (1924). "Tissue culture and cell physiology." *Physiol. Rev.*, **4**, 1.   [371]

Carrel, A. and Baker L. E. (1926). "The chemical nature of substances required for cell multiplication." *J. exp. Med.*, **44**, 503.   [363, 366]

Cater, D. B., Basergar, R. and Lisco, H. (1959). "Studies on the induction of bone and soft tissue tumours in rats by gamma radiation and the effect of growth hormone and thryoxyn." *Br. J. Cancer*, **13**, 214.   [404]

Chapman, D. (1968). "Physical studies of biological membranes and their constituents." *Membrane Models and the Formation of Biological Membranes* (L. Bolis and B. A. Pethica, eds), p. 6, North-Holland, Amsterdam.   [366]

Chapman, J. M., Reeder, L. G., Massey, F. J., Borun, E. R., Picklen, B., Browning, G. G., Coulson, A. H. and Zimmerman, D. H. (1966). "Relationships of stress, tranquilizers, and serum cholesterol levels in a sample population under study for coronary heart disease." *Am. J. Epidem.*, **83**, 537.   [112, 277]

Christian, J. J. and Davis, D. (1957). "Relation of adrenal weight to social rank of mice." *Proc. Soc. exp. Biol. Med.*, **94**, 728.   [282]

Clark, E. R. and Clark, E. L. (1935). "Observations on changes in blood vascular endothelium in the living animal." *Am. J. Anat.*, **57**, 385.   [371]

Clark, G. M. and Mills, D. (1962). "Corticosteroid therapy of rheumatoid arthritis supplemented with methandrostenolone." *Arthritis Rheum.* **5**, 156.   [292]

Clarke, W. J., Howard, E. B. and Hackett, P. L. (1969). "Strontium-90 induced neoplasia in swine." *Delayed Effects of Bone-seeking Radionuclides* (C. W. Mays, ed.), p. 263. University of Utah Press, Salt Lake City.   [422]

Clayson, D. B. (1962). *Chemical Carcinogenesis* J. and A. Churchill, Ltd., London.   [380]

Clayton, B. P. (1959). "The action of fixatives on the unmasking of lipid. *Q. J. microsc. Sci.*, **100**, 269.   [361, 364]

Cochran, C. H., Jee, W. S. S., Stover, B. J. and Taylor, G. N. (1962). "Liver injury in beagles with ^{239}Pu distribution, dosage and damage." *Hlth Phys.*, **8**, 699.   [403]

Cooke, R. T. (1966). "Hashimoto's thyroiditis and Paget's disease of bone." *Lancet*, **ii**, 751.   [325]

Copp, H. C. (1964). "Parathyroids, calcitonin and control of plasma calcium." Recent *Prog. Horm. Res.*, **20**, 59.   [231]

Corni,, A., Coster, A. del Copinshi, G. and Franckson, J. R. (1965). "Effect of muscular exercise on the plasma level of cortisol in man." *Acta endocr.*, **48**, 163.   [109, 117, 282, 283, 290]

De Coursey, E. (1948). "Human pathologic anatomy of ionizing radiation effects of the atomic bomb explosions." *Milit. Surg.*, **102**, 427.   [421]

Courts, A. and Little, K. (1963). "Citrate-promoted helix formation in gelatin: 2. The structure of some precipitated gelatins." *Biochem. J.*, **87**, 383.   [35]

Cunliffe, W. J., Black, M. M., Hall, R., Johnson, I. D. A., Hudgson, P., Shuster, S., Gudmundsson, T. V., Joplin, G. F., Williams, E. D., Woodhouse, N. J. Y., Gelante, L. and MacIntyre, I. (1968). "A calcitonin—secreting thyroid carcinoma." *Lancet*, **ii**, 63.   [231, 232]

Daniel, D. G., Bloom, A. L., Giddings, J. C., Campbell, H. and Turnbull, A. C. (1968). "Increased Factor IX levels in puerperin during administration of diethyl stilboestrol." *Br. med. J.*, **i**, 801.   [290]

Daniel, D. G., Campbell, H. and Turnbull, A. C. (1962). "Oestrogens and puerpural thrombosis." *Lancet*, **2**, 287.   [275, 290]

Danielli, J. F. (1954). *Recent Developments in Cell Physiology* (J. A. Kitching, ed.), Butterworth Scientific Publications, London.   [360]

Darling, A. I. (1956). "Studies of the early lesion of enamel caries with transmitted light, polarized light and radiography." *Br. dent. J.*, **101**, 289.

Darling, A. I. (1958). "Studies of the early lesion of enamel caries: Its nature, mode of spread, and point of entry." *Br. dent. J.*, **105**, 119.   [300]

Davidson, E. A. (1964). "Hormonal control of connective tissue metabolism." *Proc. 2nd. Int. Congr. Endocrinology*, p. 398. Publ. Exerpta Medica Foundation.   [35, 232]

Davidson, E. A. and Small W. (1963). "Metabolism *in vivo* of connective tissue polysaccharides." *Biochim. Biophys. Acta*, **69**, 445.   [35, 181]

Davis, J., Morrill, R., Fawcett, J., Upton, U., Bondy, P. K. and Spiro, H. M. (1962). "Apprehension and elevated serum cortisol levels." *J. psychosom. Res.*, **6**, 83.   [113, 277]

Dawson, I. M., Hocsack, J. and Wyburn, G. M. (1955). "Observations on the Nissl's substance, cytoplasmic filaments and the nuclear membrane of spinal ganglion cells." *Proc. R. Soc. B.*, **144**, 132.   [360, 365]

Dempster, W. J. (1969). "Renal transplantation and leucocyte migration." *Br. med. J.*, **4**, 428.   [378]

Diamant, B., Karlsson, J. and Nachenson, A. (1968). "Correlation between lactate levels and pH in discs of patients with lumbar rhizopathies." *Experientia*, **24**, 1195.   [343]

Doak, P. B., Montgomerie, J. Z., North, J. K. D. and Smith F. (1968). "Reticulum cell sarcoma after renal homotransplantation and azathioprine and prednisone therapy." *Br. med. J.*, **iv**, 747.   [397]

Dodds, C. (1961). "Rime and reason in endocrinology." *J. Endocr.*, **23**.   [290]

Dodgson, C. L. (1896). "Symbolic Logic." Part 1. *Elementary*. 3rd Ed. Macmillan Co., London.   [276]

Dogherty, D. G., Congdon, C. C., Makinodan, T. and Hollaender, A. (1958). "Modification of the biological response of mammals to whole-body irradiation." In *Radiation Biology and Medicine* (W. D. Claus, ed.), p. 370–374. U.S.A.E.C. Addison–Wesley Publishing Co, New York.   [421]

Dooren, A. van and Dougherty, T. F. (1957). "Steroid hormone conversions by osteosarcoma cells of beagle dogs." *Proc. Am. Ass. Cancer Res.*, **2**, 257.   [396]

Dorfman, H. F., Norman, A. and Wolff, K. (1966). "Fibrosarcoma complicating bone rarefaction in a caisson worker." *J. Bone Jt Surg.*, **48A**, 528.   [384]

Dougherty, J. H. (1962). "Some hematological responses to internal irradiation in the beagle." In *Some Aspects of Internal Irradiation*, p. 79. Pergamon Press, Oxford.   [422]

Dougherty, J. H. and Taylor, G. N. (1968). "Hemopoietic disorders in beagles injected with ^{90}Sr", p. 90. COO–119–237. Abstract in *Nuclear Science Abstracts*.   [422]

Dougherty, T. F. (1952). "Effect of hormones on lymphatic tissue." *Physiol. Rev.*, **32**, 379.   [116, 182, 183, 261]

Dougherty, T. F. and White, A. (1944). "Influence of hormones on lymphoid tissue structure and function. Role of pituitary adrenotrophic hormone in regulation of lymphocytes and other cellular elements of blood." *Endo-crinology*, **31**, 1.   [116, 290, 402]

Dougherty, T. F. and White, A. (1946). "Pituitary—adrenal cortical control of lymphocyte structure and function as revealed by experimental X-radiation." *Endocrinology*, **39**, 370.   [116]

Dougherty, T. F. and Dougherty, J. H. (1953). "Blood: formed elements." *Ann. Rev. Physiol.*, **15**, 195.   [113, 116]

Dougherty, T. F. and Schneebeli, G. L. (1955). "The use of steroids as anti-inflammatory agents." *Ann. N.Y. Acad. Sci.*, **61**, 328.   [370]

Dougherty, T. F. and Mays, C. W. (1969). "Bone cancer induced by internally deposited emitters in beagles." *Radiation-Induced Cancer*, p. 361. IAEA Vienna.   [419]

Dougherty, T. F., Berliner, M. L. and Berliner, D. L. (1960). "Hormonal influence on lymphocyte differentiation from RES cells." *Ann. N.Y. Acad. Sci.*, **88**, 78.   [370, 396]

Dougherty, T. F., Berliner, D. L. and Berliner, M. L. (1961). "Corticosteroid—Tissue Interactions." *Metabolism*, **10**, 966.   [28, 30, 182, 194, 238, 370, 396]

Dougherty, T. F., Berliner, M. L. and Berliner, D. L. (1962). "Hormonal control of lymphocyte production and destruction." *Prog. Hemat.*, **3**, 155. [283, 396]

Dougherty, T. F., Berliner, M. L., Schneebeli, G. L. and Berliner, D. L. (1964). 'Hormonal control of lymphatic structure and function." *Ann. N.Y. Acad. Sci.*, **113**, 825.   [396]

Drinker, C. K., Field, M. E. and Homans, J. (1934). "The experimental production of oedema and elephantiasis as a result of lymphatic obstruction." *Am. J. Physiol.*, **108**, 509.   [160, 161]

Du Hammel, M. (1737–38). "Observations and experiments with Madder-root, which has the faculty of tinging the bones of living animals of a red colour." *Phil. Trans. R. Soc.*, **40**, 390.   [16]

Dungworth, D. L., Goldman, M., Switzer, J. W. and McKelvie, D. H. (1969). "Development of a myeloproliferative disorder in beagles continuously exposed to ^{90}Sr." *Blood*, **34**, 610.   [422]

Dyson, E. D. (1966). "A specific activity method for derived working limits of phosphorus 32." *Hlth Phys.*, **12**, 1521.   [404]

Edington, G. M., Ward, A. H., Judd, J. M. and Mole, R. H. (1956). "The acute lethal effects in monkeys of radiostrontium." *J. Path. Bact.*, **71**, 277. [420]

Elkeles, A. (1953). "Peptic ulcers in the aged and gastric carcinoma in their relationship to arteriosclerosis: A roentgenological study." *Am. J. Roentg.*, **70**, 797. [354]

Elkeles, A. (1957). "A comparative radiological study of calcified atheroma in males and females over 50 years of age." *Lancet*, **ii**, 714.   [353, 354]

Elkeles, A. (1964). "Gastric ulcer in the aged and calcified atherosclerosis." *Am. J. Roent.*, **91**, 774.

Elkeles, A. (1966a). "Sex differences in the calcification of the costal cartilages." *J. Am. Geriat. Soc.*, **14**, 456.   [351]

Elkles, A. (1966b). "Sex differences in the ageing process of the larger arteries." *Proc. 7th Int. Cong. Gerontol.* Paper 329, p. 461.   [353, 354, 355]

Erf, L. A. and Herbert, P. H. (1944). "Primary and secondary myelofibrosis (a clinical and pathological study of 13 cases of fibrosis of the bone marrow). *Ann. Int. Med.*, **21**, 863.   [422]

Evans, R. D., Koane, A. T., Kolenkow, R. J., Neal, W. R. and Sharaham, M. M. (1969). "Radiogenic tumours in the radium and mesothorium cases studied at M.I.T." *Delayed Effects of Bone-seeking Nuclides* (C. W. Mays, ed.), p. 157. University of Utah Press, Salt Lake City.   [402]

Ewing, J. (1926). "Radiation Osteitis." *Acta radiol.*, **6**, 399.   [404]

Ewing, J. (1940). *Neoplastic Diseases.* 4th Ed. W. B. Saunders Company, London and New York.   [380 397]

Eyre-Brook, A. L. and Price, C. H. G. (1969). "Fibrosarcoma of bone: Review of fifty consecutive cases from the Bristol Bone Tumour Registry." *J. Bone Jt Surg.*, **51B**, 20.   [386]

Eyre-Brook, A. L., Bailey, R. A. J. and Price, C. H. G. (1969). "Infantile pseudarthrosis of the tibia: Three cases treated successfully by delayed autogenous by-pass graft, with some comments on the causative lesion." *J. Bone Jt Surg.*, **51B**, 604.   [376, 377]

Faccini, J. M. (1969). Fluoride-induced hyperplasia of the parathyroid glands." *Proc. R. Soc. Med.*, **62**, 241.   [173]

Farmer, J. and Little, K. (1969). "Preparation of sections of plastics and polymers for the electron microscope." *Br. Polymer J.*, **1**, 259.   [43]

Farquhar, M. G., Wissig, S. L. and Palade, G. E. (1961). "Glomerular permeability 1. Ferratin transfer across the normal glomerular capillary wall." *J. exp. Med.*, **113**, 47.   [238]

Fell, H. (1933). "Chondrogenesis in cultures of endosteum." *Proc. R. Soc. B.*, **112**, 417.   [26]

Finkel, A. J., Miller, C. E. and Hasterlik, R. J. (1969). "Radium-induced malignant tumours in man. *Delayed Effects of Bone-seeking Radionuclides.* (C. W. Mays, ed.), p. 227. University of Utah Press, Salt Lake City.   [403]

Fischman, D. A. and Hay, E. D. (1962). "Origin of osteoclasts from mononuclear leucocytes in regenerating newt limbs." *Anat. Rec.*, **143**, 329.   [174]

Fisher, S. H. (1963). "Psychological factors and heart disease." *Circulation*, **27**, 113.   [112]

Forbes, J. C., Rudolph, R. A. and Petterson, O. M. (1966). "Effect of hydrocortisone feeding on concentration of free fatty acids and other lipids of rabbit serum." *Proc. Soc. exp. Biol. Med.*, **122**, 299.   [114]

Frank, J. A. and Dougherty, T. F. (1953). "Cytoplasmic budding of human lymphocytes produced by cortison and hydrocortisone in *in vitro* preparations." *Proc. Soc. exp. Biol. Med.*, **82**, 17.   [370]

Friedman, M. and Rosenman, P. H. (1957). "Comparison of fat intake of American men and women. Possible relationship to incidence of clinical coronary artery disease." *Circulation*, **16**, 339.   [111]

Friedman, M., Rosenman, R. H. and Carrol, V. (1958). "Changes in the serum cholesterol and blood clotting time in men subjected to cyclic variation of occupational stress." *Circulation*, **17**, 852.   [112, 279]

Fryer, D. I. (1969). "Subatmospheric Decompression Sickness in Man." NATO AGARD, No. 125.   [316, 319]

Gaillard. P. J. (1955). "Parathyroid gland and bone *in vitro* I." *Expl. Cell Res.*, suppl. **3**, 154.   [168, 232]

Gaillard, P. J. (1959). "Parathyroid gland and bone *in vitro* VI." *Devel. Biol.*, **1**, 152.   [186, 232]

Gardner, E. V. and Heslington, H. V. (1946). "Osteosarcomas from intravenous beryllium compounds in rabbits." *Fedn Proc. Fedn Am. Socs exp. Biol.*, **5**, 221.   [380, 382]

Geizer, M. and Trueta, J. (1958). "Muscle action, bone rarefaction and bone formation." *J. Bone Jt Surg.*, **40B**, 282.   [167, 302]

Gey, G. O. and Thalhimer, W. (1924). "Observations on the effect of insulin introduced into the medium of tissue culture." *J. Am. Med. Ass.*, **82**, 1609.   [370]

Gibbons, H. L., Plechus, J. L., Chandler, E. H. and Ellis, J. W. (1966). "Alcohol-induced hypoglycemia as a factor in aircraft accidents." *Aerospace Med.*, **37**, 959.   [293]

Gibbons, J. R. P., Alladine, F. F. and Little, K. (1969). "Cholesterol deposition on aortic prostheses." *Br. Med. J.*, **1**, 709.   [114]

Gilbert, R. S. and Johnson, H. A. (1966). "Stress fractures in military recruits: a review of twelve years' experience." *Milit. Med.*, **131**, 716.   [217]

Goldhaber, P. (1963). "Some chemical factors influencing bone resorption in tissue culture," in *Mechanisms of Hard Tissue Destruction*. Am. Ass. Adv. Sci., Washington.   [180]

Goldman, M., Della Rosa, R. J. and McKelvie, D. H. (1969). "Metabolic, dosimetric and pathological consequences in the skeletons of beagles fed ^{90}Sr." *Delayed Effects of Bone-seeking Radionuclides* (C. W. Mays, ed.), p. 61. University of Utah Press, Salt Lake City.   [420]

Goodlad, G. A. and Munro, H. N. (1959). "Diet and the action of cortisone on protein metabolism." *Biochem. J.*, **73**, 343.   [235]

Goodman, A. H. and Sherman, M. S. (1963). "Post-irradiation fracture of femoral neck." *J. Bone Jt Surg.*, **45A**, 723.   [414, 422]

Grant, E. C. G. (1968). "Relation between headaches from oral contraceptives and development of endometrial arterioles." *Br. Med. J.*, **3**, 402.   [285]

Grant, E. C. G. and Pryse-Davies, J. (1968). "Effect of oral contraceptives on depressive mood changes and on endometrial mono-amine oxidase and phosphatases." *Br. Med. J.*, **3**, 777.   [283]

Grosser, B. I., Sweat, M. L., Berliner, D. L. and Dougherty, T. F. (1962). "Comparison of cortisol metabolism by two variants of cultured fibroblasts." *Archs Biochem.*, **96**, 259.   [396]

Groves, E. W. H. (1913–14). "Experimental study of operative treatment of fractuers." *Br. J. Surg.*, **1**, 438.   [376]

Gruner, W. and McConnell (1937). "The problem of the carbonate-apatites." *Z. Kristallogr. Miner.*, **97**, 208.   [76]

Guicciardi, E. and Little K. (1967). "Some observations on the effects of blood and a fibrinolytic enzyme on articular cartilage in the rabbit." *J. Bone Jt Surg.*, **49B**, 342.   [49, 327]

Haam, E. von and Cappel, L. (1940). "Effect of hormones upon cells grown *in vitro*. II The effect of the hormones from the thyroid, pancreas and adrenal gland." *Am. J. Cancer.*, **39**, 354.   [375]

Ham, A. W. (1932). "Cartilage and Bone" *Special Cytology* (E. V. Cowdry, ed.), Vol. 2, p. 979. Hoeber, New York.   [150]

Ham, A. W. (1965) *Histology*, 5th Ed. Pitman Medical Publishing Co. and J. B. Lippincott Co., London.   [259]

Hammack, B. L. and Enneking, W. F. (1960). "Comparative vascularization of autogenous and homogenous bone transplants." *J. Bone Jt Surg.*, **42A**, 811.   [378]

Hancox, N. M. (1949). "Motion picture observations on osteoclasts *in vitro*." *J. Physiol., Lond.*, **110**, 205.   [174]

Hancox, N. (1956). "The Osteoclast." *The Biochemistry and Physiology of Bone*. (G. H. Bourne, ed.). Academic Press, London and New York.   [166, 169]

Harper, R. M. J. (1962). *Evolution and Illness*. E. & S. Livingstone, Edinburgh.   [283, 397]

Harrison, C. V. and Lennox, B. (1948). "Heart block in Osteitis Deformans." *Brit. Heart J.*, **10**, 167.   [356]

Harrison, M. H., Schajowicz, F. and Trueta, J. (1953). "Osteoarthritis of the hip:

a study of the nature and evolution of the disease." *J. Bone Jt Surg.*, **3 5B**, 598.   [327]

Harvey, W. H. (1907). "Experimental bone formation in arteries." *J. med. Res.*, **17**, 25.

Hasse, K. E. (1841). "Special pathological anatomy: An anatomical description of the diseases of the organs of circulation and respiration." Trans. from the German (W. E. Swaine, ed.). London Sydenham Soc. 1846.   [149, 350]

Hechter, O. (1955). "Hormone action at the cell membrane." *Mechanisms of Hormone Action* (P. Karlson, ed.). Academic Press, London and New York.   [230, 293]

Henneman, P. H. and Wallack, S. (1957). "A review of prolonged use of estrogens and androgens in postmenopausal and senile osteoporosis." *Arch. int. Med.*, **100**, 715.   [307]

Hicks, J. F. (1965). "The health of children's feet: the manufacturers problem—how to compromise." *Br. med. J.*, Suppl. (May), 182.   [327]

Hippocrates (B.C.*a*). *The Genuine works of Hippocrates*. Translated by Francis Adams (1849). London Sydenham Soc.   [14, 15, 17]

Hippocrates (B.C.*b*). *The Presages of Divine Hippocrates*. The whole collected and translated by Peter Lovve, Scottish-man (1634). Printed by Thomas Purfoot, London.   [14]

Hökfelt, B. (1961). "The effect of smoking on the production of adreno-cortical hormones." *Acta Med. scand.* Suppl., **170**, 123.   [276]

Howell, W. H. (1890). "Observations upon the occurrence, structure and function of the giant cells of the marrow." *J. Morph.*, **4**, 117.   [166, 259]

Hurley, J. V., Ham, K. N. and Ryan, G. B. (1969). "The mechanism of the delayed response of the skin of hairless mice and of rats to X-irradiation." *Pathology*, **1**, 3.   [412]

Irey, N. S., Manion, W. C. and Taylor, H. B. (1970). "Vascular lesions in women taking oral contraceptives." *Archs Path.*, **79**, 1.   [285, 286]

Irving, J. T. (1960). "Histochemical changes in early stages of ossification." *Clin. Ortho.*, **17**, 92.

Irving, J. T. and Handelman, C. S. (1963). "Bone destruction by multinucleated giant cells." In *Mechanisms of hard tissue destruction*. p. 515. Am. Ass. Adv. Sci., Washington.   [178]

Isaacs, W. A. and Hayhoe, F. G. J. (1967). "Steroid hormones in sickle-cell disease." *Nature, Lond.*, **215**, 1139.   [270]

Isaacs, W. A., Little, K., Currey, J. D. and Tarlo, L. B. H. (1963). "Collagen and a cellulose-like substance in fossil dentine and bone." *Nature, Lond.*, **197**, 192.   [37]

Jacobowitz, D., Marks, B. H. and Vernikus-Danellis (1963). "Effect of acute stress on the pituitary gland: Uptake of serine–1–C^{14} into ACTH." *Endocrinology*, **72**, 592.   [116]

Jacoby, F. (1938). "On the identity of blood monocytes and tissue macrophages; their growth rates *in vitro*." *J. Physiol., Lond.*, **93**, 48P.   [173]

Jee, W. S. S. (1962). "Histopathological endpoints in compact bones receiving alpha irradiation." *Some Aspects of Internal Irradiation*, p. 95. Pergamon Press, Oxford.   [403, 418]

Jee, W. S. S. and Arnold, J. S. (1960). "Effect of internally deposited radioisotopes upon blood vessels of cortical bone." *Proc. Soc. exp. Biol. Med.*, **105**, 351.   [419]

Jee, W. S. S. and Arnold, J. S. (1961). "The toxicity of plutonium deposited in skeletal tissues of beagles: 1. The relation of the distribution of plutonium to the sequence of histopathologic bone changes." *Lab. Invest.*, **10**, 797. [412]

Jee, W. S. S., Stover, B. J., Taylor, G. N. and Christensen, W. R. (1962a). "The skeletal toxicity of ^{239}Pu in adult beagles." *Hlth Phys.*, **8**, 599. [418]

Jee, W. S. S., Arnold, J. S., Cochran, T. H., Twente, J. A. and Mical, R. S. (1962b). "Relationship of microdistribution of alpha particles to damage." *Some Aspects of Internal Irradiation*, p. 27. Pergamon Press, Oxford. [403, 405]

Jee, W. S. S. and Nolan, P. D. (1963). "Origin of osteoclasts from the fusion of phagocytes." *Nature, Lond.*, **200**, 325. [170, 233]

Jee, W. S. S., Bartley, M. H., Dockum, N. L., Yee, J. and Kenner, G. H. (1969). "Vascular changes in bones following bone-seeking radionuclides." *Delayed Effects of Bone-seeking Radionuclides* (C. W. Mays, ed.), p. 437. University of Utah Press, Salt Lake City [419, 421]

Jellinek, S (1909) *Atlas der Elektropathologie* Urban & Schwarzenberg, Germany. [368]

Jellinek, S (1955) *Atlas zur Spurenkunde der Elektrizitat* Plate VI, figs 25 to 27. Springer-Verlag, Wein, Berlin. [198]

Jenkins, J. S. and Sampson, P. A. (1966). "The conversion of cortisone to cortisol and prednisone to prednisolone in man." *Proc. R. Soc. Med.*, **59**, 603. [234, 291]

Jenkins, J. S., Lowe, R. D. and Titterington, E. (1964). "Effect of adrenocortical hormones on release of free fatty acids and uptake of glucose in human peripheral tissues." *Clin. Sci.*, **26**, 421. [114, 291]

Johnson, C. C., Deics, W. P. and French, R. S. (1965). "Effects of changes in parathyroid status and calcium equilibrium on bone matix metabolism." *Proc. Soc. exp. Biol. Med.*, **118**, 551. [233]

Johnson, L. C. (1953). "A general theory of bone tumours." *Bull. N.Y. Acad. Med.*, **29**, 164. [388, 393]

Johnson, L. C. (1964). "Morphological Analysis in Pathology." *Bone Biodynamics* (H. M. Frost, ed.), p. 543. Little, Brown & Co., Boston.
[51, 87, 169, 176, 177, 212, 217, 303, 317, 318, 324, 392]

Johnson, L. C., Vettner, H. and Putschar, W. G. J. (1962). "Sarcomas arising in bone cysts." *Virchows Arch. path. Anat. Physiol.*, **335**, 428. [384]

Johnson, L. C., Todd Stradford, H., Geis, R. W., Dineen, J. R. and Kerley, E. (1963). "Histogenesis of stress fractures." *J. Bone Jt Surg.*, **45A**, 1542. [217]

Johnson, L. C., Hobbs, C. S., Merriman, G. M., Sharpe, J. L., Greenwood, D. A. and Largent, L. (1964). "Histogenesis and mechanisms in the development of osteofluorosis." *Fluorine Chemistry* (J. H. Simmons, ed.), Vol. IV. Academic Press, London and New York. [135]

Jones, J. P. (1971). "Alcoholism, hypercortisonism, fat embolism and osseous avascular necrosis." *Idiopathic Ischemic Necrosis of the Femoral Head in Adults* (W. Zinn, ed.), pp. 112–32. University Park Press, Baltimore, Md., USA. [285]

Jowsey, J. (1966). "Bone formation and resorption in bone disorders." *Calcified Tissues* (Fleisch et al., eds), p. 67. Springer-Verlag, Berlin. [303]

Jowsey, J. and Orvis, A. L. (1967). "Comparative deposition of ^{45}Ca, ^{65}Zn, and ^{91}Y in bone." *Radiation Res.*, **31**, 693. 402

Jowsey, J., Kelly, P. J., Riggs, B. L., Bianco, A. J., Scholz, D. A. and Gershon-Cohen, J. (1965). "Quantitative microradiographic studies of normal and osteoporotic bone." *J. Bone Jt Surg.*, **47A**, 785. [303]

Kaplan, A. S. (1959). "The nature of the neoplastic transformation in lymphoid tumour induction." *CIBA Foundation Symposium on Carcinogenesis*, p. 233.[415]

Katzman, H., Waugh, T. and Berdon, W. (1969). "Skeletal changes following irradiation of childhood tumours." *J. Bone Jt Surg.*, **51A**, 825. [412]

436 REFERENCES AND AUTHOR INDEX

Kayanga, F., Scott, M. G. and Scott, P. P. (1965). "Vascular changes in bone in calcium deficient kittens." *Proc. Nutr. Soc.*, **24**, iv. [184, 231]

Kemp, H. B. S. (1965). "Some observations on Perthe's disease." *J. Bone Jt Surg.*, **47B**, 193. [93, 95, 165, 179]

Kemp, H. B. S. (1965-6). "Factors influencing cellular proliferation in fracture repair." *Biorheology*, **3**, 174. [219]

Kemp, H. B. S. (1968). "Avascular necrosis of the femoral head in dogs." *J. Bone Jt Surg.*, **50B**, 431. [95]

Knigge, K. M. and Hoar, R. M. (1963). "A procedure for measuring plasma binding of adrenal corticoids." *Proc. Soc. exp. Biol. Med.*, **113**, 623. [282]

Kolliker, A. (1873). *Die normal Resorption des Knochengewehes und ihre Bedeutung fur die Entsehung de typischen Knochenformen.* Vogel, Leipzig. [174]

Lacoste, A. (1923). "Sur l'origine et l'evolution des osteoclastes. *C.r. Séanc. Soc. Biol.* **88**, 704. [174]

Lansing, A. I., Blumenthal, H. J. and Gray, S. H. (1948). "Ageing and calcification of the human coronary artery." *J. Geront.*, **3**, 87. [353]

Latta, J. S. and Bucholz, D. J. (1939). "The effects of insulin on the growth of fibroblasts *in vitro.*" *Arch. exp. Zellforsch.* **23**, 146. [370]

Lee, J. and Knowles, F. G. W. (1965). *Animal Hormones.* Hutchinson & Co. Ltd., Nashville. [275]

Leslie, I. and Davidson, J. N. (1951). "The effect of insulin on cellular composition and growth of chick-heart explants." *Biochem. J.*, **49**, xli. [370]

Lewis, W. H. (1935). "Normal and malignant cells." *Science, N.Y.*, **81**, 545. [393, 394]

Lick (1908). "Heteroplastische Knochenbildung in Nieren." *Arch. klin. Chir.*, **85**, 118. [353]

Lima, C. (1963). "Enxertos osseus." *IV Congresso Luso-Espanhol de Ortopedie e Traumatologia.* Barcelona. [376]

Lind, J. (1753). *Treatise of the Scurvy.* Edinburgh. Reprinted *Treatise of the Scurvy-Bicentenary Volume* 1953 (C. P. Stewart and D. Guthrie, eds). Edinburgh University Press. [183]

Lindbolm, K. (1957). "Intervertebral disc degeneration considered as a pressure atrophy." *J. Bone Jt Surg.*, **39A**, 933. [343]

Little, K. (1954). "The action of electrons on high polymers." *Proc. Conf. on Electron Microscopy (London)*, p. 165. Publ: Royal Micr. Soc. [420]

Little, K. (1957). "The effect of high doses of ionizing radiations on organic high polymers." *AERE GP/R* 1402. HMSO. [420]

Little, K. (1959). "Electron microscope studies on human dental enamel." *J. R. Micr. Soc.*, **78**, 58. [300]

Little, K. (1962). "The matrix in caries-resistant teeth." *J. R. Micr. Soc.*, **80**, 199. [300]

Little, K. (1965-6). "Some effects of cortisone and anabolic agents on cells and vessels." *Biorheology*, **3**, 173. [182]

Little, K. (1969a). "Nature of osteopetrosis." *Br. med. J.*, **ii**, 49. [13]

Little, K. (1969b). "Bone marrow and ageing." *Gerontologia*, **15**, 155.

Little, K. (1970a). "Interactions between catabolic and anabolic steroids." *Cur. ther. Res.*, **12**, 658. [143, 182, 251, 306]

Little, K. (1970b). "The production of platelet thrombi." *Cur. ther. Res.*, **12**, 677. [115, 266]

Little, K. (1970c). "Some effects of sterilizing doses of radiation on biological tissues." IAEA–PL–333/5 in *Sterilization and Preservation of Biological Tissues by Ionizing Radiation.* IAEA, Vienna. [378]

Little, K. (1970d). "Mechanisms of incorporation of homografts and herografts." *Proc. R. Soc. Med.*, **62**, 999.   [378]

Little, K. and Edwards, J. H. (1962). "Electron microscope examination of whole fibroblasts." *J. R. Micr. Soc.*, **81**, 23.   [365]

Little, K. and Edgington, T. S. (1963). "Tetracycline splenomegaly in young rabbits." *Am. J. Dis. Child.*, **106**, 521.   [13]

Little, K. and Valderrama, J. A. F. de (1968). "Some mechanisms involved in the osteoporotic process." *Gerontologia*, **14**, 109.   [167, 303]

Little, K. and White, A. M. (1968). "Stimulation of megakaryocyte formation in rabbits by anabolic and progestational steroids administered in conjunction with cortisone." *Biorheology*, **5**, 185.   [115, 183]

Little, K. and Munuera, L. (1970). "Some mechanisms of action of stanozolol (Stromba) and its interactions with cortisone." *Cur. ther. Res.*, **12**, 291.
                                                                                 [142]

Little, K., Pimm, L. H. and Trueta, J. (1958). "Osteoarthritis of the hip: an electron microscope study." *J. Bone Jt Surg.*, **40B**, 123.   [329]

Lovve, Peter (1634). *A Discourse of the Whole Art of Chyrurgerie.* Compiled by Peter Lovve, Scottishman. 3rd Ed.; corrected and much amended. Printed by Thomas Purfoot, London.   [13, 14, 15, 17, 301, 302]

Luxton, R. W. (1957). "Paget's disease of bone associated with Hashimoto's stroma lymphomatosa." *Lancet*, **i**, 441.   [325]

Lynch, S. R., Berelowitz, I., Seftel, H. C., Miller, G. B., Krawitz, P., Charlton, R. W. and Bothwell, T. H. (1967). "Osteoporosis in the Johannesburg Bantu, S.A." *J. Med. Sci.*, **32**, 59.   [312]

McClellan, R. O. and Jones, R. K. (1969). "⁹⁰Sr-induced neoplasia: a selective review." *Delayed Effects of Bone-Seeking Radionuclides* (C. W. Mays, ed.), p. 293, University of Utah Press, Salt Lake City.   [419, 420]

McConkey, B., Fraser, G. M. and Bligh, A. S. (1965). "Transparent skin and osteoporosis: a study in patients with rheumatoid disease." *Ann. rheum. Dis.*, **24**, 219.   [283, 307]

McConnell, D. (1938). "A structural investigation of the isomorphism of the apatite group." *Am. Mineralogist*, **23**, 1.   [76]

Macht, D. I. (1952)."Influence of some drugs and of emotions on blood coagulation. *J. Am. Med. Assoc.*, **148**, 265.   [114, 279]

Mack, P. B., Vose, G. P., Vogt, F. B. and LaChance, P. A. (1966). Gemini Midprogramme Conference. Experiment M–6, "Bone demineralization," p. 407. NASA SP–121.   [255, 305]

Malawski, S. and Serafin, J. (1969). "The use of dry-freezed bone grafts, sterilized by gamma rays, in orthopaedic surgery." *Chirurgja narz. Ruchu Ortop. pol.* **34**, 61. (Abstracted in *Nuclear Science Abstracts*.)   [378]

Mallams, J. T., Balla, G. A. and Finney, J. W. (1965). "Malignant tumours of the head and neck treated by regional oxygenation and irradiation." *Oral Surg.*, **20**, 757.   [181]

Manchester, K. L. and Young, F. G. (1961). "Insulin and protein metabolism." *Vitams Horm*, **19**, 95.   [230, 293]

Mankin, H. J. and Conger, K. A. (1966). "The effect of cortisol on articular cartilage of rabbits: 1, Effect of single dose of cortisol on glycine–C¹⁴ incorporation." *Lab. Invest.*, **15**, 784.   [270]

Marmor, L. (1960). "Bone banks. A new concept in procurement and storage for homologous grafts." *Calif. Med.*, **92**, 407.   [378]

Mason, J. K. (1963). "Asymptotic disease of coronary arteries in young men." *Br. med. J.*, **ii** 1234.   [118, 280]

Mason, J. W. (1959). "Viseral functions of the nervous system." *A. Rev. Physiol.*, **21**, 353.   [113, 277]

Mason, J. W., Sachar, E. J., Fishman, J. R., Hamburg, D. A. and Handlam, T. H. (1965). "Corticosteroid response to hospital admission." *Archs gen. Psychiat.*, **13**, 1.   [113, 277]

Mays, C. W., Dougherty, T. F., Taylor, G. N., Lloyd, R. D., Stover, B. J., Jee, W. S. S., Christensen, W. R., Dougherty, J. H. and Atherton, D. R. (1969). "Radiation-induced bone cancer in beagles." *Delayed Effects of Bone-seeking Radionuclides* (C. W. Mays, ed.), p. 387. Salt Lake City, University of Utah Press.   [405]

Melcher, A. H. (1969). "Histologically demonstrable bound lipid apparently associated with relatively stable mature collagen fibres." *Gerontologia*, **15**, 217.   [178]

Mellanby, E. (1950). *A Story of Nutritional Research: the effect of some dietary factors on bones and the nervous system.* The Williams & Wilkins Co., Baltimore.   [184]

Mellanby, M. (1930). "Experiments on dogs, rabbits and rats, and investigations on man, which indicate power of certain food factors to prevent and control dental disease." *J. Am. dent. Ass.*, **17**, 1456.   [299]

Mellanby, M. (1934). *Diet and Teeth, an Experimental Study.* Part 3. MRC Special Report Series, no. 191.   [299]

Metz, R. (1960). "The effect of blood glucose concentration on insulin output." *Diabetes*, **9**, 89.   [230, 293]

Meyer, J. (1852). "Uber die Neubildung von Blutgefassen in plastischen Exudaten seroser Membranes und in Hautwunden." *Ann Charite* (Berlin), **4**, 41.   [371]

Miles, H. (1740/1). "Some remarks concerning the circulation of the Blood, as seen in the Tail of a Water-Eft, through a Solar Microscope." *Phil. Trans. R. Soc.*, **41**, 725.   [15]

Mills, I. H. (1962). "Transport and metabolism of steroids." *Br. med. Bull.*, **18**, 127.   [116]

Mills, I. H., Schedl, H. P., Chen, P. S. and Bartler, F. C. (1960). "The effect of estrogen administration on the metabolism and protein binding of hydrocortisone." *J. clin. Endocr., Metab.*, **20**, 515.   [291]

Mills, J. N. (1938). "The effects of prolonged muscular exercise on the metabolism." *J. Physiol. Lond.*, **93**, 144.   [116]

Mitchell, J. R. A., Schwartz, C. J. and Zingler, A. (1964). "Relationship between aortic plaques and age, sex and blood pressure." *Br. med. J.* **i**, 205.   [118, 121, 280, 284]

Mohr, O. L. (1934). *Heredity and Disease.* W. W. Norton & Co., New York.   [394]

Morgan, J. D. (1959). "Blood supply of the growing rabbit's tibia." *J. Bone Jt Surg.*, **41B**, 185.   [136]

Morris, J. N. (1968). "Report of a Research Committee. Control trial of soya-bean oil in myocardial infarction." *Lancet*, **ii**, 693.   [111]

Morris, J. N., Heady, T. S., Raffle, R. A. B., Roberts, C. G. and Parks, J. W. (1953) "Coronary heart disease and physical activity of work." *Lancet*, **ii**, 1053 and 1111.   [117, 282]

Moschi, A. and Little, K. (1966). "Fluorescent properties of the non-collagenous components of the intervertebral disc." *Nature, Lond.*, **212**, 722.   [40]

Mottram, J. C. (1927). "The role of carbon dioxide in the growth of normal and tumour cells." *Lancet*, **ii**, 1232.   [343, 369, 395]

Mottram, J. C. (1928). "On the division of cells under varying tensions of carbon dioxide." *Br. J. exp. Path.*, **9**, 240.   [394]

Mount, D. and Brusce, W. R. (1964). "Local plasma volume and vascular permeability of rabbit skin after irradiation." *Radiat. Res.*, **23**, 430.   [411]

Nachemson, A. (1969). "Intradiscal measurements of pH in patients with lumbar
rhizopathies." *Acta orthop. scand.*, **40**, 23.   [342]

Nachemson, A. L. (1971). "Low back pain: It's etiology and treatment." *Clin.
Med.*, **18**.   [342]

NASA (1967). "Gemini summary conference." NASA SP–138.   [277]

Neuman, W. F. and Neuman, M. W. (1953). "Nature of the mineral phase in bone."
Chem. Rev., **53**, 1.   [66]

Nisbet, J. and Nordin, B. E. (1969). "Some hormonal effects on bone in tissue
culture." *Proc. R. Soc. Med.*, **62**, 239.   [233]

Nordin, B. E. C. (1961). "Effects of malabsorption syndrome on calcium metabolism." *Proc. R. Soc. Med.*, **54**, 497.   [308]

Nordin, B. E. C. (1964). "Osteoporosis." *Adv. Metabol. Dis.* **1**, 125.   [307]

Nordin, B. E. (1966). "International patterns of osteoporosis." *Clin. Orthop.*, **45**,
17.   [278]

O'Bannon, R. P. and Grunow, O. H. (1954). "The larynx and pharynx radiologically considered." *Sth. med. J.*, **47**, 310.   [351]

O'Connell, J. E. A. (1951). "Protrusions of the lumbar intervertebral discs." *J.
Bone Jt Surg.*, **33B**, 8.   [103]

Okado, M. (1943). "Hard Tissues of Animal Body." *Shanghai Evening Post*
(Sept.), pp. 26–31. (A copy of this is in the Museum of the History of Science,
Oxford.)   [367, 369]

Oliver, M. F. and Boyd, G. S. (1961). "Influences of reduction of serum lipids on
prognosis of coronary heart disease." *Lancet*, **2**, 499.   [118, 275, 290]

Oppenheimer, B. S., Oppenheimer, E. T., Stout, A. P., Willhite, M. and Danishef-
sky, I. (1958). "The latent period in carcinogenesis by plastics in rats and its
relation to the presarcomatous stage." *Cancer*, **11**, 204.   [198]

Osler, W. (1874). "An account of certain organisms occurring in the liquor sanguis."
Proc. R. Soc., **22**, 391.   [268]

Paget, J. (1877). "On a form of chronic inflammation of bones (Osteitis deformans)." *Med.-chir. Trans.*, **60**, 37.   [317, 325]

Palade, G. E. (1961). "Blood capillaries of the heart and other organs." *Circulation*, **24**, 368.   [238]

Parsons, J. A. and Robinson, C. J. (1969). "A rapid indirect hypercalcaemia action
of parathyroid hormone demonstrated in isolated blood-perfused bone."
Proc. R. Soc. Med., **62**, 239.   [233]

Paul, F. T. (1886). "A note on calcarious degeneration of arteries." *Trans. path.
Soc. Lond.*, **37**, 216.   [350]

Peshef, L. and Shapiro, B. (1960). "Effect of epinephrine, cortisone and growth
hormone on release of unesterified fatty acids by adipose tissue *in vitro*."
Metabolism, 9, 551.   [114]

Peterson, J. E., Keith, R. A. and Wolcox, A. A. (1962). "Hourly changes in serum
cholesterol concentration. Effects of the anticipation of stress." *Circulation*,
25, 798.   [112, 117, 280]

Peterson, R. E., Nokes, G. N., Chem, P. S. and Black R. L. (1960). "Estrogens and
adrenocortical function in man." *J. clin. Endoc. Metab*, **20**, 495.

Pierie, W. R., Hancock, W. D., Koorajian, S. and Starr, A. (1968). "Materials and
heart valve prostheses." *Ann. N.Y. Acad. Sci.*, **146**, 345.   [114]

Pitot, H. C. (1966). "Some bichemical aspects of malignancy." *A. Rev. Biochem.*
35, 335.   [395]

Playfair, L. (1843). "On the changes in composition of the milk of a cow, according to its exercise and food." *J. chem. Soc.*, **1**, 174.   [235]

Plechus, J. L., Chandler, E. H. and Ellis, J. W. (1966). "Alcohol-induced hypoglycemia as a factor in aircraft accidents." *Aerospace Med.*, **37**, 956. [230, 293]

Plotz, C. M., Howes, E. L., Meyer, K., Blunt, J. W., Lattes, R. and Ragan, C. (1950). "The effect of the hyperadrenal state on connective tissue." *Am. J. Path.*, **26**, 709.   [283]

Poal-Manresa, J., Little, K. and Trueta, J. (1970). "Some observations on the effects of vitamin C deficiency on bone." *Br. J. exp. Path.*, **51**, 372.   [133]

Pommer, G. (1883). "Ueber die Ostokasten Theorie." *Virchows Arch. path. Anat. Physiol.*, **92**, 296 and 449.   [174]

Poscharissky, J. F. (1905). "Ueber heteroplastische Knockenbildung." *Beitr. path. Anat.*, **38**, 135.   [350]

Posner, A. S. and Duychaerts, G. (1954). "Infra-red study of the carbonate in bone, teeth and francolite." *Experientia*, **10**, 424.   [74]

Price, C. H. G. (1961). "Osteogenic Sarcoma: An analysis of survival and its relationship to histological grading and structure." *J. Bone Jt Surg.*, **43B**, 300.   [385, 389]

Price, C. H. G. (1962). "The incidence of osteogenic sarcoma in south-west England and its relationship to Paget's disease of bone." *J. Bone Jt Surg.*, **44B**, 366.   [278, 324, 325, 354]

Price, C. H. G. and Goldie, W. (1969). "Paget's sarcoma of Bone: a study of eighty cases from the Bristol and Leeds Bone Tumour Registries." *J. Bone Jt Surg.*, **51B**, 205.   [179, 324, 384, 386]

Pritchard, J. J. (1956). "The Osteoblast." *The Biochemistry and Physiology of Bone* (G. H. Bourne, ed.). Chapter 8. Academic Press, New York and London.   [150]

Prop, F. J. A. (1961). "Effects of hormones on mouse mammary glands *in vitro*. Analysis of the factors that cause lobulo-alveolar development." *Path. Biol., Pams*, **9**, 640.   [230, 271, 293, 370]

Prop, F. J. (1965). "Effect of insulin on mitotic rate in organ cultures of total mammary glands of the mouse." *Expl Cell Res.*, **40**, 277.   [230]

Purvis, M. J. (1962). "Some effects of administering sodium fluoride to patients with Paget's disease." *Lancet*, **ii**, 1188.

Ratcliffe, H. L. and Cronin, M. I. T. (1958). "Changing frequency of arteriosclerosis in mammals and birds at the Philadelphia Zoological Gardens." *Circulation*, **18**, 41.   [112, 117]

Reifenstein, E. C. (1957). "The relationships of steroid hormones to the development and the management of osteoporsis in ageing people." *Clin. Ortho.* p. **10**, 206.   [80, 120, 304, 305]

Rigal, W. M. (1961a). "Uptake and incorporation of tritiated thymidine in *in vitro* culture." *Nature, Lond.* **192**, 768.   [363]

Rigal, W. M. (1961b). "A study of bone development using tissue culture as the main technique." D. Phil. Thesis., Oxford.   [152, 210, 369]

Rigal, W. M. (1962). "The use of tritiated thymidine in studies of chondrogenesis." *Radioisotopes and Bones*, p. 197. Blackwell Scientific Publications, Oxford.   [90, 126, 130]

Rigal, W. M. (1964). "Sites of action of growth hormone in cartilage." *Proc. Soc. exp. Biol. Med.*, **117**, 794.   [129, 181, 232, 271, 369]

Rigal, W. M. and Little, K. (1962). "Some observations on nuclear structure in cartilage cells." *Jl. R. microsc. Soc.*, **80**, 279.   [361]

Rigal, W. M. and Hunter, W. M. (1966). "Sites and mode of action of growth hormone." *Calcified Tissues* **1965** (Fleisch *et al.*, eds), p. 250. Springer-Verlag, Berlin.   [130]

Robin, G. C., Bar-Maor, A. and Winberg, H. (1963). "Morbidity and mortality rates for internal fixation of femoral neck fractures." *J. Am. Geriat Soc.*, **11**, 560. [315]

Roeser, W. H. P., Powell, L. W. and O'Brien, R. F. (1968). "Red cell survival after heterograft valve surgery." *Br. med. J.*, **4**, 806.   [114]

Rosenburg, E. F. (1958). "Rheumatoid arthritis: Osteoporosis and fractures related to steroid therapy." *Acta. med. scand.* Suppl. 211.   [308]

Ross, M. H., Furth, J. and Bigelow, R. R. (1952). "Changes in cellular composition of the lymph caused by ionizing radiations." *Blood*, **7**, 417.   [421]

Rowland, R. E. (1963a). "Some aspects of human bone metabolism deduced from studies of radium cases." *Clin. Orthop.*, **28**, 193.   [403]

Rowland, R. E. (1963b). "Local distribution and retention of radium in man." *Diagnosis and Treatment of Radioactive Poisoning*, p. 57. IAEA, Vienna.
                                                                                     [403, 405]

Rowles, S. L. (1968). "The precipitation of whitlockite from aqueous solutions." *Bull. Soc. chim. Fr.*, p. 1797.   [56, 59]

Rubenstein, A. H., Seftel, H. C., Bersohn, I., Miller, K. and Wright, A. D. (1967). "Serum insulin and growth hormone responses to oral glucose loading in South African whites, Indians and Africans." *S.Afr. J. med. Sci.*, **32**, 132. [294]

Ruhmann, A. G. and Berliner, D. L. (1965). "Effect of steroids on growth of mouse fibroblasts *in vitro*." *Endocrinology*, **76**, 916.   [292, 370]

Sabanas, A. O., Dahlin, D. C., Childs, D. S. and Ivins, J. C. (1956). "Post-radiation sarcoma of bone." *Cancer*, **9**, 258.   [412]

Sabet, T. Y., Hidvegi, E. B. and Ray, R. D. (1961). "Bone immunology. II. Comparison of embryonic mouse isografts and homografts." *J. Bone Jt Surg.*, **43A**, 1007.   [377, 378]

Sachar, E. T., Cobb, J. C. and Stor, R. E. (1966). "Plasma cortisol changes during hypnotic trace." *Archs gen. Psychiat.*, **14**, 482.   [113, 291]

Saffran, M. (1962). "Mechanisms of adreno-cortical control." *Br. med. Bull.*, **18**, 122.   [116]

Salmon, M. L., Winkelman, J. Z. and Gay, A. J. (1968). "Neuro-ophthalmic sequelae in users of oral contraceptives. *J. Am. med. Ass.*, **206**, 85.   [285]

Sandford, K. K., Likely, G. D. and Earle, W. R. (1954). "The development of variations within a clone of mouse fibroblasts transformed to sarcoma-producing cells *in vitro*." *J. natn. Cancer Inst.*, **15**, 215.   [379]

Sandison, J. C. (1928). "A method for the microscopic study of the growth of transplanted bone in the transparent chambers of the rabbit's ear." *Anat. Rec.* **40**, 41.   [166]

Scapinelli, R. (1960a). "Interspinous ligaments in man and their apophyseal attachments: Structural changes in relation to age." *Archo ital. Anat. Embriol.*, **65**, 364.   [198]

Scapinelli, R. (1960b). "Il sesamoide della nuca." *Clinica ortop.*, **12**, 445.   [198]

Scapinelli, R. (1963). "Sesamoid bones in the ligamentum nuchae of man." *J. Anat.* **97**, 417.   [198, 356]

Scapinelli, R. and Little, K. (1970). "Observations on the mechanically induced differentiation of cartilage from fibrous connective tissue." *J. Path. Bact.*, **101**, 85.   [197]

Schajowicz, F. (1961). "Giant-cell tumours of bone (osteoclastoma). A pathological and histochemical study." *J. Bone Jt Surg.*, **43A**, 1.   [389]

Schlettwein-Gsell, D. (1966). "Geographical differences in fracture incidence of aged persons." *7th Int. Congr. of Gerontology* (Vienna). Paper No. 562. [278]

Schmorl, G. and Junghanns, H. (1932). *The Human Spine in Health and Disease.* Translated 1959: Grune & Stratton, London.   [346]

Schoefl, G. I. (1963). "Studies on Inflammation. III. Growing capillaries: their structure and permeability." *Virchows Arch. path. Anat. Physiol.*, **337**, 97.   [371, 374]

Scott, P. P. (1968). "Effect of calcium and vitamin A deficiency on the thyroid gland." *Proc. R. Soc. Med.*, **62**, 240.   [184, 231]

Scott, P. P., Greaves, J. P. and Scott, M. G. (1961). "Nutrition of the cat: 4. Calcium and iodine deficiency on a meat diet." *Br. J. Nutr.*, **15**, 35.   [184, 231, 294]

Scrimshaw, N. S., Habicht, J. P., Piche, M. L., Cholakos, B. and Arroyane, G. (1966). "Protein metabolism of young men during university examinations." *Am. J. clin. Nutr.*, **18**, 321.   [255, 277]

Seftel, H. C., Malkin, C., Schnaman, A., Abrahams, C., Lynch, S. R., Charlton, R. W. and Bothwell, T. H. (1966). "Osteoporosis, scurvy and siderosis in Johannesburg Bantu." *Br. med. J.*, **1**, 642.   [312]

Shackleford, J. M. and Wyckoff, R. W. G. (1964). "Collagen in fossil teeth and bones." *J. Ultrastruct. Res.*, **11**, 173.   [35]

Shannon, I. L., Isbell, G. M., Prigmore, J. R. and Hester, W. R. (1962). "Stress in dental patients: The serum free 17-hydroxycorticosteroid response in routinely appointed patients undergoing simple exodontia." *Oral Surg.*, **15**, 1142.   [277]

Shapir, E. and Steinberg, D. (1960). "The essential role of the adrenal cortex in the response of plasma free fatty acids, cholesterol and phospholipids to epinephrine injection." *J. clin. Invest.*, **39**, 310.   [114, 295]

Sharp, A. A. (1961). "Platelet (viscous) Metamorphosis." Henry Ford Hospital Symposium "Blood Platelets". p. 67. Little, Brown & Co. Inc., Boston. [115, 266]

Shaw, N. E. (1966). "The influence of muscle blood-flow on the circulation in bone.' *Calcified Tissues* 1965 (Fleisch *et al.*, eds), p. 104. Springer-Verlag, Berlin. [212]

Shenkin, H. A. (1964). "The effect of pain on the diurnal pattern of plasma corticosteroid levels." *Neurology, Minneap.*, **14**, 1112.   [113, 276]

Shine, I. B. (1965). "Incidence of Hallux Vulgus in a partially shoe-wearing community." *Br. med. J.*, 1648.   [327]

Sholiton, L. J., Werk, E. E. and Marnell, R. T. (1961). "Diurnal variations of adrenocortical function in non-endocrine disease states." *Metabolism*, **10**, 632.   [113, 247, 276]

Siffert, R. S. and Barash, E. S. (1961). "Delayed bone transplantation. An experimental study of early host-transplant relationships." *J. Bone Jt Surg.*, **43A**, 407.   [376]

Simonetta, B. (1949). "Chronic cholesteatomatous and chronic cholesterimic otitis." *Acta oto-lar.*, **37**, 509.   [280]

Smith, A. U. (1965). "Survival of frozen chondrocytes isolated from cartilage of adult mammals." *Nature, Lond.*, **205**, 782.   [28]

Smithers, D. W. (1960). *Clinical Prospects of the Cancer Problem.* Introductory Volume. Monographs on Neoplastic Disease. E. & S. Livingstone Ltd., Edinburgh and London.   [379 ,393]

Sokoloff, L. (1969). *The Biology of Degenerative Joint Disease.* University of Chicago Press, Chicago, USA.   [326]

Song, C. W. and Levitt, S. H. (1970). "Effect of X-irradiation on vascularity of normal tissue and experimental tumour." *Radiology*, **94**, 445.   [412]

Spiess, H. (1969). "^{224}Ra-induced tumours in children and adults." *Delayed Effects of Bone-seeking Radionuclides* (C. W. Mays, ed.) p. 227. University of Utah Press, Salt Lake City.   [402, 412]

Spiess, H. and Mays. C. W. (1970). "Bone cancers induced by ^{224}Ra (ThX) in children and adults." *Hlth Phys.*, **19**, 713.   [402]

Spuler, A. (1898). "Ueber die Verbindungskanalcher der Hohler der Knockenzellen." *Anat. Anz.*, **14**, 289.   [154]

Storey, E. (1957). "The effect of continuous administration of cortisone and its withdrawal on bone." *Aust. N.Z. J. Surg.*, **27**, 19. [103, 238, 292, 305]

Storey, E. (1958). "The effect of intermittent cortisone administration in the rabbit." *J. Bone Jt Surg.*, **40B**, 103.   [306]

Storey, E. (1961). "Cortisone-induced bone resorption in the rabbit." *Endocrinology*, **68**, 533.   [238]

Sutton, P. R. N. (1965). "The early onset of acute dental caries in adults following mental stress." *N.Y. St. dent. J.*, **31**, 450.   [300]

Swan, C. H. J. and Cook, W. T. (1971). "Nutritional osteomalacia in immigrants in an urban community." *Lancet*, **ii**, 456.   [279]

Tarlo, L. B. H. (1963). "Aspidin: the precursor of bone." *Nature, Lond.*, **199**, 46.   [158]

Tarsoly, E., Ostrowski, K., Moskalewski, S., Lojek, T., Kurnatowski, W. and Krompecher, S. (1969). "Incorporation of lyophilized and radiosterilized perforated and unperforated bone grafts in dogs." *Acta Chir. Acad. Sci. Hung.*, **10**, 55. (Abstracted in *Nuclear Science Abstracts*.)   [378]

Taylor, G. N., Dougherty, T. F., Shabestai, L. and Dougherty, J. H. (1969). "Soft tissue tumours in internally irradiated beagles." *Delayed Effects of Bone-seeking Radionuclides* (C. W. Mays, ed.), p. 323. University of Utah Press, Salt Lake City.   [403]

Taylor, T. K. F. (1964). "Some aspects of the structure, growth and degeneration of the intervertebral disc." D. Phil. Thesis, Oxford. (76, 101, 342, 344, 345]

Taylor, T. K. F. and Little K. (1963). "Calcification in the intervertebral disc." *Nature, Lond.*, **199**, 612.   [76]

Taylor, T. K. F. and Little, K. (1965). "Intercellular matrix of the intervertebral disc in ageing and in prolapse." *Nature, Lond.*, **208**, 384.   [207]

Tesse, J. J., Friedman, S. B. and Mason, J. W. (1965). "Anxiety, defensiveness and 17-hydroxycorticosteroid excretion." *J. nerv. ment. Dis.*, **141**, 549.   [113, 277]

Thewlis, J. (1940). "The structure of the teeth." MRC Special Report No. 238. HMSO, London.   [37]

Thewlis, J., Glock, C. E. and Murray, M. M. (1939). "Chemical and X-ray analysis of dental mineral and synthetic apatites." *Trans. Faraday. Soc.*, **35**, 358. [76]

Thoma, R. (1894). *Textbook of General Pathology and Pathological Anatomy.* Vol. 1. Translated by A. Bruce, 1896.   [62, 85, 149, 350, 351]

Tillis, H. H. (1961). "Clinical effects of methandrostenolone in osteoporosis." *Clin. Med.*, **8**, 274.   [307]

Tonna, E. A. and Cronkite, E. P. (1961). "Use of tritiated thymidine for the study of the origin of the osteoclast." *Nature, Lond.*, **190**, 459.   [166]

Tovborg-Jensen, A. and Moller, E. (1944). "Investigations in the properties of tooth enamel by means of X-rays." *Acta odont. scand.*, **6**, 7.   [76]

Tovborg-Jensen, A. and Rowles, S. L. (1957a). "Lattice constants and magnesium content of some naturally occurring whitlockite." *Nature, Lond.*, **179**, 912.   [56]

Tovborg-Jensen, A. and Rowles, S. L. (1957b). "Magnesian whitlockite: a major constituent of dental calculus." *Acta. odont. scand.*, **15**, 121.   [56]

Trautz, O. R. (1960). "Crystallographic studies of calcium carbonate phosphate." *Ann. N.Y. Acad. Sci.*, **85**, 145.   [76]

Trueta, J. (1958). "La vascularization des os et l'osteogenese." *Revue Chir orthop.* **44**, 3.   [150]

Trueta, J. (1961). "The housing problem of the osteoblast." *J. Traumat. Mal. prof.*, **1**, 5.   [150]

Trueta, J. (1962a). "The vascular role in calcification and osteogenesis." *Radio-isotopes and Bone*, p. 371. Blackwell Scientific Publications, Oxford.   [150]

Trueta, J. (1962b). "A theory of bone formation." *Acta orthop. scand.*, XXXII, 190.   [150]

Trueta, J. (1963). "The role of the vessels in osteogenesis." *J. Bone Jt Surg.*, **45B**, 402.   [150]

Trueta, J. (1964). "The Dynamics of Bone Circulation." *Bone Biodynamics* (H. M. Frost, ed.), p. 245. Little, Brown & Co., Boston.   [302]

Trueta, J. (1968). *Studies of the Development and Decay of the Human Frame*, Heinemann, London.   [179, 339]

Trueta, J. and Amato, V. P. (1960). "The vascular contribution to osteogenesis. 3. Changes in the growth cartilage caused by experimentally induced ischaemia." *J. Bone Jt Surg.*, **42B**, 571.   [125, 133, 150]

Trueta, J. and Morgan, J. D. (1960). "The vascular contribution to osteogenesis. 1. Studies by the injection method." *J. Bone Jt Surg.*, **42B**, 97.

Ullberg, S. and Bengtsson, G. (1963). "Autoradiographic distribution studies with natural oestrogens." *Acta endocr., Copenh.*, **43**, 75.   [281]

Valderrama, J. A. F. de and Trueta, J. (1965). "The effect of muscle action on the intra-osseous circulation." *J. Path. Bact.*, **89**, 179.   [212]

Virchow, R. C. K. (1863–7). *Die Krankhaften Geschwulste*. Berlin.   [379]

Walker, A. R. P. and Seftel, H. C. (1962). "Coronary heart-disease, strokes and diabetes in South African Indians." *Lancet*, **ii**, 786.   [277]

Ward, F. O. (1838). *Outlines of Human Osteology*. Henry Renshaw, London.   [2, 4, 6, 16, 18, 158]

Weiser, M. M. and Rothfield, L. (1968). "Reassociation of phospholipid, lipopoly, saccharide and enzyme components of bacterial cell envelopes." *Membrane Models and the Fomation of Biological Membranes* (L. Bolis and B. A. Pethica, eds), p. 149, North Holland, Amsterdam.   [365]

Wells, F. R. (1963). "The lymphatic vessels in radiodermatitis: a clinical and experimental study." *Br. J. plast. Surg.*, **16**, 243.   [412]

Wells, H. G. (1910). "Calcification and ossification." Harvey Lecture 1910–11, p. 102. J. B. Lippincott & Co., Chicago.   [61, 149, 350]

Werk, E. E., MacGee, J. and Sholiton, L. J. (1964). "Altered cortisol metabolism in advanced cancer and other terminal illnesses: excretion of 6-hydri-cortisol." *Metabolism*, **13**, 1425.   [113, 277]

White, A. M. (1966). "The anti-catabolic effects of synthetic anabolic/androgenic steroids." *Excerpta medica Int. Congr.* Ser. No. 132, p. 576   [235]

Willis, R. A. (1960). *Pathology of Tumours*. 3rd Ed. Butterworths, London.   [380, 385, 393, 395]

Willmer, E. N. (1960). *Cytology and Evolution*. Academic Press, London and New York   [24, 26]

Willmer, E. N. (1970). *Cytology and Evolution*, 2nd Ed. Academic Press, London and New York.   [24, 26, 366]

Winchell, H. S., Anderson, A. C. and Pollycove, M. (1964). "Radiation-induced haemorrhagic diathesis in dogs unassociated with thrombocytopenia: Association with an intravascular protein-polysaccharide particle." *Blood*, **23**, 186.   [421]

Witte, C. L. (1966). "Thyrotropic factor in the Viet Nam war." *Milit. Med.*, **131**, 736.   [116, 282]

Wolbach, S. B. and Howe, P. R. (1926). "Intercellular substance in experimental scorbutus." *Archs Path.*, **1**, 1.   [183]

Wolf, S., McCabe, W. R., Yamamoto, J, Adsett, D. and Schottstaedt, W. W. (1962). "Changes in serum lipids in relation to emotional stress during rigid control of diet and exercise." *Circulation*, **26**, 379.   [112, 280, 295]

Woodruff, M. F. A., Nolan, B., Robson, J. S. and MacDonald, M. K. (1969). "Renal transplantation in man." *Lancet*, **i**, 6.   [378, 397]

Woods, M., Hunter, J. and Burk, D. (1955). "Regulation of glucose utilization in tumours by a stress-modified insulin: anti-insulin system." *J. natn. Cancer Inst.*, **16**, 351.   [370, 395]

Wool, I. G., Goldstein, M. S., Ramey, E. R. and Levine, R. (1954). "Role of epinephrine in the physiology of fat metabolism." *Am. J. Physiol.*, 178, 427.

Wright, H. B., Pincheri, G. and Murray, A. (1968). *Fit for Life*. Evans Brothers, Ltd., London.   [120, 282.]

Wuthier, R. E. (1968). "Lipids of mineralizing epiphyseal tissues in the bovine foetus." *J. Lipid Res.*, **8**, 68.   [51]

Wynn, V. (1968). "The anabolic steroids." *Practitioner*, **200**, 509.   [247, 283, 307]

Wynn, V. and Landon, J. (1961). "A study of the androgenic and some related effects of methandienone." *Br. med. J.*, **i**, 998.   [247, 283, 307]

Zonneveld, R. J. van (1962). "A national health examination survey of the elderly of the Netherlands. *Geront. clin.*, **4**, 198.   [120]

Zweifach, B. W., Shorr, E. and Black, M. M. (1953). "Influence of adrenal cortex on behaviour of terminal vascular bed." *Ann. N.Y. Acad. Sci.*, **56**, 626.
                                                                          [283]

Additional Bibliography on Calcium Phosphates

Arnold, P. W. (1950). "The nature of precipitated phosphates." *Trans. Faraday Soc.*, **46**, 1061.

Bale, W. F. (1936). "Uber den anorganischen Aufbau der Zahne." *Naturwissenschaften*, **24**, 636.

Bale, W. F., Hodge, H. C. and Warren, S. L. (1934). "Roetgen-ray diffraction studies of enamel and dentine." *Am. J. Roentg.*, **32**, 369.

Bale, W. F., Bonner, J. F., Hodge, H. C., Adler, H., Wreath, A. R. and Bell, R. (1945). "Optical and X-ray diffraction studies of certain calcium phosphates." *Ind. Engng analyt. Edn*, **17**, 491.

Bassett (1917), "The phosphates of calcium." Pt. 4 The Basic Phosphates. *J. chem. Soc.*, **111**, 620.

Beevers, C. A. and McIntyre, D. P. (1946). "The atomic structure of fluor-apatite and its relation to that of tooth and bone material." *Mineralog. Mag.*, **27**, 254.

Brown, W. E., Lehr, J. R., Smith J. R. and Frazier, A. W. (1957). "Crystallography of ostacalcium phosphate." *J. Am. chem. Soc.*, **79**, 5318.

Cape, A. T. and Kitchin, P. C. (1930). "Histological phenomena of tooth tissues as observed under polarized light, with note on roentgen-ray spectra of enamel and dentine." *J. Am. dent. Ass.*, **17**, 193.

Daubeny, C. (1845). "On the occurrence of fluorine in recent as well as in fossil bones." *J. chem. Soc.*, **2**, 97.

De Jong, W. F. (1926). "Le substance minerale dans les os." *Recl Trav. chim. Pays-Basl Belg.*, **45**, 445.

Ericsson, Y. (1949). "Enamel-apatite solubility: investigations into the calcium phosphate equilibrium between enamel and saliva and its relation to dental caries." *Acta odont. scand.*, **8**, Supple., **3**, 47.

Gross, R. (1926). *Die kirstalline Structur von Dentin und Zahnschmetz.* p. 59. Festshr. Zahnartzl. Inst., Greifswald (Berlin),

Hayek, E. and Stadlmann, W. (1955). "Darstellung von reinem Hydroxylapatit fur Adsorptionzwecke." *Angew. Chemie.*, **67**, 327.

Hayek, E. and Newesely, H. (1958). "Uber die Existenz von Tricalcium phosphat im wassriger Losung." *Mh. Chem.*, **89**, 88.

Heintz, W. (1850). "On the chemical composition of bones." *Annln Phys.*, LXXVII, 267.

Hendricks, S. B. and Hill, W. L. (1950). "The nature of bone and phosphate rock." *Proc. natr. Acad. Sci.*, USA, **36**, 731.

Hodge, H. C., LeFevre, M. L. and Bale, W. F. (1938). "Chemical and X-ray diffraction studies of calcium phosphates." *Ind. Engng. analyt. Edn.*, **10**, 156.

King, J. D., Rowles, S. L., Little, K. and Thewlis, J. (1955). "Chemical and X-ray examination of deposits removed from the teeth of golden hamsters and ferrets." *J. dent. Res.*, **34**, 650.

Klement, R. (1937). "Der Carbonatgehalt der anorganischen Knochensubstanz und ihr Synthese." *Ber. dt. chem. Ges.*, **70**, 468.

Klement, R. (1938). "Die anorganische Skeletsubstanz: Ihre Zusammensetzung, naturliche und kunstliche Bildung." *Naturwissenschaften*, **26**, 145.

Logan, M. A. and Taylor, H. L. (1938). "Solubility of bone salt: factors affecting its formation." *J. biol. Chem.*, **125**, 377.

Logan, M. A. and Taylor, H. L. (1938). "Solubility of bone salt: Partial solution of bone and carbonate-containing calcium phosphate precipitates." *J. biol. Chem.*, **125**, 391.

Logan, M. A. and Kane, L. W. (1939). "Solubility of bone salt: solubility of bone in biological fluids." *J. biol. Chem.*, **127**, 705.

Middleton, J. (1845). "On fluorine in recent and fossil bones, and the sources from whence it is derived." *J. chem. Soc.*, **2**, 134.

Mooney, R. W. and Aia, M. I. (1961). "Alkaline earth phosphates." *Chem. Rev.*, **61**, 433.

Naray-Szabo, St. (1930). "Structure of fluorapatite." *Z. Kristallogr.*, **75**, 387.

Pedersen, K. J. (1949). "Relations between vapour pressures and solubilities of hydrates." *Acta. chem. scand.*, **3**, 65.

Posner, A. S. (1960). "The nature of the inorganic phase in calcified tissues," in *Calcification in Biological Systems.* Am. Ass. Adv. Sci., Washington.

Posner, A S., Perloff, A. and Diorio, A. F. (1958). "Refinement of the hydroxy-apatite structure." *Acta crystallogr.*, **11**, 308.

Roseberry, H. H., Hastings, A. B. and Morse, J. K. (1931). "X-ray analysis of bone and teeth." *J. biol. Chem.*, **90**, 395.

Schleede, A., Schmidt, W. and Kindt, H. (1932). "Zur Kenntnis der Calciumphos-phate und apatite." *Z. Elektrochem.*, **35**, 633.

Taylor, N. W. and Sheard, C. (1929). "Microscopic and X-ray investigations on the calcification of tissues." *J. biol. Chem.*, **81**, 479.

Thewlis, J. (1932). "The structure of teeth." *Br. dent. J.*, **53**, 655.

Thewlis, J. (1932). "X-ray analysis of teeth." *Br. J. Radiol.*, **5**, 353.

Tovborg-Jensen, A. and Thygesen, J. E. (1943). "Chemical composition of 'calcium deposits' from calcinosis patients." *Acta. med. scand.*, **113**, 392.

Tovborg-Jensen, A. and Dano, M. (1952). "X-ray crystallographic examination of calculi from salivary glands." *J. dent. Res.*, **31**, 620.

Tovborg-Jensen, A. and Dano, M. (1954). "Cyrstallography of dental calculus and the precipitation of certain calcium phosphates." *J. dent. Res.*, **33**, 741.

Trautz, O. R. and Fessenden, E. (1958). "Formation and stability of whitlockite and octacalcium phosphate, two components of salivary calculi." *J. dent. Res.*, **37**, 78.

Trautz, O. R., Fessenden, E. and Newton, M. G. (1952). "Magnesian whitlockite in ashed dental tissue—an identification by X-ray diffraction." *J. dent. Res,* **31**, 620.

Trautz, O. R., Fessenden, E. and Newton, M. G. (1954). "Magnesian whitlockite." *J. dent. Res.*, **33**, 687.

Trautz, O. R., Fessenden, E. and Zapanta, R. R. (1959). "Effect of sodium fluoride on calcium salts and dental enamel." *J. dent. Res.*, **38**, 691.

Trautz, O. R., Klein, E., Fessenden, E. and Addleston, H. K. (1953). "The interpretation of the X-ray diffractograms obtained from human dental enamel." *J. dent. Res.*, **32**, 420.

Tromel, G. (1932). "Beitrage zur Kenntnis des Systems Kalziumoxyd-Phosphorus pentoxyd." Mitteilungen aus dem Kaiser-Wilhelm Institut for Eisenforschung zu Dusseldorf, **14**, 25.

Tromel, G. and Moller, H. (1932). "Die Bildung schwe loslicher Klaziumphosphate aus wassriger Losung und die Beziehungen dieser Phosphate zur Apatitgruppe." *Z. anorg. allg. Chem.*, **206**, 237

Van Wazer, J. R. (1958). *Phosphorus and Its Compounds.* Vol. 1. Interscience Publishers, Inc., New York.

Warington, R. (1866). "Researches on the phosphates of calcium, and upon the solubility of tricalcic phosphate." *J. chem. Soc.*, **19**, 296.

Warington, R. (1873). "On the decomposition of tricalcic phosphate by water." *J. chem. Soc.*, **24**.

Zipkin, I., Posner, A. S. and Eanes, E. D. (1962). "The effect of fluoride on the X-ray diffraction pattern of the apatite of human bone." *Biochem. biophys. Acta.*, **59**, 255.

SUBJECT INDEX